Periodization

Theory and Methodology of Training

Sixth Edition

Tudor O. Bompa, PhD

Carlo A. Buzzichelli

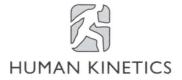

HUMAN KINETICS

Library of Congress Cataloging-in-Publication Data

Names: Bompa, Tudor O., author. | Buzzichelli, Carlo, 1973- author.
Title: Periodization : theory and methodology of training / Tudor O. Bompa, PhD, Carlo A. Buzzichelli.
Description: Sixth edition. | Champaign, IL : Human Kinetics, [2019] | Includes bibliographical references and index.
Identifiers: LCCN 2017060513 (print) | LCCN 2017041811 (ebook) | ISBN 9781492544814 (ebook) | ISBN 9781492544807 (print)
Subjects: LCSH: Periodization training. | Weight training.
Classification: LCC GV546 (print) | LCC GV546 .B546 2019 (ebook) | DDC 613.7/11--dc23
LC record available at https://lccn.loc.gov/2017060513

ISBN: 978-1-4925-4480-7 (print)

Copyright © 2019 by Tudor O. Bompa and Carlo A. Buzzichelli
Copyright © 2009 by Tudor O. Bompa and G. Gregory Haff
Copyright © 1999 by Tudor O. Bompa
Copyright © 1994, 1994, 1983 by Kendall/Hunt Publishing Company

All rights reserved. Except for use in a review, the reproduction or utilization of this work in any form or by any electronic, mechanical, or other means, now known or hereafter invented, including xerography, photocopying, and recording, and in any information storage and retrieval system, is forbidden without the written permission of the publisher.

The web addresses cited in this text were current as of February 2018, unless otherwise noted.

Acquisitions Editor: Roger W. Earle
Developmental Editor: Julie Marx Goodreau
Managing Editor: Ann C. Gindes
Copyeditor: Jackie Walker Gibson
Indexer: Nan Badgett
Permissions Manager: Martha Gullo
Graphic Designer: Denise Lowry
Cover Designer: Keri Evans
Cover Design Associate: Susan Allen
Photographs (interior): © Human Kinetics, unless otherwise noted.
Photo Asset Manager: Laura Fitch
Photo Production Manager: Jason Allen
Senior Art Manager: Kelly Hendren
Illustrations: © Human Kinetics, unless otherwise noted
Printer: Versa Press

Printed in the United States of America   10 9 8 7 6 5

The paper in this book is certified under a sustainable forestry program.

Human Kinetics
1607 N. Market Street
Champaign, IL 61820
USA

United States and International
Website: **US.HumanKinetics.com**
Email: info@hkusa.com
Phone: 1-800-747-4457

Canada
Website: **Canada.HumanKinetics.com**
Email: info@hkcanada.com

Contents

Preface vii
Acknowledgments ix

Part I Training Theory 1

Chapter 1 Basis for Training 3

Scope of Training 3
Objectives of Training 4
Classification of Skills 5
System of Training 6
Adaptation 8
Supercompensation Cycle and Adaptation 12
Sources of Energy 19
Summary of Major Concepts 27

Chapter 2 Principles of Training 29

Multilateral Development Versus Specialization 29
Individualization 36
Development of the Training Model 40
Load Progression 42
Sequence of the Training Load 48
Summary of Major Concepts 49

Chapter 3 Preparation for Training 51

Physical Training 51
Exercise for Physical Training 54
Technical Training 55
Tactical Training 58
Theoretical Training 68
Summary of Major Concepts 69

Chapter 4	**Variables of Training**	**71**
	Volume	71
	Intensity	73
	Relationship Between Volume and Intensity	78
	Frequency	84
	Complexity	85
	Index of Overall Demand	86
	Summary of Major Concepts	86

Part II Planning and Periodization — 89

Chapter 5	**Periodization of Biomotor Abilities**	**91**
	Brief History of Periodization	91
	Periodization Terminology	93
	Applying Periodization to the Development of Biomotor Abilities	99
	Simultaneous Versus Sequential Integration of Biomotor Abilities	101
	Periodization of Strength	103
	Periodization of Power, Agility, and Movement Time	106
	Periodization of Speed	107
	Periodization of Endurance	109
	Integrated Periodization	110
	Summary of Major Concepts	113
Chapter 6	**Planning the Training Session**	**115**
	Importance of Planning	115
	Planning Requirements	116
	Types of Training Plans	119
	Training Session	119
	Daily Cycle of Training	132
	Modeling the Training Session Plan	134
	Summary of Major Concepts	136
Chapter 7	**Planning the Training Cycles**	**137**
	Microcycle	137
	Macrocycle	159
	Summary of Major Concepts	164

Contents

Chapter 8	**Periodization of the Annual Plan**	**165**
	Annual Training Plan and Its Characteristics	165
	Classifying Annual Plans	177
	Chart of the Annual Training Plan	184
	Criteria for Compiling an Annual Plan	192
	Summary of Major Concepts	205
Chapter 9	**Peaking for Competition**	**207**
	Training Conditions for Peaking	207
	Peaking	208
	Defining a Taper	209
	Competition Phase of the Annual Plan	215
	Identifying Peaking	223
	Maintaining a Peak	224
	Summary of Major Concepts	225

Part III Training Methods   227

Chapter 10	**Strength and Power Development**	**229**
	The Relationship Between the Main Biomotor Abilities	229
	Strength	231
	Methods of Strength Training	238
	Manipulation of Training Variables	238
	Implementation of a Strength Training Program	253
	Periodization of Strength	259
	Summary of Major Concepts	263
Chapter 11	**Endurance Training**	**265**
	Classification of Endurance	265
	Factors Affecting Aerobic Endurance Performance	267
	Factors Affecting Anaerobic Endurance Performance	275
	Methods for Developing Endurance	276
	Methods for Developing High-Intensity Endurance	284
	Periodization of Endurance	294
	Summary of Major Concepts	300

Chapter 12	**Speed and Agility Training**	**301**
	Speed Training	301
	Agility Training	311
	Program Design	313
	Periodization of Speed and Agility Training	319
	Summary of Major Concepts	323

Glossary   325
References   331
Index   371
About the Authors   381

Preface

The classic text *Theory and Methodology of Training* by Tudor Bompa played a large role in shaping the training practices of many coaches and athletes throughout the world. This seminal text eventually became known as *Periodization: Theory and Methodology of Training*. Since its first publication in 1983, *Periodization* has presented the latest research and practices related to training theory. The text has been translated into many languages and has become one of the major resources on periodization for sport scientists, coaches, and athletes throughout the world. For the sixth edition of *Periodization: Theory and Methodology of Training*, Bompa has teamed with Carlo Buzzichelli to cover the science and practice of the theory and methodology of training. The sixth edition offers information central to understanding the training process while providing scientific support for the principles fundamental to periodization.

Organization of the Text

In the sixth edition, Bompa and Buzzichelli organize the text into the three major content areas found in the previous editions: training theory, planning and periodization, and training methods. Part I, Training Theory, contains four chapters that delve into the major concepts central to training, such as the basic concepts of the training process (chapter 1), the principles of training (chapter 2), the tactical, technical, and physical components of the training process (chapter 3), and the variables associated with developing a training plan (chapter 4). These four chapters give the coach, sport scientist, and athlete the concepts necessary for understanding and developing periodized training plans, which are addressed in part II.

Part II, Planning and Periodization, contains five chapters that discuss the methodological concepts that concern training planning. These chapters provide the historical context within which the concept of periodization was developed and the methodological tools for the periodization of the annual plan and biomotor abilities (chapter 5). They also cover how to conceptualize and plan training sessions (chapter 6), methods for constructing different training cycles (chapter 7), expanded discussions on the designing of the annual training plan (chapter 8), and methods for elevating performance at appropriate times (chapter 9). Chapter 9 couples the current scientific knowledge about the interrelation between training stress and performance with practical information that will allow coaches and athletes to manipulate training to ensure optimal performance during competition.

The chapters in part III, Training Methods, discuss the development of strength and power (chapter 10), endurance (chapter 11), and speed and agility (chapter 12). In its examination of strength and power training, chapter 10 presents information on the interrelationships of force, velocity, rate of force development, and power, along with information on variables that can be manipulated in the construction of a strength training program. The chapters on endurance (chapter 11) and speed training (chapter 12) have been expanded to include the latest information on testing and developing these important sport performance characteristics.

Updates to the Sixth Edition

The sixth edition of *Periodization: Theory and Methodology of Training* maintains several of the components of the fifth edition, including sample annual training plans, microcycle loading structures, and charts for designing periodized training plans. New to the sixth edition of *Periodization* are these features:

- Discussions on the importance of the designing of a sport-specific annual plan that is specific to competition-level athletes. This helps overcome the misconception that planning and programming can use a one-size-fits-all approach.
- An expanded chapter on the integration of biomotor abilities within the training process.
- A historical contextualization of the concept of periodization of training as well as the clarification of several terms and concepts commonly used in the field of theory and methodology.
- A comprehensive, coaching-derived update on the concepts of session, microcycle, and macrocycle organization.
- An expanded chapter on the methods for developing muscular strength. This chapter discusses such concepts as the manipulation of loading variables and the conversion to specific strength, and how those concepts can be used to maximize strength gains and transfer to sport-specific performance.
- A more detailed explanation of speed and agility training, differentiating between individual and team sports.
- Expanded discussions about the development of sport-specific endurance and its individualization, again differentiating between individual and team sports. In this context different types of endurance and specific methods for testing and developing endurance are presented. The physiological bases for these methods are also presented to explain how training can affect the athlete's physiology.

The sixth edition of *Periodization: Theory and Methodology of Training* builds on the tradition established in previous editions of this text and expands on the current understanding of training theory and the application of periodization.

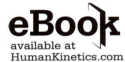

Acknowledgments

The team at Human Kinetics did a wonderful job putting together this book, a book that is so important for everyone who wants to become comfortable with the theory of training, periodization, and planning. My sincere thanks to Roger Earle for his constant guidance and to Julie Marx Goodreau for her diligence and competent editorial work. Carlo and I are also deeply indebted to Ann Gindes for her assiduity and her deliberate work. It was an incredible journey to eliminate many errors from the original manuscript. Thanks Ann.

I would also like to sincerely thank my coauthor, Carlo Buzzichelli, who made an essential contribution to the final form of this book. Grazie, Carlo.

Finally, to my readers: Once I was young and full of dreams, like so many of you. Success came to me far too early. I started to believe how great I was! But after an important fiasco, I realized that the road to success is also full of frustrations. I have learned much more from my failures than from my athletes' victories. I owe a great deal to my habit of being well organized. Planning became my greatest preoccupation and attribute. If you want to achieve success, I highly recommend being the best planner you can be.

—Tudor Olimpius Bompa

I want to thank Tudor Bompa for his mentorship and for giving me, once again, the chance to coauthor a book with him—especially a very important text like this one, probably the most adopted book among theory and methodology courses around the world. Mulțumesc!

I want to extend my gratitude to the athletes and coaches I have worked with in the last two decades. Their contribution to my understanding of the training process as it pertains to sports is inestimable. The concept of periodization has evolved through its application in the context of a multitude of sports; reverse engineering the best practices allows us to bridge the gap between science and practice.

—Carlo A. Buzzichelli

PART I
TRAINING THEORY

Basis for Training 1

The science of sport and the preparation of athletes is continuously evolving. This evolution is based largely upon an ever-expanding understanding of how the body adapts to different physical and psychological stressors. Contemporary sport scientists continue to explore the physiological and performance effects of different training interventions, recovery modalities, nutritional countermeasures, and biomechanical factors in order to increase the performance capacity of the modern athlete. As our understanding of the body's response to different stressors has grown, contemporary training theorists, sport scientists, and coaches have been able to expand upon the most basic concept of training.

Central to training theory is the idea that a structured system of training can be established that incorporates training activities that target specific physiological, psychological, and performance characteristics of individual sports and athletes. It follows that it is possible to modulate the adaptive process and direct specific training outcomes. This process of modulation and direction is facilitated by an understanding of the bioenergetic functions (how the body supplies energy) required to meet the physical demands of various physical activities. The coach who understands the **bioenergetics** of physical activity and sport—as well as the impact of the timing of the presentation of training stimuli on the timeline for physical adaptation—will have a greater chance of developing effective training plans.

Scope of Training

Athletes prepare to achieve a specific goal through structured and focused training. The intent of training is to increase the athlete's skills and work capacity to optimize athletic performance. Training is undertaken across a long period of time and involves many physiological, psychological, and sociological variables. During this time, training is progressively and individually graded. Throughout training, human physiological and psychological functions are modeled to meet demanding tasks.

Per the traditions of the ancient Olympic Games, athletes should strive to combine physical perfection with spiritual refinement and moral purity. Physical perfection signifies multilateral, harmonious development. The athlete acquires fine and varied skills, cultivates positive psychological qualities, and maintains good health. The athlete learns to cope with highly stressful stimuli in training and competitions. Physical excellence should evolve through an organized and well-planned training program based on practical experience and application of scientifically supported methods.

Paramount to training endeavors for novices and professionals is a realistic and achievable goal, planned according to individual abilities, psychological traits, and social environments. Some athletes seek to win a competition or improve previous performance; others consider gaining a technical skill or further developing a **biomotor ability**. Whatever the objective, each goal needs to be as precise and measurable as possible. In any plan, short or long term, the athlete needs to set goals and determine procedures for achieving these goals before beginning training. The deadline for achieving the final goal is the date of a major competition.

Objectives of Training

Training is a process by which an athlete is prepared for the highest level of performance possible (59, 107). The ability of a coach to direct the optimization of performance is achieved through the development of systematic training plans that draw upon knowledge garnered from a vast array of scientific disciplines, as shown in figure 1.1 (107).

The process of training targets the development of specific attributes correlated with the execution of various tasks (107). These specific attributes include multilateral physical development, sport-specific physical development, technical skills, tactical abilities, psychological characteristics, health maintenance, injury resistance, and theoretical knowledge. The successful acquisition of these attributes is based upon utilizing means and methods that are individualized and appropriate for the athletes' age, experience, and talent level.

- *Multilateral physical development:* Multilateral development, or general fitness (107) as it is also known, provides the training foundation for success in all sports. This type of development targets the improvement of the basic biomotor abilities, such as endurance, strength, speed, flexibility, and coordination. Athletes who develop a strong foundation will be able to better tolerate sport-specific training activities and ultimately have a greater potential for athletic development.
- *Sport-specific physical development:* Sport-specific physical development, or sport-specific fitness (107) as it is sometimes referred to, is the development of physiological or fitness characteristics that are specific to the sport. This type of training may target several specific needs of the sport such as strength, skill, endurance, speed, and flexibility (105, 107). However, many sports require a blending of key aspects of performance, such as **power**, **muscle endurance**, or **speed endurance**.
- *Technical skills:* This training focuses on the development of the technical skills necessary for success in the sporting activity. The ability to perfect technical skills is based upon both multilateral and sport-specific physical development. For example, the ability to perform the iron cross in gymnastics appears to be limited by strength, one of the biomotor abilities (36). Ultimately the purpose of training that targets the development of technical skills is to perfect technique and allow for the optimization of the sport-specific skills necessary for successful athletic performance. The development of

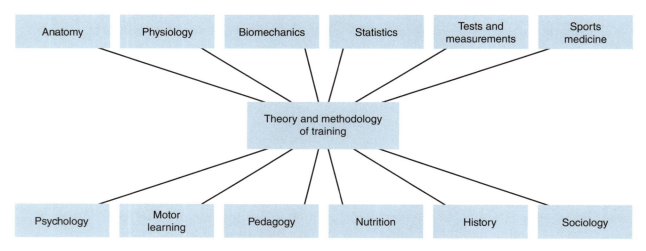

FIGURE 1.1 Auxiliary sciences.

technique should occur under both normal and unusual conditions (e.g., weather, noise, etc.) and should always focus on perfecting the specific skills required by the sport.
- *Tactical abilities:* The development of tactical abilities is also of particular importance to the training process. Training in this area is designed to improve competitive strategies and is based upon studying the tactics of opponents. Specifically, this type of training is designed to develop strategies that take advantage of the technical and physical capabilities of the athlete so that the chances of success in competition are increased.
- *Psychological factors:* Psychological preparation is also necessary to ensure the optimization of physical performance. Some authors have also called this type of training personality development training (107). Regardless of the terminology, the development of psychological characteristics such as discipline, courage, perseverance, and confidence are essential for successful athletic performance.
- *Health maintenance:* The overall health of the athlete should be considered very important. Proper health can be maintained by periodic medical examinations and appropriate scheduling of training, including alternating between periods of hard work and periods of regeneration or restoration. Injuries and illness require specific attention, and proper management of these occurrences is an important priority to consider during the training process.
- *Injury resistance:* The best way to prevent injuries is to ensure that the athlete has developed the physical capacity and physiological characteristics necessary to participate in rigorous training and competition and to ensure appropriate application of training (61). The inappropriate application of training, which includes excessive loading, will increase the risk of injury. With young athletes it is crucial that multilateral physical development is targeted, as this allows for the development of biomotor abilities that will help decrease the potential for injury. Additionally, the management of fatigue appears to be of particular importance. When fatigue is high, the occurrence of injuries is markedly increased (101); therefore, the development of a training plan that manages fatigue should be considered to be of the utmost importance.
- *Theoretical knowledge:* Training should increase the athletes' knowledge of the physiological and psychological basis of training, planning, nutrition, and regeneration. It is crucial that the athlete understands why certain training activities are being undertaken. This can be accomplished through discussing the training objectives established for each aspect of the training plan or by requiring the athlete to attend seminars and conferences about training. Arming the athlete with theoretical knowledge about the training process and the sport improves the likelihood that the athlete will make good personal decisions and approach the training process with a strong focus, which will allow the coach and athlete to better set training goals.

Classification of Skills

There are many suggested methods for classifying physical activity skills. Aside from the traditional method of classifying sport activities into individual sports (track and field, gymnastics, boxing) and team sports (soccer, football, basketball, volleyball, rugby), a widely accepted classification uses biomotor abilities as a criterion. Biomotor abilities include strength, speed, endurance, and coordination (53). While classifying sports by biomotor abilities is very useful, coaches also use other methods. One popular method is to classify sporting skills as **cyclic skills**, **acyclic skills**, or **acyclic combined skills**:

- *Cyclic skills* are used in sports such as walking, running, cross-country skiing, speedskating, swimming, rowing, cycling, kayaking, and canoeing. The main characteristic of these sports is that the motor act involves repetitive movements. Once the athlete learns one cycle of the motor act, he can duplicate it continuously for long periods. Each cycle consists of distinct, identical phases that are repeated in succession. For example, the four phases of a rowing stroke—the catch, drive through the water, finish, and recovery—are part of a whole. The athlete performs them over and over in the same succession during the cyclic motion of rowing. Each cycle the athlete performs is linked; it is preceded and followed by another one.

- *Acyclic skills* show up in sports such as shot putting, discus throwing, most gymnastics, team sports, wrestling, boxing, and fencing. These skills consist of integral functions performed in one action. For instance, the skill of discus throwing incorporates the preliminary swing, transition, turn, delivery, and reverse step, but the athlete performs them all in one action.
- *Acyclic combined skills* consist of cyclic movements followed by an acyclic movement. Sports such as figure skating, diving, jumping events in track and field, and tumbling lines and vaulting in gymnastics use acyclic combined skills. Although all actions are linked, we can easily distinguish between the acyclic and cyclic movements. For instance, we can distinguish the acyclic movement of a high jumper or vaulter from the preceding cyclic approach of running.

The coach's comprehension of these skill classifications plays an important role in the selection of appropriate teaching methods. Generally, teaching the skill as a whole appears to be effective with cyclic skills, while breaking the skill into smaller pieces appears to be more effective with acyclic skills. For example, when working with javelin throwers, the standing throw should be mastered prior to the three-step stride approach, the six-step approach, and the full approach (38).

System of Training

A system is an organized, methodically arranged set of ideas, theories, or speculations. The development of a training system is based upon scientific findings coupled with accumulated practical experience. A training system should not be imported, although it may be beneficial to study other training systems before developing one. Furthermore, in creating or developing a better training system, you must consider a country's social and cultural background.

Bondarchuk (9) suggested that a system of training is constructed by observing three basic principles:

1. *Uncovering the system's forming factors:* Factors that are central to the development of the training system can stem from general knowledge about the theory and methods of training, scientific findings, experiences of the nation's best coaches, and the approaches used by other countries.
2. *Determining the system's structure:* Once the factors central to the success of the training system are established, the actual training system can be constructed. A model for both short- and long-term training should be created. The system should be able to be applied by all coaches, but it should also be flexible enough that coaches can enrich the system's structure based upon their own experiences. The sport scientist plays a crucial role in the establishment of a training system. Research, especially applied research, increases the knowledge base from which the training system is developed and further evolved. Additionally, the sport scientist can aid in the development of athlete-monitoring programs and talent-identification programs, the establishment of training theories, and the development of methods for dealing with fatigue and stress. While the importance of sport science to the overall training system seems apparent, this branch of science is not embraced with equal enthusiasm throughout the world. For example Stone and colleagues (108) suggested that the use of sport science in

the United States is on the decline, which may explain, at least in part, the decrease in performance levels evidenced by some U.S. track and field athletes at some of the recent Olympic Games.

3. *Validating the efficacy of the system:* Once a training system is initiated, it should be constantly evaluated. The evaluation of the efficacy of a training system can be undertaken in a multidimensional manner. The most simplistic assessments used to validate a training system are the actual performance improvements achieved in response to the system. More complex assessments can also be used, including direct measurements of physiological adaptation such as hormonal or cell signaling adaptations. Additionally, mechanical assessments can be quantified to determine whether the training structure is working effectively; examples include the evaluation of maximal anaerobic power, maximal aerobic power, maximal force generating capacity, and peak rate of force development. Sport scientists can play a very important role in this capacity, using their expertise to evaluate the athlete and provide insight into the effectiveness of a training system. If the training system is not optimal, then the performance enhancement team can reevaluate and modify the system.

As a whole, the quality of the training system depends on direct and supportive factors (figure 1.2). Direct factors include those related to both training and evaluation, while supportive factors are related to administrative and economic conditions and to professional styles and lifestyles. Although each factor in the overall system plays a role in the success of the system, it appears that the direct factors are most significant. The importance of the direct factors further strengthens the argument that the sport scientist is an important contributor to the development of a quality training system.

The development of a quality training system is essential to the optimization of performance. Training quality does not solely depend upon the coach, but upon the interaction of many factors that can impact the athlete's performance (figure 1.3). Hence, all factors that could affect the quality of training need to be effectively implemented and constantly evaluated and, when necessary, adjusted to meet the ever-changing demands of modern athletics.

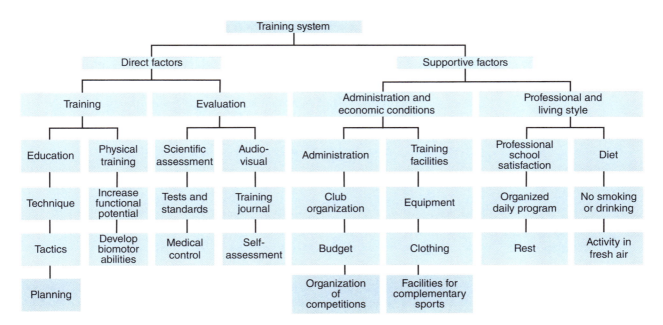

FIGURE 1.2 Components of a training system.

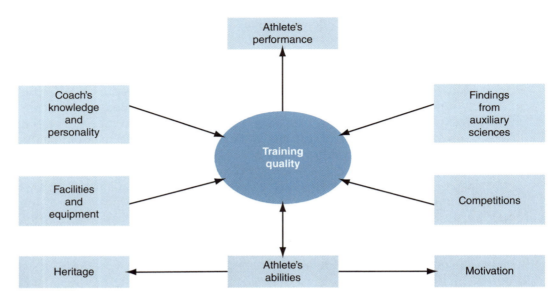

FIGURE 1.3 Factors that affect training quality.

Adaptation

Training is an organized process whereby the body and mind are constantly exposed to stressors of varying volume (quantity) and intensity. The ability of an athlete to adapt and adjust to workloads imposed by training and competition is as important as the ability of a species to adapt to the environment in which it lives: No adaptation, no survival! For athletes, an inability to adapt to constantly varying training loads and the stressors associated with training and competition will result in critical levels of **fatigue**, **overreaching**, or even **overtraining**. In such circumstances, the athlete will be unable to achieve training goals.

A high level of performance is the result of many years of well-planned, methodical, and challenging training. During this time, the athlete tries to adapt her physiology to the specific requirements of her sport. The greater the degree of adaptation to the training process, the greater the potential for high levels of performance. Therefore, the objective of any well-organized training plan is to induce adaptations that improve performance. Improvement is possible only if the athlete observes this sequence:

Increasing stimulus (load) → Adaptation → Performance improvement

If the load is always at the same level, adaptation occurs in the early part of training, followed by a plateau (stagnation) without any further improvement (figure 1.4):

Lack of stimulus → Plateau → Lack of improvement

If the stimulus is excessive or overly varied, the athlete will be unable to adapt, and maladaptation will occur:

Excessive stimulus → Maladaptation → Decrease in performance

Therefore, the objective of training is to progressively and systematically increase the training stimulus (the intensity, volume of training loads, and frequency of training) to induce superior adaptation and, as a result, improve performance. These alterations in the training stimulus must include training variation to maximize the athlete's adaptation to the training plan (figure 1.5).

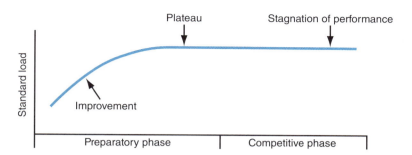

FIGURE 1.4 A standard load results in improvements only during the early part of the plan.

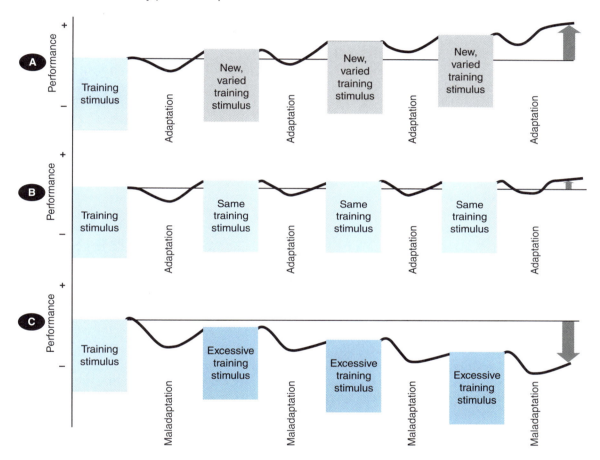

FIGURE 1.5 Training stimulus and adaptation.
A = increasing stimulus (load) → adaptation → performance improvement; B = lack of stimulus → plateau → lack of improvement; C = excessive stimulus → maladaptation → decrease in performance; ↑ = increased performance; ↓ = decreased performance.

Training adaptations are the sum of the transformations brought about by systematically repeating bouts of exercise. These structural and physiological changes result from the specific demands that athletes place on their bodies by the activities they pursue, depending on the volume, intensity, and frequency of training. Physical training is beneficial only as long as it overloads the body in such a way that adaption is stimulated. If the stimulus does not induce a sufficient physiological challenge, no increase in adaptation can be expected. On the other hand, if the training load is very high, intolerable, and undertaken for an excessively long period of time, injury or overtraining may occur.

Specificity of Adaptation

Because adaptation is highly specific to the type of training undertaken, training must be based on the energy systems dominant in the sport, the skills of the sport, and the motor abilities required by the sport. The time required to reach a high degree of adaptation depends on the skill complexity and the physiological and psychological difficulty of the sport. The more complex and difficult the sport, the longer the training time required for the human body to adapt.

If an athlete expects superior performance, he must be exposed to a systematic and progressive increase in training stimuli that is designed to elevate the athlete's physiological and performance capacity (i.e., cross the threshold of adaptation). Therefore, it is of utmost importance that a systematic and well-organized training program be followed to induce superior adaptations of the main functions of the body, such as the following:

- *Neuromuscular:* Increase the efficiency of movements and coordination, increase the reflex activity of the nervous system, synchronize motor unit activity, increase recruitment of motor units, increase **motor unit** firing rate (**rate coding**), increase muscle **hypertrophy**, increase mitochondrial biogenesis, and alter cell signaling pathways (19).

- *Metabolic:* Increase the muscular stores of **adenosine triphosphate (ATP)** and **phosphocreatine (PCr)**, increase the capacity of muscle to store glycogen, increase the capacity of muscle to tolerate **lactic acid** buildup and delay the onset of fatigue, increase the capillary network for a superior supply of nutrients and oxygen, increase the use of fat as energy for long-duration activities, increase the efficiency of the **glycolytic energy system**, increase efficiency of the **oxidative system**, and alter specific enzymatic processes associated with the various bioenergetic systems noted on page 19 (87).

- *Cardiorespiratory:* Increase lung volume; increase hypertrophy of the left ventricular wall; increase volume of the left ventricle to increase **stroke volume** and, as a result, facilitate delivery of oxygenated blood to the working muscles; decrease heart rate; increase capillary density; increase the lactate threshold so that the athlete can perform at a higher rate of oxygen consumption; and increase $\dot{V}O_2\text{max}$ to enhance aerobic capacity for prolonged exercises.

The focus of any training program is to improve performance. This is only possible by breaking the threshold of the present level of adaptation by exposing the athlete to higher training demands (e.g., using high training loads, greater than 80% in strength training; increase duration of training or its intensity in endurance sports; or increase the percentage of maximum speed and agility through training). When an athlete achieves a new level of adaptation, his performance will improve (figure 1.6).

Adaptation is a long-term, progressive physiological response to general and sport-specific training programs with the goal of readying the athlete for the specific demands of competition. Adaptation occurs through positive changes of the main functions of the body. Training phases—preparatory and competitive—are combined with different types of adaptations:

- *Preadaptation* is gradual and temporary adaptation to training during the early part of a training plan (in this case an annual plan). If the training load and the physiological stressors that result from it are not excessive, these early weeks of training will progressively lead to a more durable adaptation visible via increased work capacity and improved tolerance to higher training demand.

- *Compensation* can be defined as the body's reactions to a training program before reaching a stable adaptation. During this phase, still in the early part of the preparatory phase, the athlete experiences positive reactions to the training demand and thus improved results in testing and skills proficiency. At this time, the body can

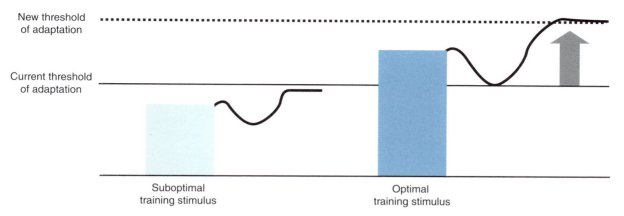

FIGURE 1.6 Breaking the threshold of adaptation should improve performance.
↑ = increase in the threshold of adaptation.

compensate for high training demands as a demonstration of the athlete's improved training potential and increased physiological efficiency.
- *Stable or precompetitive adaptation* is a phase of improved equilibrium between work and compensation, between high stressors and the ability to tolerate and recover from them. Many training loads and social or psychological stressors have to be planned and applied at the same levels as during competition so that the athletes can learn to react to and cope with them. Exhibition games and competitions should be used to test both technical and tactical proficiency and physiological and psychological efficiency. High levels of stability of all training factors indicate that athletes are in, or are close to reaching, the state of readiness to compete in the competitions that are scheduled for the next phase.
- *State of readiness for competitions* is the result of the athlete's training. The athlete is ready to compete with high technical efficacy, demonstrates high levels of athletic effectiveness, displays sport-specific motor skills and physical qualities, and is able to tolerate stress and adapt to it.

Training Effect

Any training program creates a certain reaction to the adaptive responses of the body; this is called a **training effect**. Since the 1960s several authors have discussed this subject, among them H.K. Cooper with his very influential work *The New Aerobics* (22). Training effect can be classified into three categories:

1. *Immediate training effect* can be detected during and immediately after a training session in the form of physiological reaction to a training load, such as increased heart rate, increased blood pressure, decreased force production as a result of fatigue, increased fatigue, and depletion of muscle glycogen, depending on the intensity and volume of the training bout.
2. *Delayed training effect* is the final outcome of a training session that can be long lasting. Although the immediate posttraining effect is reduced because of fatigue, the delayed training effect (i.e., the positive training benefits) is apparent after the fatigue associated with training dissipates. The onset of the delayed training effect depends on the training bout: The more intense the training session, the longer the time frame before performance gains are realized (42, 43).
3. *Cumulative effect* is the result of several sessions or even phases of training, which can include sessions with very challenging loads that are meant to break the threshold of

adaptation of a given training phase. The occurrence of the cumulative training effect often surprises coaches and athletes alike, who may not be able to anticipate or explain it ("We have worked hard and suddenly it just happened!"). Good planning of training sessions, altering high loads and intensities with compensation sessions, will allow the athlete to benefit from the cumulative training effect.

Zatsiorsky and Kraemer (119) proposed that the relationship between fatigue and training gains is a factor of 3:1, meaning that fatigue is three times shorter in duration (e.g., 24 h) than the positive training effect (e.g., 72 h). Certainly, the type of training can change this ratio because anaerobic training is more demanding and thus more fatiguing. In any case, the positive effects of a training session are visible after fatigue is eliminated; adaptation then can take place, accompanied by improved performance.

Cooper (22) used five categories to assess the postexercise training effect. He suggested that the athlete accumulate 30 points a week to achieve a good training effect (e.g., 2 × category 5 = 10 points; 2 × category 3 = 6 points) (table 1.1).

TABLE 1.1 Cooper's Training Effect Categories

Category	Training effect	Results
1	1.0-1.9 Minor	Develops base endurance. No improvement in maximum performance. Enhances recovery.
2	2.0-2.9 Maintenance	Maintains aerobic fitness. Does little to improve maximum performance.
3	3.0-3.9 Improvement	Improves aerobic fitness if repeated two to four times weekly.
4	4.0-4.9 Rapid improvement	Rapidly improves aerobic fitness if repeated one or two times weekly. Needs few recovery sessions.
5	5.0-up Overreaching	Dramatically increases aerobic fitness if combined with good recovery.

Adapted from Cooper 1968 (22a).

Thus, training effects are complex phenomena with short- and long-lasting influences that can be determined by the following:

- One's current functional or training state
- The effects of previous training bouts
- The sum of all training stimuli (loads) or their combinations, their order of application, and the interval between them

Supercompensation Cycle and Adaptation

The training phenomenon called **supercompensation**, also known as Weigert's law of supercompensation, was first described by Folbrot in 1941 (105) and later was discussed by Hans Selye (102), who called it the **general adaptation syndrome (GAS)**. Several Russian, East German, and American (40) researchers and authors have also shed light on this essential training concept.

Selye's general adaptation syndrome (GAS) theory (figure 1.7) is the basis of **progressive overloading**, which, if applied inappropriately, can create high degrees of undesirable stress.

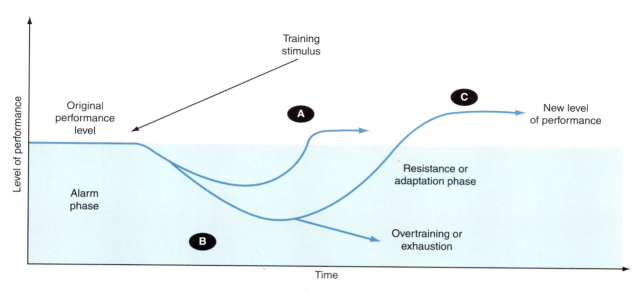

FIGURE 1.7 Illustration of Selye's general adaptation syndrome theory.
A = typical training; B = overtraining; C = overreaching or supercompensation.

Adapted, by permission, from A.C. Fry, 1998, The role of training intensity in resistance exercise overtraining and overreaching. In *Overtraining in sport*, edited by R.B. Kreider, A.C. Fry, and M.L. O'Toole (Champaign, IL: Human Kinetics), 114.

These concepts suggest that for the best training adaptations to occur, training intensities, training volumes, and bioenergetic specificity have to be systematically and rationally alternated in a sequence of phases. For example, the coach should plan training **microcycles** that alternate high, moderate, and low training intensities. These alternations of intensities allow for recovery between training sessions; the addition of recovery time between carefully **sequenced training phases** is the basis for cyclical planning (known as **periodization**) and supercompensation.

Supercompensation, therefore, is a relationship between work and regeneration that leads to superior physical adaptation as well as metabolic and neuropsychological arousal before a competition. Applying the concept of supercompensation in training has many benefits:

- Helps the athlete manage stress and cope with high training intensities
- Helps coaches create structured training systems
- Avoids the onset of critical levels of fatigue and overtraining
- Makes a coach cognizant of the need to alternate intensities to facilitate the best adaptations
- Justifies the use of different types of posttraining and postcompetition recovery techniques (e.g., passive and active rest, nutrition, physiotherapy, psychological techniques)
- Facilitates precompetition training to achieve peak performance
- Uses both physiological and psychological techniques in training

When athletes train, they are exposed to a series of stimuli that alter their physiological status. These physiological responses can include acute metabolic (28, 40, 96, 111), hormonal (46, 52), cardiovascular (88), neuromuscular (32, 48, 49), and cell signaling alterations (5). Such responses are mitigated by the volume, intensity, frequency, and type of training undertaken by the athlete. The greater the volume, intensity, or duration of training, the greater the magnitude of the physiological responses to training.

The acute physiological responses to a training session will result in the accumulation of fatigue (33, 84), which can manifest itself as an inability to produce or maintain maximal voluntary force output (48, 49, 92, 93). The postexercise period also is associated with a reduction in muscle **glycogen** stores (56), lactic acid accumulation (110, 115), reductions

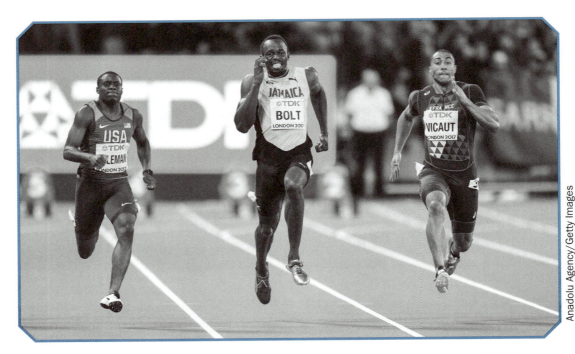

World-record holder and 11-time world champion Usain Bolt spent many years training as a sprinter. The cumulative training effect for Bolt was winning eight Olympic gold medals.

in PCr stores (64, 72), and an increase in circulating **cortisol** levels (3, 54, 94). These physiological responses temporarily reduce the athlete's performance capacity.

Following the training session, the athlete must dissipate fatigue, restore muscle glycogen and phosphagen stores, reduce circulating cortisol levels, and deal with the lactic acid that has accumulated. The time that the athlete needs to recover is affected by many factors, which can include the training status of the athlete (49), the muscular contraction type encountered during the training session (92), the use of restoration techniques, and the nutritional status of the athlete (12). Nutritional status is of particular importance: An inadequate diet can increase the time needed for recovery (13).

The fatigue induced by exercise results in an abrupt drop in the athlete's homeostasis curve (figure 1.8), which is coupled with a reduction in functional capacity. Following the exercise bout, the return of the athlete to homeostasis can be considered a period of compensation. The return to homeostasis, or a normal biological state, is slow and progressive, requiring

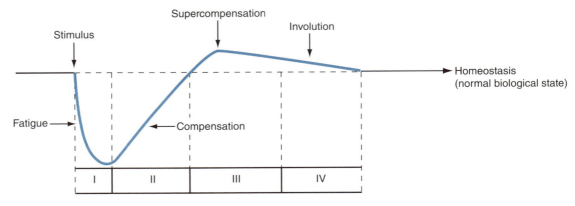

FIGURE 1.8 Supercompensation cycle of a training session.

Modified from Yakovlev 1967 (116).

several hours to several days (93). If the time between high-intensity training sessions is sufficient, the body dissipates fatigue and fully replaces the energy sources (especially glycogen), allowing the body to rebound into a state of supercompensation.

Every time supercompensation occurs, the athlete establishes a new, increased homeostatic level with positive benefits for training and performance. Consider supercompensation as the foundation of a functional increase of athletic efficiency, resulting from the body's adaptation to the training stimulus (load) and the replenishment of glycogen stores in the muscle. If the resulting phase or the time between two stimuli is too long, supercompensation will fade, leading to **involution,** or a reduction in performance capacity.

Phases of Supercompensation

The supercompensation cycle (figure 1.9) has four phases and occurs in the following sequence.

Phase I: Duration of One to Two Hours

After training, the body experiences fatigue. Exercise-induced fatigue occurs via either central or peripheral mechanisms (32). Fatigue is a multidimensional phenomenon caused by several factors:

- Reductions in neural activation of the muscle, which are generally associated with central fatigue, can occur in response to exercise (49).
- Exercise-induced central fatigue can also increase brain serotonin levels, which can lead to mental fatigue (32). This accumulated mental fatigue can affect the athlete's willingness to tolerate high levels of discomfort or pain associated with training and competition.

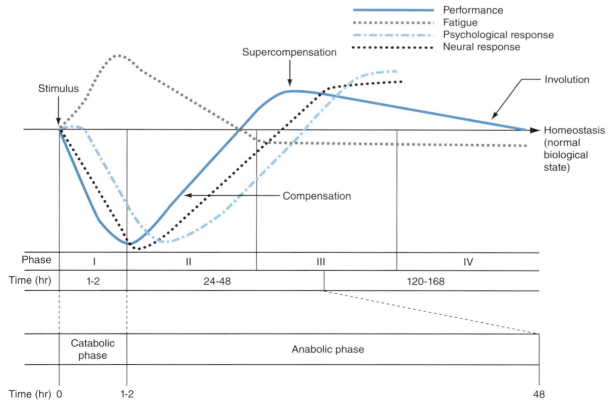

FIGURE 1.9 Supercompensation cycle response to a training session.

- Exercise can result in impairments in neuromuscular transmission and impulse propagation, impaired Ca^{2+} handling by the **sarcoplasmic reticulum**, substrate depletion, and other factors that disrupt the contractile process and are associated with exercise-induced peripheral fatigue (31).
- Exercise-induced substrate utilization occurs in response to the intensity, volume, and duration of the exercise bout. Substrates that can be significantly affected include muscle glycogen and phosphocreatine stores. Muscle glycogen can be significantly reduced in response to high-intensity interval training (11, 106), resistance training (55, 83), and endurance training (23, 27). Phosphocreatine stores can be significantly reduced in as little as 5 to 30 s and can be completely depleted after exhaustive exercise (64, 73, 74).
- The classic literature suggests that lactic acid accumulation as a result of exercise is a major player in the formation of fatigue (115). It is theorized that higher levels of lactic acid formation cause a state of **acidosis**, which may decrease force-generating capacity as a result of alterations in contractile properties (112, 115). Contemporary literature suggests that inorganic phosphate (P_i), which is formed from the breakdown of PCr, rather than acidosis, may be the major cause of muscle fatigue that occurs in response to exercise (115). Increased P_i concentrations appear to affect sarcoplasmic reticulum handling of Ca^{2+} (6, 30). It has also been suggested that P_i can reduce **cross-bridge** attachment force as a result of a decrease in myofibrillar Ca^{2+} sensitivity (115).
- During prolonged exercise there is an increase in **glucose** uptake, despite a decrease in the amount of circulating **insulin** (75). Glucose uptake is thought to be facilitated during exercise as a result of **glucose transporter-4 (GLUT4)** (109). GLUT is contraction sensitive and facilitates the uptake of glucose by the working tissue (109).
- During exercise, whether endurance training or resistance training, significant eccentric exercise components can result in muscle damage (18). Examples of exercises that have the potential to increase muscle damage—resulting in **delayed-onset muscle soreness (DOMS)**—are downhill running and lowering weights in resistance training. Impairments in exercise performance in response to muscle damage and DOMS can last for up to 24 h, depending on the degree of muscle damage (47, 85). It has been hypothesized that the **inflammation** associated with muscle damage plays a role in muscle repair (18).

Phase II: Duration of 24 to 48 Hours

As soon as training is terminated, the compensation (rest) phase begins. During the compensation phase the following occur:

- Within 3 to 5 min of the cessation of exercise, ATP stores are completely restored (60, 66), and within 8 min PCr is completely resynthesized (60). Very high-intensity exercise may require up to 15 min of recovery after exercise for PCr to be completely restored (89). Depending on the volume, intensity, and type of training, the ATP and PCr pool may increase above normal levels (1, 2).
- Within 2 h after exercise bouts with large **stretch shortening cycle (SSC)** components, such as jumping, electromyographic (EMG) activity is partially restored as well as maximal voluntary contraction (MVC) (93). However, SSC-induced fatigue (as indicated by depressed EMG and MVC) exhibits a bimodal recovery, with the first recovery occurring within 2 h and the final recovery taking days (93). Muscle glycogen usually is restored to basal levels within 20 to 24 h (13, 29). If extensive muscle damage occurs, more time is needed for muscle glycogen recovery (25). The rate at which muscle glycogen is restored is directly related to the amount of carbohydrate consumed during the compensation period (26).
- An increase in oxygen consumption following exercise, known as **excess postexercise oxygen consumption (EPOC)**, occurs in response to the exercise bout (77).

Depending on the modality and intensity of the exercise bout, EPOC can remain elevated for 24 to 38 h after the cessation of exercise (14, 77, 90).

- Resting energy expenditure is elevated as a result of a resistance training or endurance training bout. This elevation in energy expenditure can be expected to last 15 to 48 h, depending on the magnitude of the training bout (71, 91). Although the exact mechanism for stimulating an elevation in resting energy expenditure is not known, some authors have suggested that increased **protein** synthesis (81), increased thermogenesis from the thyroid hormones (80), and increased **sympathetic nervous system** activity (100) play a role in increasing the rate of energy expenditure after exercise.
- After a resistance training bout, an increased protein synthesis rate occurs (17, 81). By 4 h postexercise the muscle protein synthesis rate is increased by 50%, and by 24 h it is elevated by 109%. The protein resynthesis rate returns to baseline by 36 h (81). Thus, it is thought that this phase of the supercompensation cycle is the initiation of the **anabolic** phase.

Phase III: Duration of 36 to 72 Hours

This phase of training is marked by a rebounding or supercompensation of performance. During this phase the following occur:

- Force-generating capacity and muscle soreness have returned to baseline by 72 h postexercise (118).
- Psychological supercompensation occurs, which can be marked by high confidence, feelings of being energized, positive thinking, and an ability to cope with frustrations and the stress of training.
- Glycogen stores are fully replenished, enabling the athlete to rebound (12).

Phase IV: Duration of 3 to 7 Days

If the athlete does not apply another stimulus at the optimal time (during the supercompensation phase), then involution occurs, which is a decrease in the physiological benefits obtained during the supercompensation phase. By 6 to 8 days after stretch shortening cycle (SSC) performance, the second rebound in electromyographic and maximal voluntary contraction strength occurs (93).

Following the optimal stimuli of a training session, the recovery period, including the supercompensation phase, is approximately 24 h. Variations in the duration of the supercompensation phase depend on the type and intensity of training. For instance, following a medium-intensity aerobic endurance training session, supercompensation may occur after approximately 6 to 8 h. On the other hand, intense activity that places a high demand on the central nervous system may require more than 24 h—sometimes as much as 48 h—for supercompensation to occur.

Elite athletes who follow training programs that do not allow 24 h between training sessions do not experience supercompensation after every training session because they must undertake a second workout before supercompensation can occur. As suggested in figure 1.10, the improvement rate is higher when athletes participate in more frequent training sessions (50). When long intervals exist between training sessions, such as when training is performed three times per week (figure 1.10a), the athlete will experience less overall improvement than when training is undertaken more frequently (figure 1.10b) (50, 97). When less time exists between training sessions, the coach or athlete must alternate the intensity of the training sessions, which effectively alters the energy demands of the session, as suggested in the planning of microcycles.

If the athlete is exposed to high-intensity training sessions too frequently, the body's ability to adapt to the training stimuli will be significantly compromised and overtraining may occur (41, 44, 45). As illustrated in figure 1.11, frequent maximal-intensity stimuli can result in exhaustion or overtraining, which will lead to a decrease in performance. Research

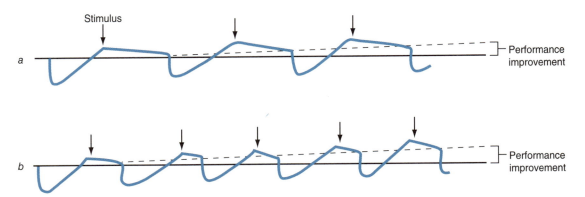

FIGURE 1.10 The sum of training effect: *(a)* long intervals between training sessions and *(b)* short intervals between training sessions.

Adapted from Harre 1982 (59).

on the training adaptations experienced in response to resistance training supports this contention (69, 97). Specifically, the research suggests that when maximal attempts are undertaken too frequently, there is a significant reduction in the athlete's ability to adapt to the training program (97). Coupling this finding with previous work on high-intensity overtraining (41, 44, 45) makes it clear that training at high intensities too frequently does not maximize the athlete's performance. Some overzealous coaches, who intend to project an image of being tough and hardworking, believe that athletes must reach exhaustion in each workout ("No pain, no gain!"). Under such circumstances, athletes never have time to compensate because such high levels of fatigue have been generated. As fatigue increases, the athlete will require longer time for regeneration. If additional hard training sessions are added too frequently, the time for restoration continues to lengthen. Thus, a better practice is to intersperse lower-intensity training sessions into the training plan so that compensation and ultimately supercompensation can occur.

To maximize the athlete's performance, the coach must regularly challenge the athlete's physiology, which elevates the ceiling of adaptation and, ultimately, performance (figure 1.12). This means that the coach must alternate high-intensity training with lower-intensity training. If done appropriately, this schedule will enhance compensation and lead to a supercompensation effect. As the athlete adapts to training, new levels of homeostasis will be achieved and higher training levels will be required for adaptation to continue (97). As the athlete adapts to new, higher levels of training, a new supercompensation cycle will begin (figure 1.13). Conversely, if the intensity of training is not planned well, the compensation curve will not surpass the previous levels of homeostasis and the athlete will not benefit from the supercompensation (figure 1.14).

High levels of fatigue resulting from continuous or too frequent high-intensity training will attenuate the supercompensation effects and prevent the athlete from achieving peak performance.

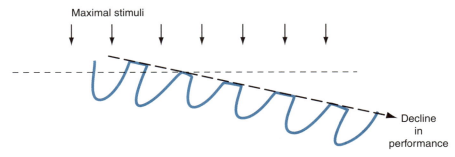

FIGURE 1.11 Decline in performance from prolonged maximal-intensity stimuli.

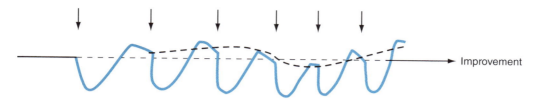

FIGURE 1.12 Alternating maximal- and low-intensity stimuli produces a wavelike improvement curve.

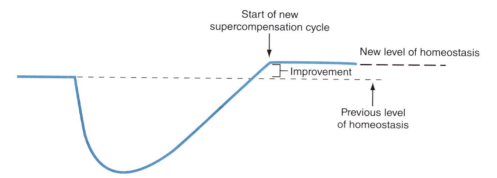

FIGURE 1.13 A new, higher level of homeostasis means that the next supercompensation cycle starts from that point.

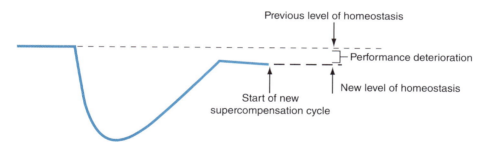

FIGURE 1.14 A decreased level of homeostasis means that the next supercompensation cycle starts at a point lower than the previous level.

Sources of Energy

Energy provides an athlete the capacity to perform work. **Work** is the application of force—that is, contracting muscles to apply force against a resistance. Energy is a prerequisite for performing physical work during training and competitions. Ultimately, we derive energy from converting foodstuff at the muscle cell level into a high-energy compound known as adenosine triphosphate (ATP), which is then stored in the muscle cell. ATP, as its name suggests, consists of one molecule of adenosine and three molecules of phosphate.

Energy required for muscular contraction is released by converting high-energy ATP into ADP + P_i (adenosine diphosphate + inorganic phosphate). As one phosphate bond is broken, causing ADP and P_i to split, energy is released. The amount of ATP stored in muscle is limited, so the body must continually replenish ATP stores to enable physical activity.

The body can replenish ATP stores by any of the three energy systems, depending on the type of physical activity: the anaerobic phosphagen (ATP-PC) system, the anaerobic glycolytic system, and the aerobic oxidative system (figure 1.15).

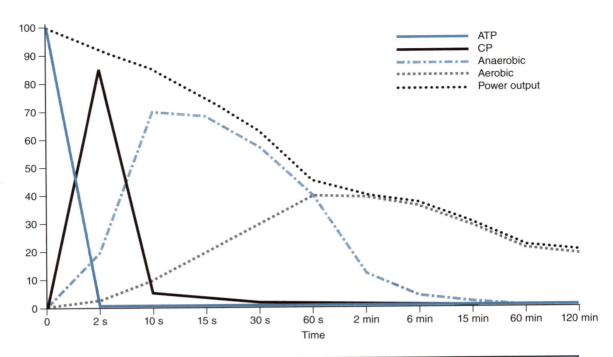

FIGURE 1.15 Energy provision of the three energy systems.

Adapted from K.A. van Someren, 2006, The physiology of anaerobic endurance training. In *The physiology of training*, edited by G. Whyte (Oxford, UK: Elsevier), 88, and E. Newsholme, A. Leech, and G. Duester, 1994, *Keep on running: The science of training and performance* (West Sussex, UK: Wiley).

Phosphagen (ATP-PC) System

The primary anaerobic energy system is the **phosphagen system (ATP-PC)**. The phosphagen system contains three basic reactions that are used in the processing of ATP. The first reaction results in the breakdown of ATP into **adenosine diphosphate (ADP)** and P_i, resulting in a release of energy. Because the skeletal muscle has limited ATP stores, further reactions are needed to maintain ATP availability. The second reaction is used to resynthesize ATP from ADP and phosphocreatine (creatine phosphate or PCr). In this scenario a phosphate is removed from the PCr, forming P_i and creatine (C). The P_i that is formed by this process is then added to ADP and an ATP molecule is formed. The final reaction that can occur breaks ADP into adenosine monophosphate and P_i, after which the P_i can again be added to ADP, resulting in the formation of ATP.

Because skeletal muscle can store only a small amount of ATP, energy depletion occurs in as little as 10 s of high-intensity work (87); PCr can be decreased by 50% to 70% of initial values in as little as 5 s of high-intensity exercise and can be almost completely depleted in response to intense exhaustive exercise (64, 73, 74). Interestingly, the highest contribution to ATP production by PCr occurs in the first 2 s of the initiation of exercise. By 10 s of exercise the ability of PCr to supply ATP is decreased by 50%, and by 30 s of exercise PCr contributes very little to the supply of ATP. At around 10 s, the glycolytic system's contribution to ATP supply begins to increase (87).

The phosphagen system appears to be the primary energy source for extremely high-intensity activities, such as short sprints (e.g., 100 m dash, 40 m dash), diving, American football, weightlifting, jumping and throwing events in track and field, vaulting in gymnastics, and ski jumping.

The replenishment of the phosphagen stores is usually a rapid process, with 70% restoration of ATP occurring in about 30 s and complete restoration occurring within 3 to 5 min of exercise (65). The restoration of PCr takes longer, with 2 min for 84% restoration, 4 min for 89% restoration, and 8 min for complete restoration (58, 65, 66). Restoration of the phosphagens occurs mostly via aerobic metabolism (60). However, the glycolytic system may also contribute to the restoration of the phosphagen pool after high-intensity exercise (34, 60).

Glycolytic System

The second anaerobic energy system is the glycolytic system, which is the prevalent energy system for activities that last from 20 s to about 2 min (87). The primary fuel for the glycolytic system comes from the breakdown of blood glucose and glycogen stores (107). Initially, the vast majority of ATP is supplied from **fast glycolysis**, and as the duration of activity approaches 2 min, the supply of ATP primarily comes from **slow glycolysis**.

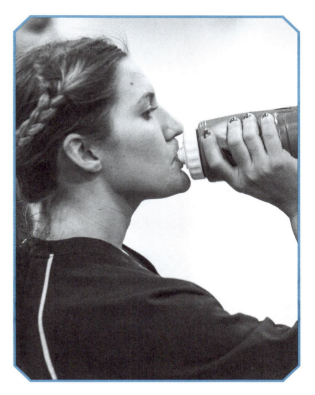

To perform well, an athlete must replenish her energy sources through proper nutrition and hydration.

Fast glycolysis results in the formation of lactic acid, which is rapidly converted to **lactate** (20). When glycolysis occurs at a very rapid rate, the body's ability to convert lactic acid to lactate may become impaired and lactic acid will begin to accumulate, which can result in fatigue and ultimately a cessation of activity (107). The accumulation of lactic acid is most prevalent in repeated high-intensity exercise bouts, especially those with short rest duration (63, 76). Thus, a high concentration of lactic acid may indicate a rapid energy supply.

As the duration of the activity increases toward the 2 min mark, the supply of ATP shifts from fast glycolysis to slow glycolysis. Theoretically, as the intensity of the bout of exercise is decreased the rate of glycolytic breakdown of glucose and glycogen is slowed, thus reducing the buildup of lactic acid and allowing the body to buffer lactic acid to lactate and form pyruvate (20, 107). Once pyruvate is formed it is shuttled into the **mitochondria**, where it is used in oxidative metabolism. Lactate is also shuttled to the liver, where it is converted into glucose, or goes to active tissue such as the skeletal and heart muscle, where it is converted to pyruvate and ultimately used in oxidative metabolism (87).

The amount of glycogen available is related to the amount of **carbohydrates** present in the diet (26). Thus, it is easy to see that low-carbohydrate diets will result in a reduction of muscle glycogen stores, which will impair the athlete's performance (57). The utilization of glycogen during exercise and competition depends on the duration and intensity of the exercise bout (56, 103, 104). Aerobic exercise (51) and anaerobic exercise such as repeated sprint intervals (3) and resistance training (56) can significantly affect muscle and liver glycogen stores. Following exercise, one of the major concerns for athletes and coaches is the time frame for glycogen resynthesis. If the athlete does not replenish glycogen stores, performance can be significantly impaired. Inadequate muscle glycogen stores have been linked to exercise-induced muscle weakness (117), decreases in isokinetic force production (70), and decreases in isometric strength (62).

After the completion of an exercise bout, it generally takes 20 to 24 h for muscle glycogen to be completely restored (29). If, however, inadequate carbohydrate is present in the diet or excessive exercise-induced muscle damage occurs, the time required for glycogen restoration can be significantly extended (24, 26). In the 2 h after the cessation of exercise, the athlete has a great opportunity to increase muscle glycogen synthesis rates. Ivy and colleagues (68) suggested that if carbohydrates are consumed within 2 h of the completion of exercise, muscle glycogen storage can increase 45%. This may be particularly important when the athlete has only a short period of time between exercise bouts or competitive bouts on the same day (56).

Oxidative System

Much like the glycolytic system, the oxidative system has the ability to use blood glucose and muscle glycogen as fuel sources for producing ATP. The major difference between the glycolytic and oxidative systems is that the enzymatic reactions associated with the oxidative system occur in the presence of O_2, whereas the glycolytic system processes energy without O_2 (10). Unlike the fast glycolytic system, the oxidative system does not produce lactic acid from the breakdown of glucose and glycogen. Additionally, the oxidative system has the ability to use fats and proteins in the production of ATP (107).

At rest, the oxidative system derives about 70% of its ATP yield from the oxidation of fats and about 30% of its ATP from the oxidation of carbohydrate (10, 107). Fuel utilization depends on the intensity of exercise. Brooks and colleagues (10) outlined what is termed the **cross-over concept**, in which lower-intensity exercise receives its ATP primarily from the oxidation of fat and some carbohydrates. As the intensity of exercise increases, the amount of carbohydrate used for ATP production increases whereas the utilization of fat to supply ATP decreases. This again gives support for the concept that higher-intensity exercise bouts use carbohydrate as a primary fuel source.

The oxidative or aerobic system is the primary source of ATP for events lasting between 2 min and approximately 3 h (all track events of 800 m or more, cross-country skiing, long-distance speedskating). Conversely, activities that are shorter than 2 min rely on anaerobic means to meet their ATP demands (88).

The coach and athlete need to understand the bioenergetic mechanisms that supply energy for exercise and sport performance. A structure can be created in which the athlete is trained based on the bioenergetics of the sporting activity. This has been termed **bioenergetic specificity** (107). Figure 1.16 illustrates the energy sources used for specific sports and events. The coach and athlete can use the bioenergetic classification of sports, which is based on the duration, the intensity, and the fuel used by the activity, to create effective training programs for specific sports.

Overlap of the Energy Systems

At all times the various energy systems contribute to the overall ATP yield. However, depending on the physiological demands associated with the exercise bout, ATP yield can be linked to a primary energy system (107). For example, very high-intensity events that occur in a short time, such as the 100 m sprint, can result in a significant reliance on the anaerobic energy systems to meet the demand for ATP (99). As the duration of the activity is extended, the reliance on oxidative mechanisms for supplying ATP increase (figure 1.17). For example, exercise bouts that last approximately 1 min will meet 70% of the body's energy demand via anaerobic mechanisms, whereas bouts of exercise that are 4 min in duration will meet 65% of the body's energy demand via the use of aerobic metabolism (99). Thus, there is a primary energy system that meets the athlete's ATP needs during a specific sporting event, and understanding this will help the coach and athlete design training programs that target specific bioenergetic needs for the sporting activity (107).

Energy pathways	Anaerobic pathways		Aerobic pathways							
	ATP-PC	Glycolytic								
Primary energy sources	ATP produced without the presence of oxygen		ATP produced in the presence of oxygen							
Fuel	Phosphagens: muscular stores of ATP and PCr	Blood glucose Liver glycogen Muscle glycogen		Glycogen completely metabolized in the presence of oxygen			Fat			Protein
Duration	0 s	10 s	40 s	60 s	2 min	4 min	10 min	30 min	1 hr	2 hr	3 hr
Sports events	Sprinting (<100 m)	Sprinting (200-400 m)		100 m swimming		Middle-distance track, swimming, speed skating	Long-distance track, swimming, speed skating, and canoeing				
	Throwing	Speed skating (500 m)		800 m track		1,000 m canoeing	Cross-country skiing				
	Throwing	Most gym events		500 m canoeing		Boxing	Rowing				
	Weightlifting	Track cycling		1,500 m speedskating		Wrestling	Cycling: road racing				
	Ski jumping	50 m swim		Floor exercise in gymnastics		Martial arts	Marathon				
	Golf (swinging)			Alpine skiing		Figure skating	Triathlon				
	Diving			Cycling: track; 1,000 m and pursuit		Synchronized swimming					
	Vaulting in gymnastics					Cycling: pursuit					
	Most team sports, racket sports, sailing										
Skills	Mostly acyclic	Acyclic and cyclic					Cyclic				

FIGURE 1.16 Energy sources for competitive sport.

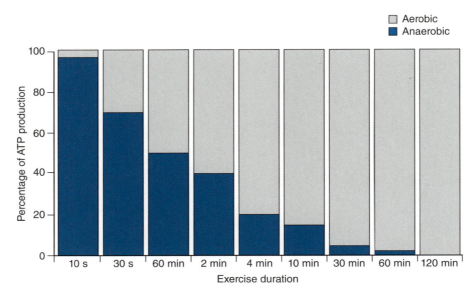

FIGURE 1.17 Relationship between time and anaerobic and aerobic energy supply.

The amount of lactate in the blood gives insight into which energy system is acting as the primary energy supplier. Higher levels of lactate formation suggest that the glycolytic system is operating at a very high rate, thus creating a buildup of lactic acid and lactate. In endurance or aerobic activities, the first point at which lactate formation begins to abruptly increase is termed the **lactate threshold (LT)** and represents a shift from aerobic energy supply to anaerobic energy supply as intensity of exercise increases (107). In untrained individuals, the LT occurs somewhere between 50% and 60% of **maximal aerobic capacity** ($\dot{V}O_2$max), whereas highly trained endurance athletes demonstrate an LT as high as 80% of $\dot{V}O_2$max (16, 88). The LT of an elite endurance athlete can occur somewhere between 83% and 93% of maximal heart rate (35, 67, 95). The second major increase in lactate accumulation occurs at about 4 mm and is termed the **onset of blood lactate accumulation (OBLA)** (88). In trained endurance athletes, the OBLA has been demonstrated to occur between 90% and 93% of maximum heart rate (35, 67, 95).

Several researchers have offered evidence that the time point at which the LT and OBLA occur is affected by the training stimulus (39, 78, 79). Recent work by Esfarjani and Laursen (39) suggests that performing high-intensity intervals can result in significant elevations in endurance performance and in the LT, allowing the endurance athlete to work at a higher intensity before experiencing lactic acid buildup.

Sprint interval training has been demonstrated to increase glycolytic and oxidative enzymatic activity, improve maximal short-term power output, and increase maximal aerobic power (82). It has been suggested that a high aerobic capacity enhances the recovery from high-intensity anaerobic exercise because this capacity enhances removal of lactate and PCr regeneration (112). These findings might falsely lead coaches and athletes to think that aerobic training is needed to enhance the athlete's ability to recover from repetitive bouts of high-intensity anaerobic exercise. However, several studies clearly demonstrate that maximal aerobic power or capacity is of little importance in the recovery from repetitive bouts of high-intensity anaerobic exercise (8, 15, 22, 114). The inclusion of high-intensity interval training by athletes who participate in sports that are predominated by anaerobic energy supply will result in an aerobic capacity that is high enough to enhance **postexercise recovery** (15). Although the inclusion of aerobic training significantly increases aerobic power and capacity, it generally decreases anaerobic performance (37). Therefore, coaches and athletes should focus on enhancing the bioenergetic profile for the sporting event.

Table 1.2 provides information regarding the bioenergetic characteristics of many sports. In interval training, the rest interval between bouts of activity can significantly affect the primary energy system stressed (107). Shorter work-to-rest intervals (such as 1:1-1:3) will selectively target the oxidative system, whereas longer work-to-rest intervals (1:12-1:20) will selectively target the phosphagen system (107). Coaches should consider modeling the intensity and time characteristics of the sporting event, design conditioning drills that model the bioenergetics of the sporting event, and incorporate the tactical and technical components of the activity. If incorporated correctly, the conditioning drill will account for the time characteristics and the intensity profile of the activity. To design effective programs, the coach or athlete needs to understand the performance characteristics and bioenergetic demands of the sporting activity.

TABLE 1.2 Energy Delivery Systems (Ergogenesis in Percentages) for Sports

Sport	Event or position	Phosphagen	Glycolytic	Oxidative	Reference
Archery		0	0	100	Mathews and Fox (86)
Athletics (track and field)	100 m	53	44	3	van Someren (113), Newsholme and Duester (92b)
	200 m	26	45	29	van Someren (113), Newsholme and Duester (92b)
	400 m	12	50	38	van Someren (113), Newsholme and Duester (92b)
	800 m	6	33	61	van Someren (113), Newsholme and Duester (92b)
	1,500 m	-	20	80	van Someren (113), Newsholme and Duester (92b)
	5,000 m	-	12.5	87.5	van Someren (113), Newsholme and Duester (92b)
	10,000 m	-	3	97	van Someren (113), Newsholme and Duester (92b)
	Marathon	-		100	van Someren (113), Newsholme and Duester (92b)
	Jumps	90	10	0	Powers and Howley (99)
	Throws	90	10	0	Powers and Howley (99)
Baseball		80	15	5	Powers and Howley (99)
Basketball		80	10	10	Powers and Howley (99)
Biathlon		0	5	95	Dal Monte (31)
Canoeing	C1: 1,000 m	25	35	40	Dal Monte (31)
	C2: 1,000 m	20	55	25	Dal Monte (31)
	C1,2: 10,000 m	5	10	85	Dal Monte (31)
Cycling	200 m track	98	2	0	Dal Monte (31)
	4,000 m pursuit	20	50	30	Dal Monte (31)
	Road racing	0	5	95	Dal Monte (31)

(continued)

TABLE 1.2 *(continued)*

Sport	Event or position	Phosphagen	Glycolytic	Oxidative	Reference
Diving		98	2	0	Powers and Howley (99)
Driving	Motor sports, luge	0	0-15	85-10	Dal Monte (31)
Equestrian		20-30	20-50	20-50	Dal Monte (31)
Fencing		90	10	0	Dal Monte (31)
Field hockey		60	20	20	Powers and Howley (99)
Figure skating		60-80	10-30	20	Dal Monte (31)
Football		90	10	0	Powers and Howley (99)
Golf (swinging)		100	0	0	Powers and Howley (99)
Gymnastics		90	10	0	Powers and Howley (99)
Handball		80	10	10	Dal Monte (31)
Ice hockey	Forward	80	20	0	Powers and Howley (99)
	Defense	80	20	0	Powers and Howley (99)
	Goalie	95	5	0	Powers and Howley (99)
Judo		90	10	0	Dal Monte (31)
Kayaking	K1: 500 m	25	60	15	Dal Monte (31)
	K2,4: 500 m	30	60	10	Dal Monte (31)
	K1: 1,000 m	20	50	30	Dal Monte (31)
	K2,4: 1,000 m	20	55	25	Dal Monte (31)
	K1,2,4: 10,000 m	5	10	85	Dal Monte (31)
Rowing		20	30	50	Powers and Howley (99)
Rugby		30-40	10-20	30-50	Dal Monte (31)
Sailing		0	15	85-100	Dal Monte (31)
Shooting		0	0	100	Dal Monte (31)
Skiing	Slalom (45-50 s)	40	50	10	Alpine Canada (4)
	Giant slalom (70-90 s)	30	50	20	Alpine Canada (4)
	Super giant (80-120 s)	15	45	40	Alpine Canada (4)
	Downhill (90-150 s)	10	45	45	Alpine Canada (4)
	Nordic	0	5	95	Dal Monte (31)
Soccer	Goalie	80	20	0	Powers and Howley (99)
	Halfback	60	20	20	Powers and Howley (99)
	Striker	80	20	0	Powers and Howley (99)
	Wing	80	20	0	Powers and Howley (99)

Sport	Event or position	Phosphagen	Glycolytic	Oxidative	Reference
Speedskating	500 m	95	5	0	Dal Monte (31)
	1,500 m	30	60	10	Dal Monte (31)
	5,000 m	10	40	50	Dal Monte (31)
	10,000 m	5	15	80	Dal Monte (31)
Swimming	50 m	95	5	0	Powers and Howley (99)
	100 m	80	15	5	Powers and Howley (99)
	200 m	30	65	5	Powers and Howley (99)
	400 m	20	40	40	Powers and Howley (99)
	800 m	10	30	60	Mathews and Fox (86)
	1,500 m	10	20	70	Powers and Howley (99)
Tennis		70	20	10	Powers and Howley (99)
Volleyball		90	10	0	Powers and Howley (99)
Water polo		30	40	30	Dal Monte (31)
Wrestling		45	55	0	Powers and Howley (99)

The coach or athlete should consider the durations of a rally in racket sports, a tactical segment of a game in basketball or ice hockey, and the rest interval between bouts of exercise. For example, when designing training programs for sports such as football, soccer, or rugby, the coach should consider the position the athlete plays on the team. In American football, the average play lasts between 4 and 6 s and players have rest intervals of 25 to 45 s; in addition, different positions have very different physiological challenges (98). When looking at soccer, the coach should consider the distance covered by the various positions (defenders ~10 km; midfield players ~12 km; forwards ~10.5 km); these distances will affect the bioenergetic stressors placed on each athlete (7). In a soccer match, high-intensity exercise that taxes the anaerobic system lasts around 7 min with an average of 19 sprints that last about 2.0 s, with the remainder of the activity taxing the aerobic system (7).

Summary of Major Concepts

The purpose of training is to increase athletes' working capacity, skill effectiveness, and psychological qualities to improve their performance in competitions. Training is a long-term endeavor. Athletes are not developed overnight, and a coach cannot create miracles by cutting corners and overlooking scientific and methodological theories.

As athletes train, they adapt or adjust to the training load. The better the athlete's anatomical, physiological, and psychological adaptation, the higher the probability of improving his or her athletic performance.

Supercompensation is the most important concept in training. The dynamics of a supercompensation cycle depend on planned training intensities. Good planning must consider supercompensation because its application in training ensures the restoration of energy and, most importantly, helps athletes avoid critical levels of fatigue that can result in overtraining.

To conduct an effective training program, coaches must understand energy systems, the fuel used by each system, and how much time athletes need to restore energy fuels used in training and competition. A good understanding of restoration time for an energy system is the foundation for calculating rest intervals between training activities during a workout, between workouts, and after a competition.

Principles of Training 2

Since athletic training began, more than 3,000 years ago (see *The Aeneid*, written by the Roman poet Virgil in the second decade BC), athletes and trainers have established and followed principles of training. These principles have evolved through the years as a result of research in the biological, pedagogical, and psychological sciences. These principles of sports training are the foundation of the theory and methodology of training.

The main objective of training is to increase the athlete's sporting skills and, ultimately, level of sporting performance. Training principles are part of a whole concept and should not be viewed in isolated units. However, they are often examined separately to better understand the basic concepts. Correct use of these training principles will result in superior training programs and well-trained athletes.

Multilateral Development Versus Specialization

The overall development of athletes involves striking a balance between multilateral development and specialized training. In general, the early development of athletes should focus on multilateral development, which targets the overall physical development of the athletes. As the athlete becomes more developed, the proportion of specialized training, which focuses primarily on the skills needed in the targeted sport, steadily increases. In order to effectively develop the athlete, the coach must understand the importance of each of these two training stages and how the training focus changes as the athlete develops.

Multilateral Development

Support for the concept of multilateral development is found in most areas of education and human endeavors. In athletics, multilateral development, or overall physical development, is a necessity (9, 25, 83). The use of a multilateral development plan is extremely important during the early stages of an athlete's development (83). Multilateral development during the athlete's formative years lays the groundwork for later periods of training when specialization becomes a greater focus of the training plan. If properly implemented, the multilateral training phase will allow the athlete to develop the physiological and psychological basis needed to maximize performance later in her career (83).

The temptation to deviate from a multilateral development plan and begin specialized training too soon can be very great, especially when a young athlete demonstrates rapid development in a sporting activity. In such cases, it is paramount that the instructor, coach, or parent resist this temptation; it has been well documented that a broad multilateral base of physical development is necessary to prepare the athlete for more specialized training later in his development (9, 25, 83). If training is sequenced appropriately and begins with a strong foundation of multilateral training early in the athlete's development, the athlete

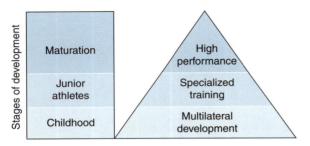

FIGURE 2.1 Sequential model for long-term athletic training.

will be able to achieve much higher levels of physical preparation and technical mastery and ultimately will achieve higher levels of performance.

A sequential approach to an athlete's development, progressing from multilateral to specialized training as the athlete matures, appears to be a prerequisite for maximizing sporting performance (25, 79, 84). Figure 2.1 illustrates a conceptual model for a long-term sequential approach to training.

The base of the pyramid in figure 2.1 represents a period of multilateral development, which is the foundation of the training program. This part of the training program includes multifaceted motor development, multisport skills, and some sport-specific skills. The variety of exercise that the athlete undertakes during this time allows for full development of the child's physiological systems. For example, in this phase of training the neuromuscular, cardiovascular, and energy systems are activated in various ways to allow for balanced development. When the athlete's development reaches an acceptable level, especially her physical development, she will progress to the second phase of development, which is marked by a greater degree of specialization.

The multilateral phase of training does not exclude specificity in the training process. On the contrary, training specificity is present in all stages of a training program but in varying proportions, as can be seen in figure 2.2. Figure 2.2 shows that during the multilateral phase of training, the percentage of specialized training is very small. As the athlete matures, the degree of specialization increases. It is believed that the multilateral base serves as a foundation for future development and helps the athlete avoid overuse injuries and staleness in training (83).

Support for the benefits of multilateral development can be seen in three longitudinal studies performed in three countries (18, 22, 46). In a 14-year study in the former East

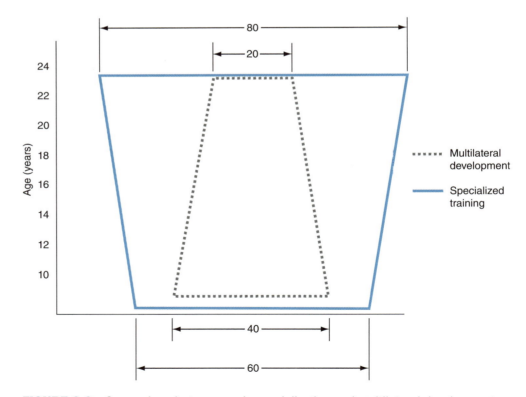

FIGURE 2.2 Comparison between early specialization and multilateral development.

Germany (46), a large number of 9- to 12-year-olds were placed into two groups. The first group trained in a manner similar to the approach taken in North America, focusing on early specialization in a given sport. These athletes used exercises and training methods that were specific to a particular sport. The second group followed a generalized program that focused on multilateral development. This group participated in a variety of sports, learned a variety of skills, and undertook overall physical training in addition to sport-specific skills training. The results of this investigation support the contention that a strong foundation, which is established by using a multilateral approach, leads to greater athletic success.

Russian sources (22) often refer to a survey that resulted in similar findings. This longitudinal study concluded that specialization should not start in most sports before the age of 15. Some of the major findings of this study are as follows:

- Most of the best Russian athletes had a strong multilateral foundation.
- Most athletes started training at 7 or 8 years of age. During the first few years, all athletes participated in various sports, such as soccer, cross-country skiing, running, skating, swimming, and cycling. From ages 10 to 13, the children also participated in team sports, gymnastics, rowing, and track and field.
- Specialized programs started at ages 15 to 17, without neglecting earlier sports and activities. Best performances were achieved after 5 to 8 years in the specialized sports.
- Athletes who specialized at a much earlier age achieved their best performances at a junior age level (<18 years). These performances were never duplicated when they became seniors (>18 years). Many retired before reaching senior levels. Only a minority of the athletes who specialized at a young age were able to improve performance at senior level.

Comparison Between Early Specialization and Multilateral Development

Early Specialization
- Quick performance improvement
- Best performances achieved at 15 to 16 years of age because of quick adaptation
- Inconsistent performance in competition
- High incidence of burnout and quitting sport by age 18
- Increased risk of injury because of forced adaptation and lack of physiological development

Multilateral Development
- Slower performance improvement
- Best performances at age 18 or older when the athlete has reached physiological and psychological maturation
- Consistent and progressive performance in competition
- Longer athletic career
- Fewer injuries as a result of more progressive loading patterns and overall physiological development

Based on Harre 1982 (46).

- Many top-class athletes started to train in an organized environment at the junior level (14-18 years of age). They had never been junior champions or held national records, but at the senior age many of them achieved national- and international-class performances.
- Most athletes considered their success attributable to the multilateral foundation built during childhood and junior age.

The third study, conducted by Carlson (18), analyzed the training background and development patterns of elite Swedish tennis players who were very successful in international competition. The subjects were divided into a study group that consisted of elite adult tennis players and a control group that was matched by age, gender, and junior rankings. The most relevant findings are shown in the summary of research on page 33. Both groups of players were equal in skills up to the age group of 12 to 14; the difference in skills between the two groups occurred after this age. Researchers also found that, in the control group, skill development was fast during early adolescence, and these players participated in an atmosphere of high demand for success. Interestingly, the control group players specialized at age 11, whereas the study group did not begin to specialize until age 14. In fact, the study group participated in a wide variety of sporting activities during early adolescence, whereas the control group performed specialized, professional-like training. Although the control group demonstrated significantly greater performances as juniors, the study group demonstrated their highest levels of performance as senior athletes. The work of Carlson (18) supports the importance of a multilateral training approach that is marked by all-around sport engagement and less professional-type training during early childhood and adolescence.

The coach should consider multilateral training in the early stages of an athlete's development as the foundation for future specialization and athletic mastery (58). Multilateral training should be used mostly when training children and juniors (9, 58). In these stages of athlete development, it is essential that a strong vocabulary of physical and psychological attributes be developed. Physical skill sets that are essential during this phase of training include natural movements like running, jumping, climbing, and throwing (58, 78). Additionally, it is important to develop speed, agility, coordination, flexibility, and overall general fitness at this phase of development. These training goals are best accomplished through diverse activities that allow for the development of several biomotor abilities. In this process, the young athlete will be taught a diverse group of exercise techniques, which include some of the technical aspects of the selected sport. All of these skill sets will be used as the athlete becomes more developed and as multilateral training becomes less of a focus.

All athletes should participate in multilateral training to some degree throughout their careers (figure 2.2). The greatest amount of multilateral training occurs during the early stages of development; as the athlete progresses, there is less focus on this type of training. Multilateral development is essential to optimize the effects of specialized training later in the athlete's career.

Specialization

Whether training on a field, in a pool, or in a gymnasium, the athlete eventually will specialize in a sport or event. Training for a sport results in physiological adaptations that are specific to the activity's movement pattern, metabolic demand, force generation pattern, contraction type, and muscle recruitment pattern (28, 82, 89). The type of training used has a very specific effect on the athlete's physiological characteristics (21). For example, endurance training has the ability to stimulate both central and peripheral adaptations, which can include altering neural recruitment patterns, modifying bioenergetic or metabolic factors, and stimulating significant skeletal muscle alterations (2, 48). Conversely, strength training results in significant alterations to the contractile machinery, neuromuscular system, and bioenergetic or metabolic pathways (1, 21). Contemporary research suggests that skeletal muscle exhibits a large amount of plasticity in response to different modalities of strength

Summary of Research Examining the Effects of Early Specialization and Multilateral Training on Athlete Development

Control Group
- Began to specialize at age 11, when multilateral training ceased
- Experienced significantly less multilateral training during early development ages
- Practiced tennis more than the study group between the ages of 13 and 15
- Tended to lose self-confidence as they progressed through training
- Developed faster than the study group during early adolescence
- Experienced greater pressure for success during early stages of development from parents and coaches

Study Group
- Began to specialize at age 14 or older
- Experienced significantly more multilateral training during early development stages
- Practiced tennis more than the control group after age 15
- Tended to gain self-confidence as they progressed through training
- Developed more slowly than the control group during early adolescence
- Experienced less pressure for success during early stages of development from parents and coaches

Adapted from Carlson 1988 (18).

---

or endurance training; this results in the activation or deactivation of different molecular signaling pathways depending on the type of training encountered (4, 6, 7, 21, 67, 68, 100). Specific adaptations are not limited to physiological responses because technical, tactical, and psychological traits are also developed in response to specialized training. It is likely that each sporting activity can develop attributes that allow the athlete to achieve a high level of mastery.

Specialization is a complex, nonunilateral process that is based on multilateral development. As an athlete progresses from a beginner to a mature athlete who has mastered his sport, the total volume and intensity of training progressively increase, as does the degree of specialization. Several authors suggest that the best training adaptations occur in response to exercises specific to the sporting activity and exercises that target given biomotor abilities only after a multilateral foundation has been developed (22, 78). The former refers to exercises that parallel or mimic the movements of the sport; the latter refers to exercises that develop strength, speed, and endurance. The ratio between these two exercise groups varies for each sport, depending on the sport's characteristics. In long-distance running, for example, approximately 90% of the volume of training consists of sport-specific exercises. In other sports, like high jumping, these exercises represent only 40%; exercises that develop leg strength and jumping power make up the rest. When working with advanced athletes, coaches should dedicate only 60% to 80% of the total training time to sport-specific exercise (figure 2.2) and should dedicate the remainder of training to developing biomotor abilities.

Coaches should carefully plan the ratio between multilateral and specialized training, taking into consideration the modern tendency to lower the age of athletic maturation. In some sports, athletes achieve a high level of performance at young ages and thus must enter the sport at a young age (25). Examples of these sports include artistic gymnastics, gymnastics, figure skating, swimming, and diving. However, recent changes to Olympic competition rules may increase the average age for high-level gymnastics performance. For example, to compete in the Olympics a female gymnast must turn 16 during the year of the Olympic Games. During the years 2005 to 2007, the average age of competitors at the gymnastics world championships was about 18 (84).

Table 2.1 presents a rough guide for the age an individual can begin to train, the age when specialization may start, and the age when the highest performance is usually reached. Some authors suggest that the optimal age to begin training is between 5 and 9 (9, 12). During these early phases of training the coach should focus on developing a physical literacy that includes basic skills such as running, jumping, and throwing (9). It is important to develop these skills at the initiation of training because young athletes seem to develop these abilities at a faster rate than more mature athletes. Once the athlete develops the basics skills, he can

TABLE 2.1 Age of Starting, Specializing in, and Reaching High Performance in Different Sports

Sport	Age to begin training	Age to start specialization	Age when highest performance is achieved
Archery	12-14	16-18	23-30
Athletics (track and field)			
Sprinting	10-12	14-16	22-26
Middle-distance running	13-14	16-17	22-26
Long-distance running	14-16	17-20	25-28
High jump	12-14	16-18	22-25
Triple jump	12-14	17-19	23-26
Long jump	12-14	17-19	23-26
Throws	14-15	17-19	23-27
Badminton	10-12	14-16	20-25
Baseball	10-12	15-16	22-28
Basketball	10-12	14-16	22-28
Biathlon	10-12	16-17	23-26
Bobsled	12-14	17-18	22-26
Boxing	13-15	16-17	22-26
Canoeing	12-14	15-17	22-26
Chess	7-8	12-15	23-35
Continental handball	10-12	14-16	22-26
Cycling	12-15	16-18	22-28
Diving			
Women	6-8	9-11	14-18
Men	8-10	11-13	18-22

Sport	Age to begin training	Age to start specialization	Age when highest performance is achieved
Equestrian	10-12	14-16	22-28
Fencing	10-12	14-16	20-25
Field hockey	11-13	14-16	20-25
Figure skating	7-9	11-13	18-25
Football	12-14	16-18	23-27
Gymnastics			
Women	6-8	9-10	14-18
Men	8-9	14-15	22-25
Ice hockey	6-8	13-14	22-28
Judo	8-10	15-16	22-26
Modern pentathlon	11-13	14-16	21-25
Rowing	11-14	16-18	22-25
Rugby	13-14	16-17	22-26
Sailing	10-12	14-16	22-30
Shooting	12-15	17-18	24-30
Skiing			
Alpine	7-8	12-14	18-25
Nordic	12-14	16-18	23-28
More than 30K	—	17-19	24-28
Jumping	10-12	14-15	22-26
Speedskating	10-12	15-16	22-26
Soccer	10-12	14-16	22-26
Squash and handball	10-12	15-17	23-27
Swimming			
Women	7-9	11-13	18-22
Men	<7-8	13-15	20-24
Synchronized swimming	6-8	12-14	19-23
Table tennis	8-9	13-14	22-25
Tennis			
Women	7-8	11-13	20-25
Men	7-8	12-14	22-27
Volleyball	10-12	15-16	22-26
Water polo	10-12	16-17	23-26
Weightlifting	14-15	17-18	23-27
Wrestling	11-13	17-19	24-27

Reprinted, by permission, from T.O. Bompa and M. Carrera, 2015, *Conditioning young athletes* (Champaign, IL: Human Kinetics), 9.

begin some specialized training for his chosen sport. This generally occurs between ages 10 and 14 (9). As stated previously multilateral training is the primary focus until around age 14, after which more specialized training occurs.

Individualization

Individualization is one of the main requirements of contemporary training. Individualization requires that the coach consider the athlete's abilities, potential, and learning characteristics and the demands of the athlete's sport, regardless of the performance level. Each athlete has physiological and psychological attributes that need to be considered when developing a training plan.

Too often, coaches take an unscientific approach to training by literally following training programs of successful athletes or sport programs with complete disregard for the athlete's training experience, abilities, and physiological makeup. Even worse, some coaches take programs from elite athletes and apply them to junior athletes who have not yet developed the physical literacy, physiological base, or psychological skills needed to undertake these types of programs. Young athletes are not physiologically or psychologically able to tolerate programs created for advanced athletes (26, 27, 39, 99). The coach needs to understand the athlete's needs and develop training plans that meet those needs. This can be accomplished by following some guidelines.

Plan According to Tolerance Level

The training plan must be based on a comprehensive analysis of the athlete's physiological and psychological parameters, which will give the coach insight into the athlete's work capacity. An individual's training capacity can be determined by the following factors:

- *Biological age:* The **biological age** of an athlete is considered a more accurate indicator of the individual's physical performance potential than his **chronological age** (25, 65). One of the best indicators of biological age is sexual maturation (15, 38) because it indicates an increase in circulating **testosterone** levels (65, 75). Athletes who are more physically mature, as indicated by a higher biological age, appear to be stronger, faster, and better at team sports than their peers who exhibit a lower biological age, even when chronological age is the same (38, 65). In general children have a greater resistance to fatigue, which may explain why they respond better to higher volumes of training (73). On the other hand, older adults appear to exhibit a decreased motivation to train intensely (91), an increased prevalence of injuries (55), and an increased occurrence of social stressors (91), all of which may contribute to a decreased ability to tolerate intense training. Most junior athletes tolerate high volumes of training with moderate loads better than high-intensity or high-load training (27, 39, 73). The combination of heavy loading and high volume is of concern with youth athletes because this practice may increase the risk of musculoskeletal injuries (39).
- *Training age:* **Training age** is defined as the number of years an individual has been preparing for a sporting activity (12), and it is considerably different than the biological or chronological age. Athletes with a high training age have developed a substantial training base and most likely will be able to participate in a specialized training plan, especially if their early training was multilateral. An athlete who has a high chronological age in conjunction with a low training age may need more multilateral and skill acquisition training because he lacks the training base to allow for a high degree of specialization in his sport.
- *Training history:* The athlete's training history influences his work capacity. An athlete who has undertaken substantial multilateral training is more likely to have developed her physical potential and **readiness** for more challenging training, compared with an athlete who has not been trained as well.

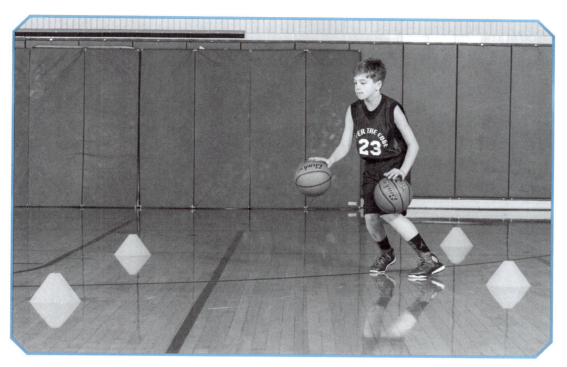

The age and skill level of an athlete, along with other factors, must be taken into consideration when planning training and practice sessions.

- *Health status:* An athlete who is ill or injured will have a reduced work capacity and often will not be able to tolerate the prescribed training loads. The type of illness or degree of injury and the physiological base converge to determine the training load that the athlete can tolerate (89). The coach must monitor the athlete's health status to determine an appropriate training load.
- *Stress and the recovery rate:* The ability to tolerate a training load is often related to all of the stressors that the athlete encounters (89). Overall stressors are considered additive, and factors that place a high demand on the athlete can alter his ability to tolerate a training load (92). For example, heavy involvement in school, work, or family activities can affect the athlete's ability to tolerate a training load. Travel to and from work, school, or training can further contribute to stress levels. Coaches should consider these factors and adjust the training load accordingly. For example, during times of high stress, such as academic examinations, a reduction in training load may be warranted.

Individualize the Training Load

The ability to adapt to a training load depends on the individual's capacity. As outlined in the preceding section, many factors contribute to the individualized response to training loads and progressions: the athlete's training history, health status, life stress, chronological age, biological age, and training age. Simply mimicking the training plans of elite athletes will not result in high levels of performance (89). Rather, the coach must address the athlete's needs and capacities by developing an individualized program; this requires detailed observations of the athlete's technical and tactical abilities, physical characteristics, strengths, and weaknesses. As will be discussed later in this chapter, in the section about training models, periodic testing of the athlete will allow for more specific and individualized training plans to be developed. If athletes are roughly at the same level of development and stage of training, less individualization of the training plan may be needed (89).

Account for Gender Differences

Gender differences can play an important role in performance and individualized training adaptations. Prepubescent boys and girls are very similar in height, weight, girth, bone width, and skinfold thickness (99). After the onset of puberty, boys and girls begin to develop substantial differences in physical attributes. After puberty girls tend to have higher levels of body fat, lower amounts of fat-free mass, and lighter total body masses (99). From a performance perspective, it is clear that men and women differ in muscle mass and strength (29, 35, 54, 93), anaerobic power and capacity (36, 64), and maximal aerobic capacity and performance (3, 19, 20, 24, 81).

Some researchers suggest that gender differences are related to anatomical or biomechanical factors (60, 66), whereas others suggest that training experiences and access to specialized training partially explain gender differences in performance (60). Support for the contention that training may partially explain the difference between the genders has been offered by Kraemer and colleagues (57), who found that differences in performance between men and women were substantially reduced when appropriate training was undertaken by women.

After looking at elite anaerobic performances (sprinting, swimming, and speedskating) from 1952 to 2006, Seiler and colleagues (80) reported that performance differences between males and females initially decreased, but more recently performances differences between the genders have ceased to narrow. Cheuvront and colleagues (19) discovered a similar trend in distance running performance when they compared performance variables between men and women.

Women are able to tolerate extensive and intensive training programs (17). In fact, Cao (17) suggested that women are capable of handling higher volumes and intensities of resistance training than their male counterparts. However, caution should be taken when examining these data because women do have specific areas that need to be addressed. For example, women tend to be weaker in the upper body (17, 28) and trunk musculature (17). The inclusion of more exercises to strengthen these areas in female athletes may be warranted.

The performance responses of female athletes during the different phases of the menstrual cycle appear to be very individualized (99). The scientific literature suggests that in most situations, maximal and submaximal aerobic performance (53) and anaerobic performance (14, 53) are not affected by the menstrual cycle. However, the scientific literature suggests that temperature regulation is compromised during the luteal phase as a result of an increase in core temperature (53). This may be an important consideration for women who are exercising or training for extended periods of time in hot and humid conditions.

Incorporate Training Variation

Variation is one of the key components needed to induce adaptations in response to training. Skill acquisition and performance increase rapidly when novel tasks are first undertaken, but the rate of skill acquisition slows with repetition of the same training plan or loading structure over time (51). Stone and colleagues (86) suggested that a lack of training variation can result in **monotonous program overtraining.** This condition occurs if the same training stimulus is introduced regularly for long periods of time, ultimately resulting in a reduction or plateau of performance, which could be defined as a form of overtraining. In support of this contention, O'Toole (69) suggested that the degree of monotony in the training plan is significantly related to poor performance.

Periodization of training not only decreases monotony or boredom in training but also sequences training phases in such a way that morphofunctional adaptations build on each other and ultimately induce greater physiological adaptations. Zatsiorsky (101) suggested that periodization is a balancing act between training variation and stability (monotony or repetition) of **training**. Thus variation of training is of paramount importance when considering periodization (72, 82, 89). Optimal training adaptations occur in response to a systematic variation in training load and content. If inadequate variation is provided and the program is monotonous, performance will not be optimized. This happens when the nervous system is not overloaded sufficiently to stimulate physiological adaptations (86, 89).

Variation can be incorporated into the training plan at many levels. For example, variation at the microcycle level can be added by altering training volume, intensity, frequency, and exercise selection. Usually, if a high variability of loading parameters is planned within the microcycle, the exercise selection stays more stable; on the other hand, if more stable loading parameters are planned within the microcycle, it is the exercise selection that varies more. Variation of exercises and loading parameters is built into the methodological concept of periodization of training. For example, to develop leg **strength** and **power** for volleyball or track and field, the athlete can practice full back squats during the general preparation phase and half squats during the specific preparation phase. During the late preparatory phase, the emphasis may shift from strength development to power-generating capacity. Thus the full or the half squat might still be used for maximum strength maintenance, whereas the quarter speed squat or the quarter jump squat can be used for power development. Therefore, the exercise program may shift as follows:

Back squat → 1/2 back squat → 1/4 speed squat → 1/4 jump squat

Another example of this concept can be seen in the preparation of cyclists. During the off-season, cyclists typically undertake training modalities such as cross-country skiing to maintain aerobic fitness and then return to training on the bike during the preparatory phase of training. The introduction–reintroduction structure (89) suggests that returning to bicycle training would rapidly increase cycling ability because the task is seminovel when reintroduced.

Training variation can be introduced within or between microcycles. For example, on some days of the microcycle the athlete trains multiple times per day, but on other days the athlete undertakes only one training session.

Multiple training sessions in the same training day have been shown to induce greater physiological adaptations than only one session per day (41). However, reducing the training frequency during the day can facilitate **recovery**, which may allow the athlete to train harder on subsequent days or microcycles.

Another way to vary the training plan is to systematically alternate the intensity of training. Alternating training intensity across the microcycle will allow for periods of stimulation and recovery, which have been suggested to induce greater physiological adaptations (89). Interestingly, alternating hard and light training sessions within the microcycle has been used to prepare both endurance athletes (69) and strength and power athletes (89). Another variation strategy is to alternate both training intensity and training frequency. For example, when manipulating the training intensity within an individual training day, a morning session may occur at a high training intensity and the subsequent afternoon session may be performed at a lower intensity. On the next training day, the number of sessions may be decreased to facilitate recovery or increased to increase the training stimulus.

Training variation is limited only by the coach's ability to apply scientific principles in a creative fashion. The implementation of training variation should be based on a complete understanding of the bioenergetics **(ergogenesis)** of the sport (28, 70, 89), movement patterns used in the sport (28), skills needed in the sport, and the athlete's level of development or training age (89). Advanced athletes will require more loading variation but less exercise variation than

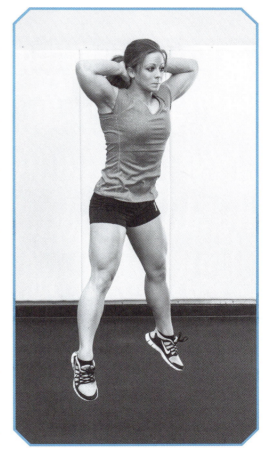

Changing the intensity of a training load, such as adding a jump to a squat, is one way to add variation to a training plan and achieve greater physiological adaptations.

novice athletes, who have a very small training base and need a multilateral approach to exercise selection. Novice athletes can achieve very good results with basic training models, even though there is significantly less variation in the training plan.

Development of the Training Model

Training models, while not always well organized and often applied randomly, have been used since the 1960s (11). Although many Eastern European sport specialists acquired knowledge and experience in the use of training models, a general trend toward the use of these tools did not occur throughout the world until the 1970s (10, 16).

It is well documented that training and performance are highly related but very individualized (5, 49). The development of a training model centers on the notion of training specificity and individualization of training programs (11, 49, 74, 90). Training models that allow for implementation, analysis, assessment, and modification of the training plan based on physiological and performance parameters are of particular use in the development of athletes (90).

The development of a training model is a long-term process that is in continual flux, because the training model will evolve in conjunction with the athlete's development. The development of a model is a labor-intensive process that relies on previous models, current athlete evaluations, and a strong scientific foundation. Although the process is time consuming, the time is well spent: The better the training model, the more likely the athlete is to achieve a high level of performance. The model must be continually evaluated and modified in response to new scientific knowledge, the athlete's level of development, and assessments of the athlete's progress. A theoretical method for developing a training model is presented in figure 2.3.

The development of a training model begins with a detailed analysis of the scientific literature regarding the sport. Understanding the physiological (e.g., bioenergetics) (74), morphological (37), anatomical, biomotor (56), and psychological characteristics (76) associated with a sport is the foundation for the second phase of developing a training model. The second phase requires the development of a targeted testing program that can be used to analyze the athlete's training state. For example, the scientific literature on throwing indicates that maximum strength and explosive power are related to high levels of performance (88). Therefore, physiological tests should be developed and implemented to evaluate the athlete's force-generating capacity (i.e., peak force-generating capacity, rate of force development, maximum strength) and explosive strength (i.e., peak power assessments, **one-repetition maximum** (**1RM**), power clean 1RM). The athlete's tactical and technical skills must also be evaluated to delineate areas of weakness, which can then be addressed by the training model. Tests should be developed that evaluate the athlete for areas of physical deficit or injury risk (e.g., range of motion, muscle imbalances). Other areas that can be evaluated include psychological traits (e.g., mood state), sleep status (e.g., quality of sleep), and nutritional practices. Finally, the athlete's **training logs** and competitive performance results should be evaluated to determine what was effective in the previous training model.

Once the evaluation of the athlete is completed, the coach interprets all the data that are collected. The training model is designed to target the athlete's needs to enhance the likelihood of a high level of performance. In this phase of the model, major training factors are established. These factors include the loading progression, training intensity, volume of training, frequency of training, and the number of repetitions necessary to stimulate the appropriate physiological and psychological adaptations. Additionally, the tactical, technical, and strategic components of the training model are established and integrated into the training model. The training model is very specific to the individual or team because the results of testing help the coach establish training parameters. After the training model is developed, it is then implemented.

During the implementation phase, the athlete must be continually monitored so the coach can detect any maladaptations. A comprehensive monitoring plan includes periodic

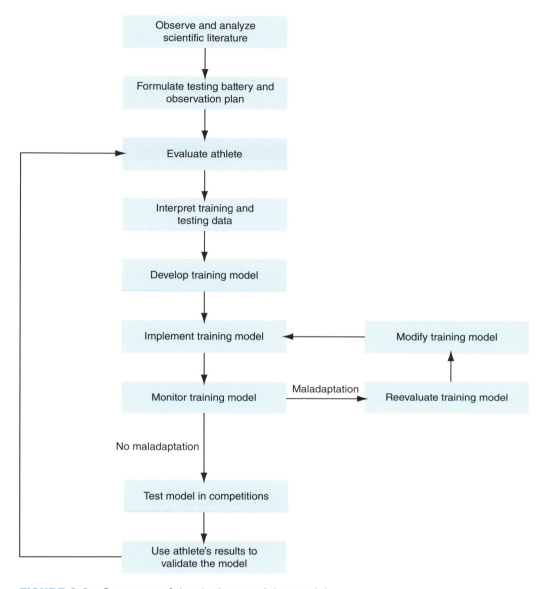

FIGURE 2.3 Sequence of developing a training model.

evaluation of physiological attributes (i.e., physiological testing similar to that conducted during the evaluation phase of model development), training log data, psychological status, nutritional status, and technical skill development. During this phase, if the coach questions the effectiveness of the training model, it should be reevaluated and modified to ensure that performance goals are reached.

The primary test of the effectiveness of the training model is the athlete's competitive results. If the athlete achieves success in competition, the training model is considered validated. After the completion of the competitive period, specifically during the transition phase, the model continues to evolve as the athlete is reevaluated. This reevaluation includes a critical and comprehensive examination of the past training year to determine whether training goals, objectives, and performance standards were achieved. All of the testing conducted throughout the training year is evaluated to determine whether trends occurred that either increased or decreased performance. How well the athlete coped with training and competitive stress should be evaluated to determine whether improvement in this area is needed. After conducting this evaluation, the coach decides whether to use a new model for the next annual plan.

Load Progression

Athletes' performance results have improved since 1975. There are many reasons for these elevations in performance, but clearly the ability to tolerate higher training loads is at the center of this phenomenon. Support for this contention is shown by the increase in training loads seen between 1975 and 2000 (table 2.2).

Improvements in performance are a direct result of the amount and quality of work the athlete achieves during training. From beginner to elite athletes, the training workload must increase gradually and be varied periodically according to each athlete's physiological capacity, psychological abilities, and work tolerance.

The training load can be thought of as a combination of intensity, volume, and frequency of training (83). The training load is determined by the degree of specificity of training and the performance development status of the athlete (82). There is a complex interaction between the athlete's **preparedness**, the training load, and the athlete's ability to tolerate training (83).

The application of a training load results in a cascade of physiological responses that allow the athlete to adapt to the training stimulus. This adaptation elevates his preparedness and leads to a greater tolerance for training as well as an increase in performance capacity (83, 102). As the athlete adapts to the training load, the load must increase for continued physiological adaptations to occur.

Training loads can be roughly classified according to their effects on physiological adaptations as stimulating, retaining, or **detraining** (101, 102). A stimulating load is a training load that is higher than the athlete's typical training load. Conversely, a detraining load is substantially lower than usual. A detraining load ultimately results in a loss of preparedness and a loss of performance capacity. In between these two loading classifications is the retaining load, which is the athlete's typical workload. The retaining load allows the athlete to maintain preparedness while undergoing recovery. As the athlete adapts to a stimulating load, that load becomes the retaining load and the previous retaining load becomes a detraining load. Thus, the loading classification is a fluid concept that changes as the athlete adapts, so the coach must pay attention to the sequence of the training loads in the periodized training plan.

A correctly sequenced training load will be increased gradually, ultimately resulting in an increase in performance capacity (83). If, however, the training load is suddenly and dramatically increased, it will take more time for the physiological adaptations to occur and performance gains to be realized (89, 95, 101, 102); with sudden increases, the risk of maladaptations and injury is high. The time frame needed for recovery and adaptation is directly proportional to the magnitude of the sudden increase in training load (89).

TABLE 2.2 Dynamics of Volume of Training From 1975 to 2000

		Year		
Sport	**Training volume**	**1975**	**1985**	**2000**
Gymnastics (women)	Elements per week	3,450	6,000	5-6,000
	Routines per week	86	86	150
Rowing (women)	Kilometers per year	4,500	6,800	6,500-7,000
Fencing	Training hours per year	980	1,150	1,100-1,200
Football (soccer)	Training hours per year	460	560	500-600
Swimming (100 m)	Training hours per year	980	1,070	1,000-1,040
Boxing	Training hours per year	960	1,040	1,000-1,100

The gradual, systematic manipulation of the training load is the basis for periodization of training and is found at all levels of the training plan (from the microcycle to the Olympic cycle) in all levels of athletes. The appropriate sequencing of the training load is directly related to the athlete's performance improvements. Loading structures vary among different sports and geographical regions of the world. A brief examination of several loading theories is presented in the following sections.

Standard Loading

Standard loading involves the use of similar training loads and frequencies throughout the preparatory phase of training. When standard loading is used regularly during the preparatory phase, performance improvements occur only during the early part of this phase.

As the athlete shifts from the preparatory phase of training to the competitive phase, the training stimulus remains very similar, with the exception of a reduction in training load. If standard loading is implemented in this fashion, performance plateaus during the competitive phase (see figure 1.4 on page 9). This plateau in performance occurs as a result of a lack of variation in the training load. If suboptimal training loads are used during the competition phase, performance will most likely deteriorate, especially during the later part of this phase (52).

Because performance improves only during the early portion of the preparatory phase, training load must be increased each training year. Contemporary training theorists suggest that this type of loading is suboptimal in almost all situations and that strategies using step loading or conjugated sequencing may result in greater performance enhancements in the long term (71). Therefore, to optimize performance adaptations in response to the training load, the load must be increased year over year to create the stimulus necessary for superior physiological adaptations. These enhancements will occur only if the training plan is sequenced appropriately and includes adequate periods of recovery.

Linear Loading

The linear loading of training is a concept that appears to violate many of the tenets of periodization (71, 89); however, this type of loading structure is very popular. According to the original proponents of this principle (50, 59), performance will increase only if the athlete trains at her maximal capacity against workloads that are gradually increased and are progressively higher than those normally encountered (8, 71, 72). Conceptually, this would lead to a loading curve that depicts a continual increase across time (figure 2.4). Although the literature has clearly demonstrated that the training load should be increased across the training cycle of the athlete's career (87, 102), this method of loading may only be useful during a short period of time, especially for beginners (23, 31, 32, 34, 45). If linear loading is undertaken for a long period of time, overtraining likely will result. If overtraining does occur, the athlete will exhibit physiological and psychological maladaptations, a decrease in markers of performance, and a high level of fatigue (69). Thus, linear loading in its purest sense is not an optimal way to train, except when implemented for short periods of time, because it does not allow enough time for recovery and because the potential for burnout and injury increases incrementally.

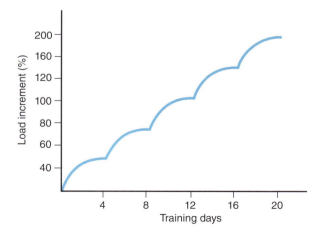

FIGURE 2.4 Load increments according to linear loading.

Based on data from Hellebrandt and Houtz 1956 (50).

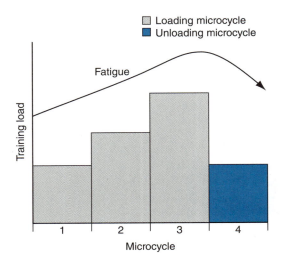

FIGURE 2.5 A 3:1 loading structure.

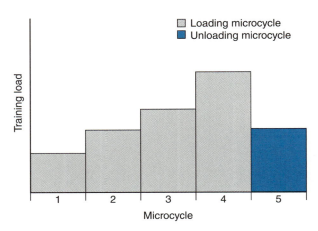

FIGURE 2.6 A 4:1 macrocycle structure, indicated for the beginning of the general preparation phase.

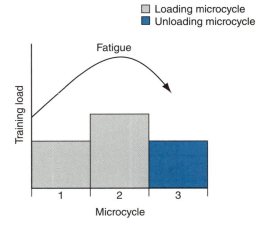

FIGURE 2.7 A 2:1 loading structure.

Step Loading

The step-loading model of training allows for a progressive overload that is interspersed with periods of unloading. It is sometimes referred to as a traditional or classic periodization model (11b, 62, 63, 71). The use of unloading phases or maintenance loads allows for regeneration, greater physiological adaptations, and periods of psychological restoration. With the step-loading model (figure 2.5), a wavelike increase in training load occurs (87, 89, 96, 102). Because one training session is insufficient to provoke noticeable physiological or psychological adaptations, it is often recommended that the same stimulus be repeated over several training sessions. This type of loading uses a 3:1 loading structure, in which the training load is increased across three microcycles and then is reduced during the fourth microcycle to allow recovery and avoid the problems typically associated with overtraining.

Figure 2.5 illustrates a classic 3:1 loading structure (11b, 11c). There is much evidence to support using a 4-week **macrocycle** of training (63, 71, 89) or a 2- to 6-week (usually 4 weeks) macrocycle of training (96, 101, 102). The load increases gradually in the first three microcycles as does the amount of accumulated fatigue, followed by an unloading phase that entails a decrease in training load and fatigue as depicted in the fourth microcycle in figure 2.5. This reduction in training load reduces fatigue, increases readiness, and induces a series of physiological adaptations that prepare the athlete for further loading in the next series of microcycles (89). A greater number of progressive loading steps can be granted at the beginning of the general preparation phase, as the starting training load will be low (figure 2.6). In some situations, it might be warranted to use only a few increasing steps. For example, a young athlete might use a 2:1 structure, with two microcycles of increasing training load followed by one microcycle of recovery (figure 2.7).

Step loading results in an intensification of workload with each progressive step, which develops a base for the next training macrocycle. This type of loading is excellent for novice athletes, athletes at the beginning of the general preparation phase, and for endurance athletes in general (71). Scientific support for including more microcycle variations and periodically including submaximal training can be found in both human (30) and animal (13) studies. This literature suggests that the periodic inclusion of light training days results in a greater potential for adaptive responses, which ultimately will increase performance.

Concentrated Loading

Short-term overloading is often classified as **concentrated loading** (91) or overreaching (61). The athlete usually can recover from this type of loading in a short period of time if she uses appropriate recovery loads (45). As a general rule, the greater the magnitude and duration of the concentrated

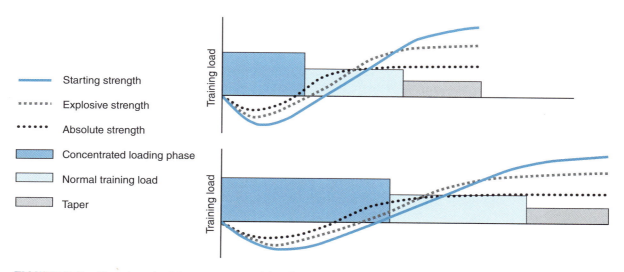

FIGURE 2.8 Time to adapt to concentrated loading.
Based upon Plisk and Stone 2003 (71) and Stone, Stone, and Sands 2007 (89).

loading phase, the more time needed for fatigue to dissipate and performance to improve (82, 89, 101, 102). Siff and Verkhoshansky (82) suggested that performance gains may occur after a period equivalent to the duration of the concentrated loading phase (figure 2.8).

Scientific support for the use of periodic concentrated loading or planned overreaching can be seen in studies that have explored the neuroendocrine responses to overreaching (40, 42, 44). Investigators have explored the hormonal and endocrine responses to short (1 week) and long (≥3 weeks) periods of concentrated loading followed by 2 to 5 weeks of recovery. The most commonly used endocrine measure is the **testosterone/cortisol ratio (T:C ratio)**, which indicates the anabolic–catabolic balance. Although the T:C ratio is not a measure of overtraining, it does indicate readiness (72, 89, 97). Thus, a high T:C ratio often corresponds to a high level of performance (33, 71).

A significant increase in training load for 3 weeks or longer results in a decrease in the basal or preexercise T:C ratio, indicating a shift toward a catabolic state that corresponds to a reduction in performance or readiness (40, 42, 44). Conversely, if after the completion of a concentrated loading period the training load is returned to normal or lower levels, the T:C ratio and performance appear to supercompensate (40, 43). This phenomenon has also been observed in response to substantial increases in training load across one microcycle (33, 85, 97). As noted previously, the duration of the concentrated loading phase corresponds to the duration of restitution needed before the supercompensation of performance occurs (figure 2.8).

Conjugated Sequence Loading Structure

The **conjugated sequence** loading structure is also referred to as the coupled successive system (94). Viru (96), Siff and Verkhoshansky (82), and Plisk and Stone (71) suggested that this method of sequence loading allows for periods of concentrated loading or overreaching followed by periods of restitution. There are a multitude of methods for implementing this type of loading structure, but the most common method is to use phases of four microcycles in which one primary emphasis is highlighted while maintenance loads are allocated to other areas of emphasis (71). Plisk and Stone (71) suggested that the primary goal of this type of loading is to give the athlete periods that are saturated with a specific training stimulus during which fatigue is elevated and some performance variables are decreased. For example, an athlete may undertake a concentrated loading phase in which strength is the major emphasis; then during the unloading phases, the athlete decreases the emphasis on strength while slightly increasing speed work. This pattern of loading will result in a supercompensation effect in which performance is increased dramatically (71). After completing this phase, the athlete undertakes a phase that imposes a progressively stronger specific stimulus, thus allowing the athlete to improve performance.

The literature notes several advantages to this type of loading structure (71, 77, 82, 85, 92, 94-96, 98, 101). Proponents of this loading structure suggest that a potent stimulus can be delivered to the athlete and performance can be elevated to a higher level than with traditional loading structures. Additionally, this type of loading may alleviate the cumulative fatigue associated with parallel or concurrent training with traditional loading structures. Finally, work volumes can be reduced over the long term (71). Plisk and Stone (71) suggested that fatigue will be substantial during the accumulation or concentrated loading phase, and the athlete must have the training capacity to tolerate these high training loads. Therefore, it is often recommended that this loading structure be used only with advanced athletes (71, 89).

A foundational concept that must be considered within the conjugated sequence theory is that training can be sequenced in such a way that performance can be elevated at given times. Plisk and Stone (71), in their seminal article on periodization strategies, offered a preseason training example in which concentrated loading phases of training are interspersed with periods of restitution. In this example, 3-week phases of concentrated loading are interspersed with 4-week phases of recovery (table 2.3). Plisk and Stone (71) suggested that by manipulating the training frequency and duration significantly, different training loads can be used without changing the basic intensity and volume parameters. Additionally, these investigators suggested that the coach or athlete can create greater contrast between concentrated loading phases and restitution phases by further reducing the distribution of training during the restitution phases.

TABLE 2.3 Conjugated Sequence Model of Training and a Modified Conjugated Sequence Model of Training for the Preseason

Training variable	Conjugated loading phase 1	Recovery phase 1	Conjugated loading phase 2	Recovery phase 2
Conjugated sequence model of training				
Duration	3 weeks	4 weeks	3 weeks	4 weeks
Strength and power training	12 total sessions 4 days/week	12 total sessions 3 days/week	12 total sessions 4 days/week	12 total sessions 3 days/week
Speed, agility, and conditioning training	6 total sessions 2 days/week	12 total sessions 3 days/week	6 total sessions 2 days/week	12 total sessions 3 days/week
Modified conjugated sequence creating more intraphase contrast				
Duration	3 weeks	4 weeks	3 weeks	4 weeks
Strength and power training	12 total sessions 4 days/week	8 total sessions 2 days/week	12 total sessions 4 days/week	8 total sessions 2 days/week
Speed, agility, and conditioning training	6 total sessions 2 days/week	12 total sessions 3 days/week	6 total sessions 2 days/week	12 total sessions 3 days/week

Adapted from Plisk and Stone 2003 (71).

Flat Loading

A flat loading structure is used mainly for the specific preparation phase and the competitive phase in power sports (11d). In this model, two microcycles with similar loading are followed by a recovery microcycle. In the flat loading model (figure 2.9), the first two microcycles create a high physiological demand as a result of the load of training (which is an optimal load to stimulate the adaptations of the trained biomotor abilities, thus no overreaching is sought after). After the first two microcycles, the athlete undertakes a third easy microcycle, called the unload or deload microcycle, during which fatigue is reduced and readiness elevates.

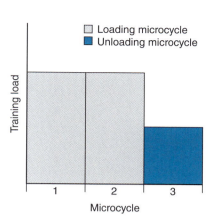

FIGURE 2.9 Example of a flat loading model.

The step-loading model can be used in conjunction with the flat loading model to progressively increase the athlete's training load. Figure 2.10 shows a preparatory phase of training in which the training load changes according to the scope of the phase of training. The program shown in figure 2.10 may also be identified as three major subphases: general, specific, and precompetitive preparation.

In the general preparation subphase, two types of macrocycle structures (3:1 and 2:1) can be used to stimulate physiological and psychological adaptations that will prepare the athlete for the next subphase, which will involve intensive training. The training goals of general preparation are accomplished through a progressive increase in training load via the use of the step-loading model. After completing the general preparation subphase, the athlete moves to the specific preparation subphase of training.

In the specific preparation subphase, the primary goal is to elevate the athlete's preparedness, technical proficiency, and tactical skills as much as possible. This is accomplished by exposing the athlete to high training loads for a short series of microcycles followed by regenerative microcycles to offset overtraining. After the completion of this subphase, the focus of training shifts to stabilization and peaking, which comprise the competitive subphase. Thus, the three phases prepare the athlete to perform at his highest possible level for his most important competition.

The dynamics of the loading pattern in the preparatory and competitive phases of training depend on the importance and frequency of competitions. The training loads in these phases are decreased to dissipate fatigue and begin to elevate the athlete's level of performance (increase of readiness). Recent research suggests that higher intensities with less volume may be needed to maintain performance during the competitive phase of training (52). However, prior to major competitions, the training load will be decreased to allow the athlete to recover and, if timed correctly, supercompensate, which will maximize performance.

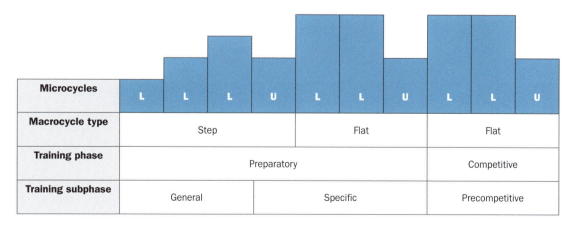

FIGURE 2.10 Step and flat macrocycles within the preparatory phase. Step loading is more appropriate for the early preparatory phase, while flat loading is suggested for the other microcycles.

Sequence of the Training Load

One of the most important aspects of periodization of training is the sequencing of the training load. If sequenced appropriately, each phase of training will increase the effect (potentiate) the next phase. For example, research evidence supporting the idea of phase potentiation has been demonstrated for strength and power development (47). Harris and colleagues (47) demonstrated that optimal strength and power performance gains occur when basic strength development precedes the development of strength and power characteristics. Siff and Verkhoshansky (82) suggested that the optimal development of medium-duration endurance for a cyclic sport occurs by sequencing training in the following fashion:

General physical preparation → strength → speed → endurance

As noted in figure 2.11, during the early portion of the training cycle, the athlete will undertake a large amount of aerobic training coupled with training to develop general physical attributes. After the first phase of training, a concentrated strength development is undertaken. After completing this period of concentrated loading, the athlete shifts emphasis to speed development, with a subsequent decrease in strength development in conjunction with a decrease in aerobic training. The collective effect of this shift in the training emphasis is a decrease in overall training stress, which allows for recovery to capitalize on the delayed training adaptations associated with concentrated loading. Finally, the athlete begins developing specialized endurance in the final phase of training; this is often accomplished through competition (82).

When choosing how to implement the different loading models presented in this chapter, the coach must consider the training status of the athlete, the goals of the training plan, the recovery interventions available to the athlete, the amount of time the athlete can dedicate to training, and the physiological responses to different loading models presented in the scientific literature. By using the scientific information available, the coach will be able to

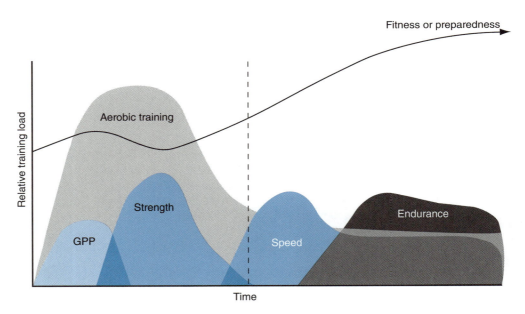

FIGURE 2.11 Sequential model for developing medium-duration endurance.

Aerobic training comprises approximately the first half of the cycle. In this example, general physical preparation (GPP) precedes a concentrated strength-loading phase. This model uses the delayed training adaptations effect while developing speed during the third block of training. The final phase is dedicated to endurance training, marked by specialized training for speed endurance, which specifically targets the competition.

Adapted, by permission, from M.C. Siff, 2003, *Supertraining* (Denver, CO: Supertraining International).

match the different loading models to the needs of the athlete, which will optimize training adaptations and lead to improved performance.

Summary of Major Concepts

Athletes must establish a strong multilateral development before specializing in a sport. If specialization occurs too soon in an athlete's development, it is likely that the athlete will achieve high levels of performance only during the junior years and will experience burnout soon after. The incorporation of a multilateral training base is especially important for young athletes. As the athlete matures, specialized training becomes more important. Such training will be dominated by drills and techniques that will lead to a faster rate of adaptation and ultimately to greater levels of performance.

A key to performance improvement is the planning of load progression. With young athletes, simple loading patterns with small amounts of loading variation can be very effective. However, advanced athletes require greater amounts of variation in loading parameters and more complex loading structures. Regardless of the athlete's level of development, regeneration and recovery must be included in the training program. Periods of recovery are essential to remove training-induced fatigue, replenish energy stores, and provide time for physiological and psychological adaptations to occur.

Preparation for Training 3

All athletic programs should address the physical, technical, tactical, psychological, and theoretical aspects of training. These factors are essential to any training program regardless of the athlete's chronological age, individual potential, level of athletic development, training age, or phase of training. However, the emphasis placed on each factor varies according to the time of year, the athlete's training age, the athlete's biological age, and the sport. Although training factors are highly interdependent, there is a specific manner in which each is developed. Physical training is the foundation on which all of the other factors related to training are developed (figure 3.1). The stronger the physical foundation, the greater the potential for developing technical, tactical, and psychological attributes.

Coaches, especially coaches of team sports, often overlook the strong relationship between physical and technical training. If the physical training base is inadequately developed, high levels of fatigue can be generated and the athlete will be unable to develop the other training factors. This often occurs when the preparatory phase (e.g., the preseason) is too short and the appropriate physiological adaptations are not developed. When this happens, the ability to effectively develop tactical, technical, and psychological skills is impaired, which increases the risk of poor performances during competition. One can consider physical training the foundation for the development of technique, whereas technique is central to the ability to develop and use tactical skills in sport. Additionally, as one's physical capacity improves, technical and tactical capacities improve as well, which will increase self-confidence and other psychological factors. Thus, physical training capacity is the cornerstone from which all training-related factors are developed, ultimately leading to the ability to excel in sport.

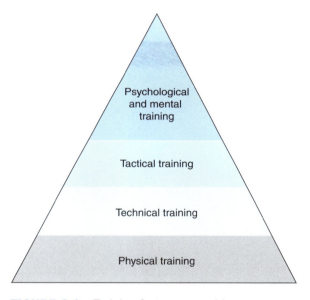

FIGURE 3.1 Training factors pyramid.

Physical Training

The physiological attributes necessary for sporting success are developed through appropriate physical training (37). These physiological adaptations are the basis from which technical and tactical advances are established. Without the development of physical abilities, the athlete's capacity to tolerate training will be significantly impaired, resulting in an inability to develop the technical and tactical attributes necessary for sporting success. Impairments in technical and tactical development usually occur as a result of accumulated fatigue, which is easily avoided through development of the appropriate physiological base via structured physical training. These concepts are among the best-kept secrets of the Eastern European training system.

Physical training has two main goals: The first is to increase the athlete's physiological potential, and the second is to maximize sport-specific biomotor abilities. In a periodized training plan, physical training is developed in a structured, sequential pattern (figure 3.2). Physical training can be broken into two interdependent parts:

- General physical training (GPT)
- Sport-specific physical training (SSPT)

General physical training and sport-specific physical training are developed during the preparatory phase of the periodized training plan. During the early part of the preparatory phase GPT is the primary emphasis, and as the athlete moves through this phase of training the emphasis shifts to SSPT. Thus GPT predominates during the early parts of the preparatory phase, whereas SSPT is dominant at the end of this phase.

Phase of training	Preparatory phase		Competitive phase
Phase of development	1	2	3
Duration (weeks)	≥3	≥6	≥4
Objective	1. Undertake general physical training	1. Undertake sport-specific physical training 2. Perfect specific sport skills (biomotor abilities)	1. Perfect specific sport skills (biomotor abilities) 2. Maintain physiological base

FIGURE 3.2 A sequential approach to the development of physical training during an annual plan.

GPT begins at the initiation of the preparatory phase, where the scope of training is to build a solid physiological foundation. This solid foundation is established via the use of high volumes of training performed at moderate intensities. The amount of time dedicated to GPT depends on many factors such as the athlete's training age, the athlete's needs, and the sport. The physiological adaptations established with GPT enable the athlete to tolerate the training loads encountered during SSPT.

As SSPT becomes more dominant, training intensity increases, depending on the requirements of the sport. In some cases, especially at the professional level, when the preparatory phase is very short (e.g., soccer in Europe), certain elements of intensity may be emphasized during the early parts of the preparatory phase. The SSPT period builds on the physiological base established during GPT and prepares the athlete for the competitive phase of the training plan. During the competitive period, the minimum objective of physical training is to maintain the sport-specific physical development established during the preparatory phase of training. However, in some instances it may be possible to improve sport-specific physical development during this phase. Conversely, if training and competition are not sequenced appropriately and adequate recovery does not occur, sport-specific physical development will begin to deteriorate (30, 41).

General Physical Training

The ultimate goal of GPT is to improve the athlete's working capacity and maximize physiological adaptations to prepare the athlete for future workloads. This phase of training targets the development of every component of physical fitness to increase work capacity. The higher the work capacity developed by the athlete during GPT, the greater the potential to adapt to the increasing physiological and psychological demands of training and competition. As stated in chapter 2, the physical development of young athletes predominantly focuses on multilateral development, which is accomplished through GPT. GPT for young athletes is rather uniform regardless of the sport being targeted in the training plan. Conversely, with advanced athletes the requirements of the sport must be addressed during GPT.

Sport-Specific Physical Training

SSPT is based on the foundation established during GPT. SSPT serves as a transition from GPT to the competitive phase. In this capacity, SSPT further develops the athlete's physical capacity in a fashion that is very specific to the demands of the sport. Targeting physiological adaptations that correspond to a specific sporting activity is of paramount importance when attempting to maximize competitive success (38, 41). If SSPT is sequenced and planned appropriately, the resultant physiological adaptations will increase the athlete's work capacity, which ultimately will result in higher levels of competitive performance. Well-planned SSPT will enhance the athlete's ability to recover from and adapt to the training load, which will ultimately enhance performance capacity.

GPT and SSPT should be clearly differentiated; the incorrect implementation of either type of training can result in inappropriate adaptations, which ultimately will decrease competitive performance. One example of an incorrect understanding of GPT and SSPT can be seen in the concept of endurance. The scientific literature indicates that different types of endurance are needed depending on the physiological demands of the sport (9, 41). A common misconception held by coaches is that aerobic exercise, resulting in what has been termed **low-intensity exercise endurance (LIEE)**, is important for all sports (40). Although aerobic training is a great way to improve LIEE or aerobic fitness, it generally compromises an athlete's ability to produce high forces or power outputs in a repetitive fashion, an ability required in most high-speed or strength and power sports (9, 40). These types of sports require a type of endurance that has been termed **high-intensity exercise endurance (HIEE)** (40). HIEE requires the athlete to sustain or repeat high-intensity exercise with exercise durations of less than 2 min (44). Therefore, for certain sports athletes must develop appropriate endurance to maximize performance. HIEE can be developed through the performance of repeated sprints (4), sprint interval training (6, 7), and resistance training (36). Recent research has shown that interval training has the potential to improve LIEE (6, 7, 19, 24) without compromising HIEE.

During the preparation phase, SSPT includes higher volumes of sprint or interval training and tactical drills that are specific to the sport. One strategy is to create scenarios during SSPT that model the conditions experienced in competition. For example, one might model an American football game by using 15 sprint intervals with a work to rest ratio of 1:10 (i.e., 5 s work, 50 s rest) to simulate what is encountered during competition (32). The implementation of SSPT in the preparatory phase of training depends on many factors including the athlete's training age, chronological age, and the requirements of the sport (figure 3.3). Physiological adaptations to SSPT can occur rapidly, in as little as 2 weeks of training (6, 7,

	Preparatory phase		
Elite/pro athletes	General physical training	• Sport-specific training • Perfecting sport-specific biomotor abilities	
Beginner to intermediate athletes	General physical training		• Sport-specific training • Perfecting sport-specific biomotor abilities
Developmental athletes	General physical training		• General physical training • Introducing sport-specific training elements

FIGURE 3.3 A basic representation of the duration of general physical training and sport-specific training between elite and professional athletes, beginners, and children.

18). SSPT may be undertaken for 2 months or more, depending on the characteristics of the sport and the athlete's level of development.

Exercise for Physical Training

An exercise is a motor act that can be used to target general physiological adaptations, movement patterns, or specific muscle groups that are related to the performance of the athletic skill. To simulate maximal amounts of physiological adaptation, the athlete must train for 8 to 12 years to optimize performance (26, 34). During these training years, exercises must be repeated systematically to stimulate adaptations that will improve performance.

Many training exercises are available to the coach when constructing a training plan. The coach should choose exercises that target the athlete's needs and the demands of the sport. Exercises can be classified as general or specific in regard to the development of precise biomotor abilities. Both general and specific exercises will be used throughout the training year, but their contribution to the training plan will vary between training cycles and depending on the athlete's training age.

Exercises for General Physical Development

Exercises for general physical development are nonspecific exercises that contribute to the athlete's physical development. These exercises develop strength, flexibility, mobility, aerobic fitness, and anaerobic capacity. Exercises for general physical development lay the foundation for further training by improving basic motor qualities that are central components of a multilateral program (34).

Exercises that focus on general physical development are central to the training plans of children and young athletes. These exercises are also important during the early part of the preparatory phase of training or with athletes who lack a solid training base. These types of exercises fall into two classifications: The first classification consists of exercises that are performed without implements (calisthenics) or are performed with objects that are not used in competition (e.g., stall bars, benches, skipping rope, medicine balls). The second classification includes exercises derived from the actual sport or related sporting events. A contemporary interpretation of this concept can be seen in cross-training: During certain parts of the training year, athletes participate in sporting activities that are related to the sport in which they compete (19). For example, a cyclist may participate in cross-country skiing in the off-season to develop cardiovascular fitness.

General physical development exercises are tools for developing overall fitness. Athletes need a balanced program in which muscular strength, flexibility, and endurance (HIEE or LIEE depending on the sport) are developed. For example, when strength training, an athlete can use high-volume, low-intensity training plans to target general physical development. This type of training, if done appropriately, can increase muscular strength, muscular endurance (HIEE and LIEE), and flexibility (if undertaken through a full range of motion), which can lay the foundation for specialized training that targets precise biomotor abilities.

Exercises for Specific Biomotor Development

Exercises for specific biomotor development target physiological adaptations, movement patterns, or muscle groups that are necessary for the sporting activity. This type of exercise is central to the concept of specificity of training. Specificity of training is the degree of similarity between the training exercise and the activities used in the sport (41). The more similar the characteristics of the training exercise are to the sport, the greater the transfer of training effects to the sport will be. When assessing the transferability of a training exercise to a sporting activity, the coach should consider the bioenergetics (29), movement patterns (35), and factors related to overload (41). The more similarities that are found between the training exercise and sport in regard to these factors, the greater the potential for the transfer of training effects.

The concept of movement pattern specificity reveals that the type of muscle action, kinematic characteristics (i.e., movement patterns), kinetic characteristics (i.e., forces, rate of force development, power output), muscle groups activated, and acceleration or velocity characteristics of the movement all contribute to the exercise's ability to transfer to the sporting activity. Particularly important to training specificity are the movement pattern and the primary muscles used in the sporting activity. For example, the primary movers related to sprinting performance are the muscles of the lower body. Therefore, a coach who works with sprinters should use exercises that target the development of lower-body muscles. However, the coach should also consider the synergistic muscles that are used in concert with the muscles of the leg. The best way to accomplish this is to target movement patterns. For example, the sprinter might use the power clean as a training exercise, because it has a power, force, and velocity profile similar to that used in sprinting. Additionally, the power clean activates the muscles of the trunk and other synergistic muscles that affect running performance. Many exercises activate the **prime movers** and synergistic muscles related to sprinting performance, including jumping (plyometrics), squatting (back squat, one-leg squat, front squat), and weighted sled pulling. In the scientific literature, sprinting performance has been significantly related to power clean performance (1), back squat performance (11), and vertical jumping performance (5, 11).

The use of exercises that are external to the athlete's sport is important, because sport performance alone will not give the athlete a great enough training stimulus to maximize performance gains (e.g., leg power, speed, or force-generating capacity). For example, the best high jumpers in the world do not perform more than 800 jumps per year, and this number of jumps is insufficient to develop leg power. To maximize performance gains, these athletes perform tens of thousands of exercises aimed at developing leg power (e.g., back squats, power cleans, plyometric exercises). However it is important to keep those exercise sport-specific; the higher the number of exercises, the lower the rate of specific adaptation.

Sport-specific exercises are essential to maximize the transfer of training effects from training to sport performance. These exercises are not only very important in the preparatory phase of training but also should be considered essential components of the competitive phase of training. Some coaches and athletes exclude sport-specific exercises during the competitive phase of the periodized training plan, choosing to only perform technical training during this time. This practice is problematic because the exclusion of sport-specific training exercises during the competitive phase may lead to a loss of preparedness that reduces performance as the season progresses. The coach and athlete should consider sport-specific exercises as essential components of every phase of the training plan because these exercises transfer directly to sporting performance.

Technical Training

One element that discriminates various sporting activities is the technique (i.e., motor skills) required. Technique encompasses all of the movement patterns, skills, and technical elements that are necessary to perform the sport. Technique can be considered the manner of performing a skill or physical exercise. Athletes must continually strive to establish perfect technique to create the most efficient movement patterns.

The more perfect or biomechanically sound the technique is, the more efficient or economical the athlete will be. For example, less energy is expended when an athlete has good running economy or technique (28). Trained runners have been reported to be more economical and to consume 20% to 30% less oxygen compared with novice runners who are running at the same submaximal speed (10, 14, 27). Biomechanists have suggested running economy is affected by stride length (8), stride rate (23), vertical stiffness (13), net vertical impulse of ground reaction forces (20), and ground contact time (28). Thus, if a runner becomes technically skilled and can optimize his stride rate, ground contact time, and stride rate, he will be more economical and thus more efficient. The relationship between technique and movement efficiency is important in all sports. Athletes must continually strive to maximize technical proficiency and therefore must incorporate technical training into their overall training plan.

Technique and Style

Every sporting activity has a technical standard or technical model that is accepted as being perfect or as close as possible to perfect and represents the accepted model of performance. A model of performance must be biomechanically sound and physiologically efficient to be widely accepted. The model is generally not developed based on the technique of elite or champion athletes because their technique may not be biomechanically or physiologically sound. Therefore, simply copying the technique of a champion is not advisable.

A technical model should exhibit some flexibility because it should be constantly updated based on new research findings. The technical model should be used as a point of comparison for an athlete's performance. This allows the coach to develop a training plan that targets deficiencies. Although the technical model is invaluable for training purposes, the athlete likely will develop her own individualized performance style. The structure of the skill is not different, but the athlete may make the skill look different as a result of her individual style of performance.

Individual technical styles are simply adaptations of an accepted model of performance that occur in response to technical problems in performing a motor act. For instance, the Fosbury flop (named after the American who won the high jump at the Mexico Olympic Games in 1968) changed the technique of high jumping dramatically. This technique requires the athlete to cross over the bar by facing it with the back rather than the front part of the body. Scientific examination revealed that this technique was more mechanically efficient than the classic technique. When first introduced, this individual high jumping style was

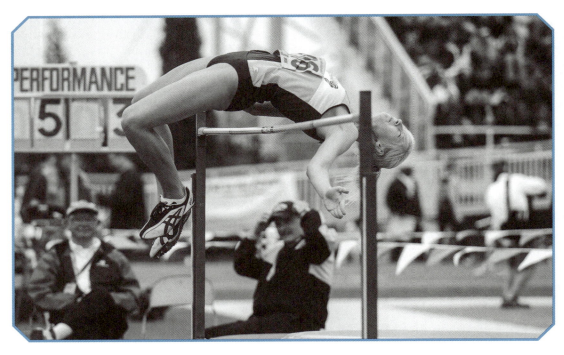

Proper technique allows an athlete to efficiently perform a skill, so technical training must be included in training plans.

not considered the optimal technique. However, in contemporary high jumping the Fosbury flop is considered the optimal model (43). This example depicts how an individual style can become a technical model.

There are also model techniques for optimal performance in team sports. For example, shot distribution, execution, and rally length in net sports can all be analyzed and used to develop a model of performance (22). In team sports, the application of a model of performance can be very team specific and related to the skill set or attributes of the team. The style of performance can have tactical implications and can affect how the team undertakes technical and tactical preparations.

Individualization of Technique

Not all techniques are useful for all athletes. For example, a novice athlete will use a more simplified technique than a world-class athlete. Therefore, when introducing technical elements to an athlete's training plan the coach must understand the individual athlete's level of development and her technical abilities and deficiencies.

In most instances technique is developed in stages, whereby simplified techniques are introduced first. After the athlete masters these basic elements, the coach then adapts the technique and adds elements that increase the technical difficulty of the training exercise. For instance, when working with a young discus thrower, a coach begins with perfecting the standing throw. Once the standing throw is mastered, the coach can add other elements, such as a 4/4 turn (i.e., step-in) or footwork drills, to begin teaching the athlete the rotational technique needed to be a successful discus thrower (16). Novice athletes generally use techniques that are vastly different than those of elite athletes as a result of their developmental status.

Variations can exist in the performance of a technical skill. Often these variations occur as a result of the complexity of the task or the biomechanical or physiological attributes of the athlete. Cyclic sports (e.g., running, cycling, rowing) often exhibit fewer interindividual technical differences, whereas acyclic sports (e.g., throwing, lifting, some team sports) have a greater potential for variations in technique. For example, Al Oerter tended to hold the discus in a lower position during his rotation than did most discus throwers, which is generally considered to be a technical flaw. However, this individual technical pattern was highly effective for Oerter because of his highly developed upper-body strength and fast leg speed (36). This example demonstrates that technique is developed based on the athlete's abilities, physiological and mechanical characteristics, and level of development.

When teaching a technical element or whole technique, the coach must understand the athlete's physical and psychological capacities. For example, if the thrower does not possess an adequate strength base, he may not be strong enough to keep his trunk vertical throughout the throwing movement (25). Therefore, it may not be warranted to work on the rotation portion of the throw until strength has been substantially increased. An inadequately developed physical base will limit the athlete's ability to learn technical aspects of the sport. This scenario strengthens the argument that physical training is the foundation of all training factors (figure 3.1).

Sometimes an athlete will be forced to interrupt his training schedule (e.g., because of illness or accidents). These interruptions in training generally affect the athlete's physical capacity, which may result in slight alterations in technique as a result of lost preparedness. When athletes experience a decline in physical capacity, a concomitant deterioration in technique often occurs. Additionally, high levels of fatigue can negatively affect an athlete's technique or ability to perfect technique. High levels of fatigue are usually related to low levels of physical work capacity. Therefore, when physical work capacity returns to normal or fatigue is dissipated, the athlete will be able to reestablish his technique. Because of the negative effects of fatigue on technique development, some suggest that technical training should occur before conditioning, and a heavy conditioning day should not precede a technique day.

Learning and Skill Formation

Learning technique is a process in which an athlete acquires mechanical skill, perfects the skill, and then ingrains the skill (34). The ability of an athlete to learn new mechanical skills depends on many factors including the athlete's current technical skill and the complexity of the skill that is being targeted (33). The athlete's physical attributes or level of development will affect the ability to learn new skills. However, many other factors such as the athlete's learning style or the teaching methods used can also affect how easily the athlete acquires the new skill set.

The learning of a new skill set has been suggested to be a three-part process (34), which may not always be broken into discrete parts because the steps are often blended. During the first part of learning a new skill, the athlete should receive a detailed explanation of the skill and observe the skill being performed. After the initial demonstration and explanation, the athlete begins to develop the rough technical aspects of the skill, paying particular emphasis to the most crucial phases of the movement pattern (34). During the second phase of the learning process, the athlete begins to refine the skill, a long-term process in which many repetitions of the movement are performed. During this phase technical errors are continually addressed and the athlete strives to perfect the movement pattern and minimize or eliminate technical deficiencies (34). In the third phase of learning the skill, the athlete begins to ingrain the movement pattern so that the skill is automated and happens naturally; this requires large amounts of repetitive practice undertaken for significant amounts of time.

Evolutional Character of Technique

Technique continues to evolve as technological and creative innovations are introduced into the sporting environment. Over time, training practices and techniques change, and what was once an advanced technique may become outdated. Technical innovations in sport can come from the coach's imagination or from scientific inquiry into the physiological and mechanical aspects of the sport. New techniques may work well in ideal situations or in practice, but they must be translated into the competitive arena before they become accepted as a technical model. Not all new techniques or ideas will translate into the competitive arena because this environment is distinctly unique, attributable to its high levels of physical and psychological stress and its random nature. When coaches and athletes attempt to improve and perfect technique, they must model the technique not only in ideal situations but also in competition.

Tactical Training

Tactics and strategy are important concepts in coaching and athletics. Both terms are derived from the military vocabulary and have a Greek origin. The word *tactics* is derived from the Greek word *taktika*, which refers to the how things are arranged. *Strategy* comes from the Greek word *strategos*, which means "general" or "the art of the general." In the theory of warfare, strategy and tactics are categorized separately because both terms have unique dimensions. When examined in the military context, strategies focus on wide spaces, long periods, and large movements of forces, whereas tactics address smaller spaces, times, and forces. When examined in a hierarchical perspective, strategies precede war planning and the actual tactics that are used on the battlefield.

Tactics and strategies can be used during training or in a competition with direct or indirect opponents. Strategy is the organization of training, play, or competition that is based on a philosophy or way of approaching a problem (e.g., training or competition). Within the strategic framework are tactics, or the training or game plans. A good example of the interrelationship between strategies and tactics can be seen in the training process, where strength and conditioning coaches induce physiological responses by using tactics that are organized into rational systems (30). When one is attempting to understand the relationship between strategies and tactics, the simplest approach is to consider strategy as the art of projecting and directing training or competitive plans, and tactics as the organization of these plans.

Tactical training refers to training offensive and defensive objectives (e.g., scoring, a specific play) that are germane to a sport. For example, in soccer, skills that are considered as part of tactical training include passing, pace of attacks, tackling, pass distribution, dribbling skills, and length of passes (22). Each sport requires certain skills, and thus tactical training may be different for each sporting activity. Tactical actions are part of the strategic framework used to train the athlete and prepare for competition. The basis of any successful tactical plan, regardless of the sporting activity, is a high level of technical proficiency. Thus, technique is a limiting factor for all tactical maneuvers, and tactics are a function of an athlete's technique. Technical abilities are based on the physiological adaptations that occur in response to physical training. Thus, physical training is the foundation for technical and tactical training (figure 3.1).

Tasks and Specificity of Tactical Training

For most elite athletes, there is very little difference between their physiological development and their technical skill (31). Often, when all other factors are held equal, the winning athlete uses more mature, advanced, and rational tactics. Even though tactical training relies heavily on physical and technical training, there appears to be an important link between psychological and tactical training (31).

Tactical mastery is founded on deep theoretical knowledge and the capacity to apply tactics appropriate for the competitive environment. Tactical training may include the following:

- Studying strategic elements of the principle sport
- Studying the rules and regulations for competition in the sport or event
- Evaluating the tactical abilities of the best athletes in the sport
- Researching the strategies used by opponents
- Evaluating the physical and psychological attributes and potential of opponents
- Evaluating the facilities and environment of competition sites
- Developing individual tactics that are based on personal strengths and weaknesses
- Critically analyzing past performances against specific opponents
- Developing an individualized tactical model with appropriate variations to meet multiple competitive demands
- Practicing a tactical model in training until it becomes ingrained

The development of tactical skills is accomplished with the same basic steps outlined earlier in this chapter, in the section titled Learning and Skill Formation. Traditionally, athletes approach tactical skills training after developing the appropriate physiological basis (physical training) and technical skills. However, it is also possible to develop all three factors simultaneously as a result of proper planning and training program **integration**.

When we examine tactical training principles, it may be helpful to classify sports into general categories. Most sporting activities can be classified into five basic groups as a result of their tactical similarities:

- *Group 1:* Sports in which athletes compete separately, with no direct contact with opponents. These sports generally require athletes to perform in a predetermined order. Examples include alpine skiing, track cycling (individual events such as the 1,000 m or 4,000 m pursuit), cycling (time trial), figure skating, gymnastics, diving, in-line skating, and weightlifting.
- *Group 2:* Sports in which athletes start the competition at the same time, in either large or small groups. In these sports, some cooperation with teammates is possible, thus adding a tactical element that requires some teamwork. Examples include running

events in track and field, cross-country skiing, cycling (track and road cycling), Nordic skiing, cross country running, and swimming.
- *Group 3:* Sports characterized by direct competition between two opponents. Examples include boxing, wrestling, tennis, fencing, and mixed martial arts.
- *Group 4:* Sports in which the opponents are in teams and the athletes have direct contact during the game or competition. These sports include baseball, soccer, American football, hockey, and rugby.
- *Group 5:* Sports that require athletic participation in a combination of different sporting activities. These sports are complex because they require tactics that are central to the individual sports and the general competitive plan. Sports in this group include the heptathlon and decathlon in track and field, the biathlon (shooting and Nordic skiing), the triathlon, and the modern pentathlon.

Classifying sports into broad groups helps us examine sport tactics. The innate similarities between the sports in each group can provide a deeper tactical understanding of sports with similar characteristics.

Uniform Distribution of Energy

The ability to maintain tactical proficiency under conditions of fatigue is an important determinant of competitive success. Therefore, the athlete's tactical training must include sessions that require the athlete to perform under conditions of fatigue. The coach can create such a condition by extending practice after the athlete has become fatigued, informing the athlete either before the session begins or at some point during the session. Another possibility is to use several rested sparring partners during training, which would force the athlete or team to constantly perform at a high level. The physical training base provides the foundation for the athlete's ability to perform under conditions of fatigue: The higher the physical training base, the greater the work capacity.

Another consideration is the athlete's ability to mobilize all of his resources to finish. In close races or games, success often depends on the athlete's capacity to mobilize all forces and give everything for the final moments of the competition. The coach can create scenarios that require the athlete to maximize effort in simulated end-of-competition situations; an example is simulating the time left in a game or competition and requiring the athlete to increase the tempo of his tactical practice.

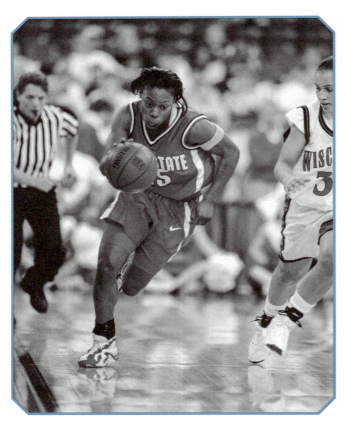

Before you can create a training program, you need to know what kinds of tactical skills are required.

Technical Solutions to Tactical Tasks

Often athletes have to perform under adverse or unusual environmental conditions, such as on a wet field, in a strong wind, in cold water, or in a noisy environment. Such conditions require special preparation. The following guidelines may help athletes adapt to these adverse conditions:

- Perform skills and tactical maneuvers correctly and efficiently under unusual or simulated conditions.
- Organize exhibition games or competitions with partners who follow the same tactics as future opponents.

- Create unique situations that demand each athlete to independently create tactical resolutions.

The ability to demonstrate tactical discipline is essential in training. However, in competition the athlete may experience a tactical problem that was not addressed or simulated by the coach. In such a case, the athlete must draw on his training and experience to create an immediate solution to the tactical problem. This process can be facilitated by exposing the athlete to various situations in training and exhibition competitions so he can create a repertoire of tactical solutions to draw on when adverse situations occur during competition.

Maximizing Teammate Cooperation

The cohesive interaction of a team is essential for success in sports classified in groups 2 and 4. Using techniques such as limiting external conditions (e.g., decreasing the available time or playing space) can force the team to interact and cooperate. Additional stress can be introduced by adding fatigue to these scenarios. This will help athletes learn how to interact and cooperate during adverse situations.

An additional strategy is to perform tactical maneuvers against a conventional opponent who is attempting to counteract the play. This scenario can be created by using an opposing team or by creating an opposing team with reserve players during training. The coach should instruct these players to behave as if they are not familiar with the applied tactics. Reserve players should participate in the preparation of game tactics because changes in the team lineup increase the potential of a breakdown in cooperation and tactics. It is useful during practices to replace key players with spare players. This allows reserve players to become familiar with the team tactics and the other players, and it allows the existing group to see how reserve players operate and how the team's tactics will change with the reserve players' presence. These techniques allow the team to develop new tactical combinations that can improve the team's competitive capabilities.

Perfecting the Team's Flexibility

To maximize team cooperation, the coach should introduce changes in the team's tactics that will increase its tactical flexibility. The team can use tactical flexibility to create scenarios that will surprise opponents. A plethora of tactical variations can be used, such as the following:

- Substitute different tactics at predetermined times or in response to signals from a coach or designated player (e.g., captain).
- Substitute players who bring a new and unexpected game change to the team.
- Expose the team to exhibition games against teams that use various styles of play. This allows the team to prepare for these scenarios in future games and develop tactical solutions to the style of play encountered.

Tactical Thinking and the Game Plan

A central component of tactical training is developing tactical thinking skills. The ability to think tactically is limited by the athlete's knowledge and repertoire of tactical skills. To think tactically, the athlete must learn to do the following:

- Realistically and correctly evaluate opponents as well as himself.
- Instantly recall technical skills and combinations of skills that can be used in game situations.
- Anticipate his opponent's tactics and use the appropriate tactics to counteract the opponent.
- Disguise or conceal tactics that may prevent the opponent from sensing and counteracting the plan of attack.
- Perfectly coordinate individual actions within the team tactics.

The competition or game plan is based on analysis of tactical trends and the opponent's strengths and weaknesses. Components of the game plan are then integrated into the tactical training portion of the training plan. The game plan usually is introduced progressively over the last two or three microcycles so that it can be perfected by the time of competition. The game or competition plan is important for several reasons:

- To instill confidence and optimism about the upcoming competition
- To inform the athlete about the place, facilities, and conditions under which the contest will be organized
- To introduce the strengths and weaknesses of future opponents into each training factor
- To use the athlete's past performance as a reference from which to build confidence (emphasizing the strong points from which to build a realistic optimism, without disregarding the athlete's weaknesses)
- To develop realistic objectives for the competition using all of the preceding factors

The implementation of the game or competition plan occurs in several phases. First, a preliminary game plan is developed. The game plan and its tactical elements are then implemented into the game situation. After the game is completed, the plan is comprehensively analyzed, allowing for further refinement of the plan and its tactical components.

Creating the Preliminary Game Plan

The first phase of game planning involves developing the preliminary game plan prior to the competition. The coach develops this plan after comprehensively analyzing potential tactical difficulties that the athlete or team is likely to encounter during the game or competition. Tactical solutions or objectives are then created in response to the potential tactical difficulties revealed during the critical analysis. In the context of the tactical plan, individual tactical objectives are assigned to players based on their strengths and weaknesses. The tactical objectives are then practiced as part of the tactical training plan.

In the days prior to the game, the athlete should avoid changing habits because this may adversely affect game-time performance. Two or three days before the competition, the coach should reinforce the game plan and the tactics that have been developed, using structured practices that allow for the development of good technical and tactical performances. When possible, the training lesson should mirror the competitive model. The coach should acknowledge good performances to develop confidence, create motivation, and increase competitive desire.

As the competition approaches, the coach should focus only on a few major points of the game plan without overwhelming the athlete with too many instructions. No matter how detailed the preliminary game plan, there is always a potential for unforeseen technical and tactical occurrences. Therefore the plan must be flexible enough to allow the athlete to respond to these challenges.

Applying the Game Plan

The second phase of the game plan is the implementation of the general plan in an actual game situation. The initial phase of the game is generally used to test the main elements of the tactical plan. In this portion of the game, the team will strive to unveil the opponent's game plan while hiding their own plan. The athlete will need to be able to analyze and comprehend the tactical situations that arise and choose a tactical action to apply. The ability to comprehend these tactical situations will depend on the athlete's tactical knowledge, experience, team dynamics, and tactical preparation. These attributes will allow the athlete to solve problems by instantaneously working through periods of analysis, synthesis (i.e., combining separate parts into a whole), comparison, and generalization. This process allows the athlete to determine the most appropriate solutions to the tactical demands of the game. The individual decision-making processes will occur in concert with the group decision-making dynamics within the team. The coordinated efforts between each individual on the team allow for rational, original, rapid, economical, and efficient solutions to the fluctuating tactical challenges that arise during the game.

Analyzing the Game Plan

The third phase of game planning requires the coach to perform a systematic, critical analysis of the game plan. The coach should closely examine how the plan was developed, the effectiveness of the individual tactical roles in the plan, the success of the tactical plan, and, if the game plan did not succeed, the reasons why. The more detailed the analysis, the more it will reveal about the strengths and weaknesses of the plan.

The most appropriate time to analyze the game plan and discuss the results of the analysis with the athletes depends on the outcome of the game or competition. If the result was favorable, analysis of the game can occur soon after the game's completion, and discussion of the results of the analysis can occur during the first practice session after the game. Conversely, if the outcome of the game is unfavorable, the analysis should be delayed to allow for a critical examination of the performance. The coach should discuss the analysis with the athletes 2 or 3 days after the competition to allow time for the psychological wounds to heal. When discussing the analysis with the athletes, the coach should be clear and reasonable and should highlight the positive aspects of the performance. The coach should also project optimism and propose a few tactical elements to emphasize in subsequent training.

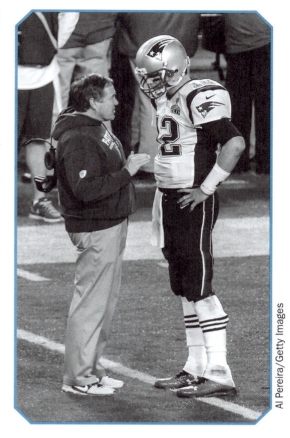

A coach needs to analyze how well a game plan is working during a competition. Is an athlete able to choose the correct tactical action to apply to a certain situation?

Perfecting Technique and Tactical Training

Both technique and strategy in sport are in continual flux. Technical and tactical knowledge is continually changing in direct response to the evolution of sport science (50) and practical experience. This increase in technical and tactical knowledge increases the effectiveness of training. To achieve technical and tactical mastery, the coach and athlete must optimize three relationships between conflicting concepts: integration–differentiation, stability–variability, and standardization–individualization (17).

Integration–Differentiation

Learning or perfecting a skill as well as training an ability is a multifactorial process, through which the athlete can develop technical and strategic mastery. Central to the process are the concepts of integration and differentiation. Integration refers to combining the individual skill or tactical maneuvers into a whole process, whereas **differentiation** involves analytically processing each component of the whole process.

When learning a new technique or skill, the athlete progresses from simple technical or tactical elements to complex elements. To master a skill or tactical maneuver that has already been learned, the process is reversed: The athlete and coach must analyze the whole skill or tactical maneuver by breaking it down into subunits to determine whether technical errors exist. If the athlete and coach determine that each subunit is free of technical faults, it is likely that errors exist in how the individual subunits are unified into the whole system (e.g., connective parts or two elements in a gymnastics routine or other sport skill). If the examination of the connections between the subunits does not reveal technical errors, further differentiation of the skill is necessary to isolate the sources of error. Once the sources of error are isolated, the coach and athlete must develop strategies to eliminate the error.

The integration–differentiation process can be used to perfect or change the technical or tactical model being used. Figure 3.4 illustrates how a skill can be perfected through the use of a systematic integration (i.e. constructing whole skills) and differentiation (i.e. dissecting skill into subunits and determining where errors are) process. The outcome of this process is mastery of the skill.

If the coach determines that a technical skill or tactical maneuver is insufficient, it may be warranted to alter the performance model. The coach must determine why an error occurred and critically analyze the model to determine which components can be removed or modified (figure 3.5). Determining technical errors occurs with the same differentiation process presented earlier. Once technical errors are isolated and the coach has decided that the model of performance must be altered, the technical error must be "unlearned" and a new technical skill or element taught. Once the athlete learns the new element or skill, she must practice the skill until it becomes automatic; then the skill is reintroduced into the whole system of performance, and the athlete practices the skill until it is mastered.

Stability–Variability

When training an athlete, there is a constant trade-off between **stability** and **variability** (45, 51). The optimal training stimulus occurs in response to a systematic variation in training load, intensity, or content (45). If, however, the training stimulus or workloads are prescribed in a monotonous fashion, the athlete will experience accommodation or stagnation problems,

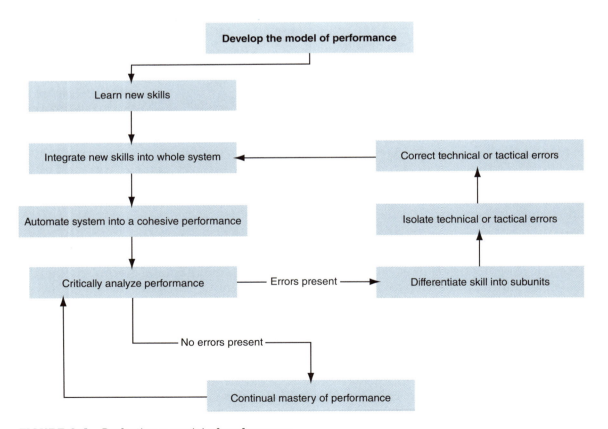

FIGURE 3.4 Perfecting a model of performance.

Adapted from Teodorescu and Florescu 1971 (44).

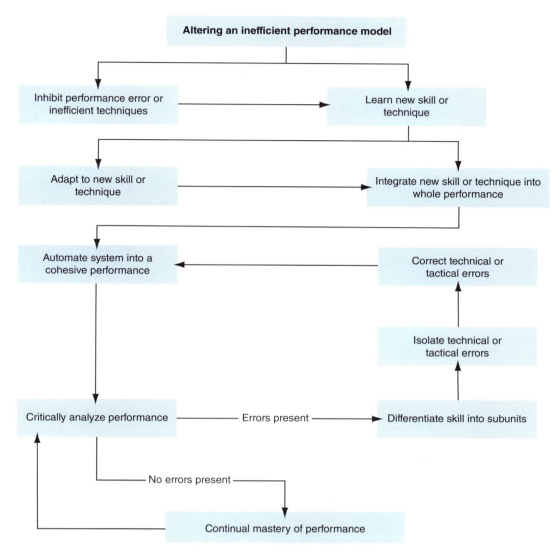

FIGURE 3.5 Altering an inefficient model of performance.
Adapted from Teodorescu and Florescu 1971 (44).

which will halt any improvement in performance (43, 45). Therefore, the training program should include planned variation, whereby novel or seminovel tasks are introduced or reintroduced periodically throughout the annual training plan. The introduction of novel or seminovel tasks will result in a greater stimulatory effect and greater adaptation (22), which will stabilize the athlete's skill and performance level. Therefore, variability in training (e.g., changes to volume, load, exercises, and workout frequency) provides a stabilizing effect in regard to performance and skill acquisition.

Standardization–Individualization

There is a constant conflict between the standardization of a skill set and the individual traits and characteristics of the athlete. The coach must develop and stabilize the athlete's technical skills while accounting for the individual's psychological and biological characteristics. In this way the coach will be able to modify the technical skill so that it becomes standardized.

Stages of Perfecting Technical and Tactical Training

The athlete's ability to perfect technique and tactics is a direct result of the coach's knowledge and teaching skill, which can include the use of preparatory and progressive drills and audiovisual aids. The athlete's ability to learn new skills is also related to her ability to process new information and her biomotor abilities. It has been suggested that athletes improve technical and tactical skills in three distinct stages (44) (figure 3.6).

In the first stage, the main objective is to perfect the individual components and technical elements of a skill (differentiation). As the components are mastered, they are integrated progressively into the whole system. Skill perfection develops in concert with the development and perfection of the dominant or supporting biomotor abilities. The development of these biomotor abilities is essential because technique is a function of physical preparation or capacity. The acquisition of new skills and techniques is best suited for the preparatory phase of the annual plan. When skill acquisition is a central focus, it is inadvisable for the athlete to participate in competitions.

The main objective in the second stage is to perfect the whole skill under standardized conditions similar to those seen during a competition. This can be accomplished by participating in either exhibition or simulated competitions. The athlete must maintain dominant biomotor abilities during this phase so he will have an adequate physical training base to continue skill development. This stage of perfecting a skill can be integrated into the annual training plan near the end of the preparatory phase.

The final stage of perfecting a skill focuses on stabilizing the whole skill and translating it to competitive performance. The coach must create an environment (e.g., including noise,

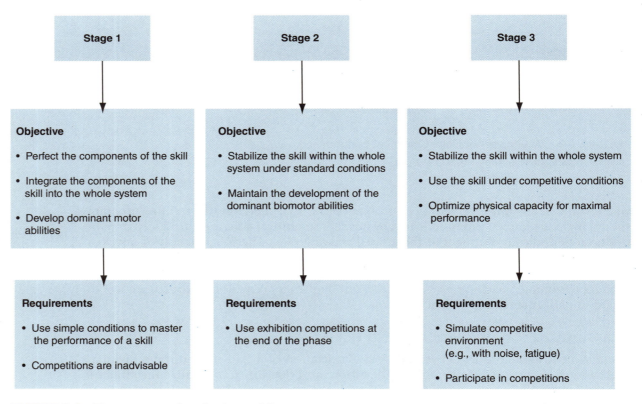

FIGURE 3.6 Three stages of perfecting a skill.

Adapted from Teodorescu and Florescu 1971 (44).

fatigue) that is as close to the actual competitive situation as possible. This stage of perfecting a skill should be implemented into the annual training plan during the competitive phase.

Correcting Technical and Tactical Errors

According to Bompa, "If a coach fails to concentrate on correcting an athlete's technical errors, all they are doing is perfecting those errors" (3). Often technical improvement or skill mastery is impaired because the athlete learns the skill incorrectly. If the technical skill is not taught correctly, the athlete's ability to correct technical errors is greatly impaired. The coach must strive to eliminate as many technical errors as possible to maximize the athlete's development. Technical or tactical errors can occur for many reasons, but generally they fall into four broad areas:

1. *The athlete is performing a skill incorrectly.* Many factors can impair an athlete's ability to learn or perfect a skill. Two interrelated factors are an insufficient physical training base and lack of correlation between biomotor abilities. A poorly developed physical training base or insufficient development of biomotor abilities can delay skill acquisition and development. For example, athletes who have not adequately developed a physical training base are more apt to develop fatigue when working on skill acquisition. Fatigue, which can result from a poor training base or a poorly implemented training plan, can impede learning or result in a deterioration of technical skills. Therefore, simply improving the athlete's physical training base may improve her ability to learn new skills. The development of biomotor abilities may also facilitate the acquisition of skills. One of the major biomotor abilities that can affect skill acquisition is strength. For example, a gymnast may not be able to learn or master a specific element (e.g., iron cross) if he does not have the appropriate level of strength to perform or practice the skill (15). Therefore, simply increasing strength as part of the physical training base will increase the athlete's ability to learn or master the targeted skill set.

2. *Psychological factors, such as self-confidence, morale, desire, and beliefs, appear to be significantly related to the athlete's ability to perform or develop skills* (12, 45). For example, athletes who set goals that are task oriented, such as working hard to perfect a skill, generally achieve greater success than athletes who are ego driven (i.e., perform for individual notoriety) (12, 45). Athletes who are ego driven tend to perceive failure as an inability to perform a task, which may result in a withdrawal from training (12). Conversely, task-oriented athletes will respond to failure by increasing their effort in training (12) because they equate success with hard work (45).

3. *The coach's teaching method causes technical faults.* The coach may use inappropriate teaching methods or demonstrate the technique incorrectly when introducing the skill or may fail to completely explain the technical aspects of the skill. Some coaches neglect to tailor skill instruction to the individual's learning capacity and biomotor ability. Additionally, the coach's personality, coaching style, and character can affect the athlete's ability to acquire technical skills. For example, if the coach does not allow the athlete sufficient time to learn a skill, the potential for developing technical errors is magnified.

4. *There are equipment, organizational, or environmental causes.* The environment must foster the acquisition of proper technique, and the training session must be properly planned. Equipment must be appropriate and must function properly during each training session. Appropriate facilities (e.g., field, court) must be available for training, because an adverse environment can impair skills acquisition.

There are many ways to correct technical errors, but it is better to prevent technical errors in the first place. The best way to prevent technical errors is through the utilization of appropriate teaching methods. If technical errors do occur, it is essential that they be addressed as soon as possible. The best time to dedicate to technical or tactical corrections is the preparatory phase of the annual plan, because the stress of competition is absent during this phase and time can be dedicated to addressing technical issues.

Learning new skills or addressing technical errors should be avoided when the athlete is fatigued; fatigue usually has a negative effect on learning. Thus, it is best to address technical errors or teach new skills immediately after the warm-up. Another strategy is to increase the amount of rest between repetitions of the drills used to address errors.

The first step in addressing a technical error is to isolate the error to be corrected from other technical skills. Once this is done the coach can introduce the correction or new element that will address the error. The athlete then practices the new skill. When the athlete has acquired or mastered the new skill it is integrated back into the system or whole skill. While this process is being undertaken, the athlete must maintain or develop the biomotor abilities that are necessary to support the skill being perfected.

Another issue that must be considered when addressing technical errors is the intensity or velocity at which the exercises are performed. In most cases, coaches concentrate on correcting technique with low-intensity or low-velocity movements. Although this is an important step in reeducating the athlete, sporting events often occur at higher velocities and intensities. Therefore, after the athlete becomes proficient at the new skill or corrected skill with low intensities and velocities, she must practice the skill at progressively higher velocities and intensities until the skill can be used in competition.

Visualization or mental practice is an excellent tool for correcting technical errors. The scientific literature has shown that athletes who use mental practice perform significantly better than those who do not (42). The coach should consider incorporating mental practice into the training plan to maximize the correction of technical errors and ultimately improve performance.

Theoretical Training

Although it is commonly accepted that athletes need to develop physical, technical, tactical, and psychological skills, whether athletes need to understand the theoretical basis of training and sport is of great debate. Some coaches are tied to the archaic belief that they need to think for their athletes and that athletes only need to concern themselves with training and competing. In fact, approaching the development of athletes in this fashion may delay the athlete's skill and performance improvement.

The coach should consider the development of the athlete, which includes educating the athlete about the sport, training theory, and why they are doing certain things in training. To effectively educate athletes, the coach must stay up-to-date with theoretical knowledge by reading sport science literature, attending sport science and coaching conferences, and interacting with other coaches. The coach should educate the athlete in the following areas:

- The rules and regulations governing the sport
- The scientific basis for understanding and analyzing the technique of the sport because understanding basic biomechanics allows the athlete to analyze movement and ensure proper mechanics, thus decreasing the risk of injury
- The scientific and methodological basis of biomotor abilities
- The planning of training and how periodization of training is used to prepare the athlete for competition
- The physiological adaptations that occur in response to training
- The causes, methods of prevention, and basic treatments for injuries
- The sociology of sport (i.e., intergroup relationships)
- The psychological aspects of sport, including communication skills, behavior modification, stress management, and relaxation techniques

- The effect of nutrition on training adaptations and how to use dietary interventions before, during, and after training or competition (with care undertaken to design nutrition strategy by consulting a nutrition specialist).

Developing the athlete's theoretical knowledge about the sport and how to prepare for the sport is an ongoing process that should include discussions before, during, and after training. The process should include activities such as film analysis, where the coach teaches the athlete how to critically analyze performance parameters. Athletes should be encouraged to become students of their sport. This can be accomplished through attending clinics, interacting with other coaches and athletes, reading periodicals and other pertinent texts, and engaging in detailed discussions with their personal coach.

Summary of Major Concepts

The preparation of athletes includes physical, technical, tactical, psychological, and theoretical training. These five factors are interrelated, with physical training being strongly linked to the development of both technical and tactical skills. Physical training is the foundation of every training program. An inadequately developed physical capacity will usually result in fatigue, which impairs technical and tactical performance during training and competition. Therefore, it is essential that the athlete's physical capacity be addressed with sound physical training.

The athlete must continually strive to attain perfect technique. The more technically proficient an athlete, the more efficient she will be and the less energy she will expend during practice and performance. Technical skills also affect the athlete's tactical capacity. Therefore, the training plan must provide for the continued development and refinement of technique.

The competitive game plan needs to be developed in advance of the competition to allow the development of the tactical training plan. The coach should integrate tactical training into the training plan to allow adequate time for the athlete to perfect the tactics prior to competition.

Variables of Training 4

The efficiency of a physical training program results from the manipulations of volume (duration, distance, repetitions, or tonnage), intensity (load, velocity, or power output), and frequency (density), which are key variables in training. These variables should be manipulated according to the physiological and psychological requirements of the training goal or competition. Thus, when designing the training program, the coach must first decide which variable to emphasize to meet the performance objective. The manipulations of these variables will establish distinct training-induced outcomes that can significantly affect the athlete's performance.

The training program should emphasize training variables in proportion to the athlete's needs. The coach must continually monitor the athlete's responses to the training program to determine whether the training variables require further adjustment.

Volume

Volume is a primary component of training because it is a prerequisite for high technical, tactical, and physical achievement. The volume of training, sometimes inaccurately called the duration of training, incorporates the following integral parts:

- The time or duration of training
- The distance covered or the **tonnage** in strength training (Tonnage = Sets × Repetitions × Load in kg)
- The number of repetitions of an exercise or technical element an athlete performs in a given time

The most simplistic definition of volume is the total quantity of activity performed in training. Volume can also be considered the sum of work performed during a training session or phase. The total volume of training must be quantified and monitored, given its impact on adaptations and the athlete's ability to recover from training.

The accurate assessment of training volume depends on the sport or activity. In endurance sports (e.g., running, cycling, canoeing, cross-country skiing, and rowing), the appropriate unit for determining training volume is the distance covered (22, 55). In weightlifting or strength training, the tonnage (60, 64, 67, 74) or metric tons of training (8, 47) expressed in kilograms (Tonnage = Sets × Repetitions × Resistance in kg) is the appropriate unit. Alternatively a very practical unit for determining training volume is the total number of **repetitions** for each intensity zone. The number of repetitions can also be used to calculate volume in activities such as plyometrics (46), throws in baseball (47), and track and field (45). Although time seems to be a common denominator for most sports, the most sensible way of expressing volume should factor in intensity zones.

Across an athlete's career, the volume of training increases (56, 77, 78) (figure 4.1). As the athlete becomes better adapted to training, greater training volumes are necessary to stimulate physiological improvement to increase performance (74, 77, 78). Once the top level has been reached, physiological adaptations are further stimulated by increasing the amount of specific training within the annual plan, rather than indefinitely increasing training volume. An increase in volume over time is particularly important for the development of aerobic athletes. An increase in technical and tactical skills training over time is also necessary because high numbers of repetitions are needed to improve performance.

There are many methods for increasing the athlete's volume of training. Three effective methods are:

- Increasing the **frequency of training** (i.e., density)
- Increasing the volume within the training session
- Increasing both the frequency of training and the volume within the training session

Researchers have suggested that it is important to increase the frequency of training as much as possible without inducing overtraining (31, 73). Other researchers have definitively stated that more frequent training results in significantly greater training-induced adaptations (31, 33, 77). Increasing the number of training sessions in a single day appears to offer a physiological benefit as well (33, 77, 78). It is not uncommon for elite athletes to perform 6 to 12 training sessions per week with multiple sessions each training day (2-5, 30, 38). The athlete's ability to recover from the training volume is the most important factor dictating how much volume is used in the training plan (60). Advanced athletes can tolerate high training volumes because they can recover more quickly from the training load. Nevertheless, the preparatory phase in particular should not be turned into a test of the athlete's work tolerance using general (not sport-specific) means, as this would lead to maladaptation.

The time that athletes spend training has consistently increased over the decades. For example, Fiskerstrand and Seiler (24) reported that between 1970 and 2001, the volume of training increased by 22% in Norwegian international-class rowers. Despite this fact, mostly due to the professionalization of sports, more and more coaches in top and elite-level power sports have started to apply the methodological concept of minimum effective volume, which implies a smaller fluctuation of volume and intensity within the annual plan (figure 4.2), in comparison to the classical models (figure 4.3). Technology now allows for the optimization of training volume according to the athlete's ability to recover and adapt; this also implies a smaller fluctuation of the athlete's readiness status within the annual plan (figures 4.4 and 4.5). It is imperative that the planned training volume takes into account the sport, training objectives, athlete's needs, athlete's training age, athlete's stage of development, and phase of the annual training plan.

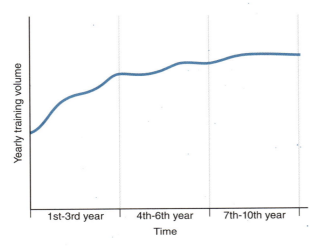

FIGURE 4.1 Theoretical increase in volume of training over time.

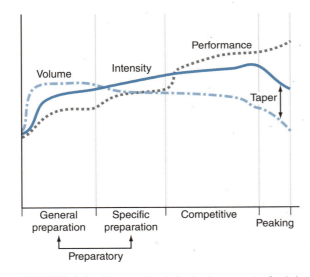

FIGURE 4.2 The methodological concept of minimum effective volume implies a smaller fluctuation of volume and intensity within the annual plan.

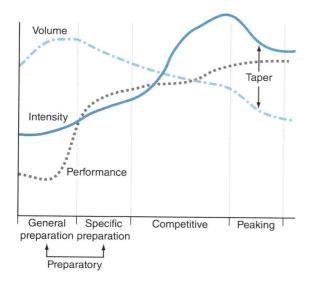

FIGURE 4.3 The traditional concept of inversely proportional volume and intensity implies a higher volume of general means during preparation and a big difference in performance within the annual plan.

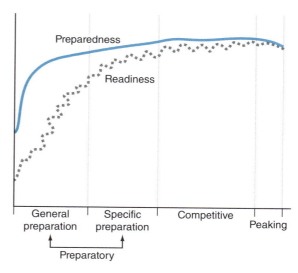

FIGURE 4.4 When a high-volume preparation is used, the athlete has a lower level of readiness that increases as the training is intensified throughout the annual plan.

Intensity

Intensity, or the qualitative component of work an athlete performs, is another important training variable. Komi (39, 40) defined intensity in relation to power output (i.e., energy expenditure or work per unit of time), opposing force, or velocity of progression. According to this definition, the more work the athlete performs per unit of time, the higher the intensity (18, 64, 74). Intensity is a function of neuromuscular activation, with greater intensities (e.g., higher power outputs, higher external loads) requiring greater neuromuscular activation (32). The neuromuscular activation pattern will be dictated by external load, speed of performance, amount of fatigue developed, and type of exercise undertaken (32). An additional factor to consider is the psychological strain of an exercise. The psychological aspect of an exercise, even in the presence of a low physical strain, can have a high level of intensity, which is manifested as a result of concentration and psychological stress.

The assessment of intensity is specific to the exercise and the sport. Exercises that involve speed usually are assessed in meters per second, rate per minute, degrees per second, or power output (watts). When resistance is used in the activity, the intensity is typically quantified in kilograms, kilograms lifted 1 m against the force of gravity (kg/m), or power output (watts). In team sports, the intensity of play is often quantified as the average heart rate, heart rate in relation to anaerobic threshold, percentage of maximum heart rate (11, 29, 71), or, more accurately, metabolic power zones (57).

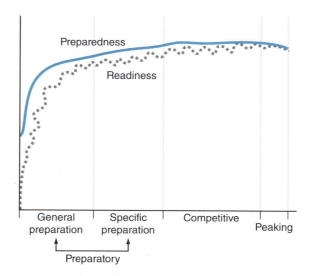

FIGURE 4.5 An optimal-volume preparation allows the athlete to maintain a higher level of readiness throughout the annual plan.

The training program should include varied intensities within the microcycle. There are many methods to quantify and establish the training intensity. For example, with exercises that are performed against a resistance or at high velocities, the training intensity can be quantified as a percentage of the best performance (63). The best performance would then represent a maximum intensity. Let's say that an athlete completes a 100 m dash in 10 s, which corresponds to a velocity of 10 m/s. If the athlete can generate a higher velocity (e.g., 10.2 m/s) over a shorter distance, the intensity would be considered supermaximal because it is more than 100% of the maximum velocity (table 4.1).

Using the intensity stratification presented in table 4.1, exercises performed with strength training loads greater than 105% of maximum would most likely be either isometric or eccentric muscle actions and thus would be considered supermaximal. When training for endurance (e.g., 5,000-10,000 m), the athlete may run shorter distances at a much faster rate and thus may perform at intensities greater than 125% of the mean velocity achieved during the actual race.

An alternative method of evaluating intensity is based on the primary energy system engaged during the activity (18, 64, 69). A six-tier intensity classification can be constructed based on the biochemical responses to different types of exercise bouts (table 4.2).

TABLE 4.1 Intensity Scale for Speed and Strength Exercises

Intensity zone	Percentage of maximum performance	Intensity
1	>100	Supermaximal
2	90-100	Maximum
3	80-90	Heavy
4	70-80	Medium-heavy
5	50-70	Medium
6	<50	Low

TABLE 4.2 Intensity Zones Based on Bioenergetics

Intensity zone	Event duration	Level of intensity	Primary energy system	Bioenergetic contributions	
				Anaerobic	Aerobic
1	<6 s	Maximum	ATP-PC	100-95	0-5
2	6-30 s	High	ATP-PC and fast glycolysis	95-80	5-20
3	30 s-2 min	Moderately high	Fast and slow glycolysis	80-50	20-50
4	2-3 min	Moderate	Slow glycolysis and oxidative	50-40	50-60
5	3-30 min	Moderately low	Oxidative	40-5	60-95
6	>30 min	Low	Oxidative	5-2	95-98

ATP-PC = phosphagen system.
Adapted from McArdle et al. 2007 (50), Brooks et al. 2000 (15), Stone et al. 2007 (74), and Conley 2000 (18).

- *Intensity zone 1:* Exercises in this zone of intensity rely almost exclusively on anaerobic metabolism and last for up to 6 s (e.g., short accelerations, Olympic lifts, shot put throw, average play in American football, discus throw). This intensity zone is marked by the highest power outputs and thus should be considered the highest intensity of exercise (18, 74). The intensity of work in this zone is substantially higher than the athlete's $\dot{V}O_2$max (maximal oxygen uptake), thus requiring any work in this zone to be supported primarily by anaerobic energy supply. The phosphagen (ATP-PC) system is the primary supplier of energy in this intensity zone. The ATP-PC system is capable of supplying energy only for very short periods of time because it relies exclusively on muscular stores of ATP and phosphocreatine (PCr) (74). The reliance on anaerobic energy supply creates a large **oxygen deficit** as a result of the rapid demand for energy that cannot be met by aerobic mechanisms (50, 74). Ultimately, an increase in oxygen consumption, or what is termed the excess postexercise oxygen consumption (EPOC), occurs following exercise to replenish the ATP and PCr stores. Exercise performed in this intensity zone usually is limited by the muscular stores of ATP and PCr (74).

- *Intensity zone 2:* The second intensity zone, which is a high-intensity zone, also relies almost exclusively on anaerobic energy supply and includes activities that last between 6 and 30 s (e.g., 100 m and 200 m sprint in track and field, 100 m sprint in swimming). In this zone, like zone 1, the rate of energy supply must be very rapid and cannot be met by aerobic mechanism. Therefore, energy demand is met by a combination of the ATP-PC and the fast glycolytic system (74). The breakdown of the muscular stores of ATP occurs very rapidly, and PCr must be used to maintain the supply of energy. Within 10 s of the initiation of high-intensity exercise, the ability of PCr to maintain ATP supply is decreased by 50%; by 30 s after initiation, PCr contributes very little to ATP supply (49). Therefore, as the exercise in this intensity zone extends from 10 to 30 s in duration, the reliance on blood glucose and muscular stores of glycogen progressively increases (49). Because of the increasing reliance on fast glycolysis, there can be a substantial increase in lactic acid accumulation depending on the duration and intensity of the exercise bout (49, 74). As a result of the increased lactic acid production stemming from exercise in this intensity zone, a substantial EPOC can occur.

- *Intensity zone 3:* Activities that last from 30 s to 2 min (e.g., 400 m run, 800 m run, 1 km in track cycling) are considered moderately high-intensity activities. These activities predominantly rely on the fast and slow glycolytic systems of energy supply. As an activity's duration shifts from 30 s toward 2 min, activation of the slow glycolytic system increases. With the activities in this zone, speed and high-intensity exercise endurance (HIEE) are of primary concern. Depending on the duration and intensity of these activities, a large amount of lactic acid is produced in response to the metabolic challenge encountered (49). The most likely limiters of performance in this intensity zone are decreases in muscular stores of ATP, PCr, and muscle glycogen. The accumulation of lactic acid may also limit performance (74).

- *Intensity zone 4:* The fourth zone of intensity includes activities that last 2 to 3 min. The intensity in this zone is considered to be moderate, and it relies on a mix of slow glycolysis and **oxidative metabolism**. When an exercise reaches this zone of intensity, the body's energy supply begins to shift from relying on anaerobic mechanisms to relying on aerobic means. Most of the activities classified in this zone rely evenly on both the anaerobic and aerobic energy systems.

- *Intensity zone 5:* Activities in this zone last from 3 to 30 min (e.g., pursuit cycling, team pursuit, 2,000 m rowing, 1,500 m run, 400 m individual medley). Activities in this zone of intensity rely predominantly on the aerobic energy system and are thus of moderately low intensity. A strong cardiovascular system is essential for success in activities in this intensity zone because oxygen supply plays a crucial role in the oxidative pathway's ability to supply energy (18). Events in this zone, especially the longer events, appear to require pacing strategies to maximize performance (74). In these events, the supply of energy (e.g., muscle and liver glycogen, fat stores) is the primary limiter of performance (74).

- *Intensity zone 6:* The final zone consists of activities that are classified as low intensity because of their predominant reliance on oxidative metabolism (e.g., marathon, triathlon, road racing in cycling) (74). Conley et al. (19) reported that power output at $\dot{V}O_2$max is about 25% to 35% of the peak power output achieved during maximal anaerobic exercise. Success in these activities relies on a strong cardiovascular system and an optimal energy supply via the oxidative system. Factors that can limit performance in these activities center on energy supply. As the activity increases in duration, there is a progressive decrease in the availability of muscle glycogen, which ultimately leads to a decrease in blood glucose levels and an increased reliance on fat stores (49). As glycogen stores become depleted, it is increasingly difficult to maintain exercise intensity; therefore, the consumption of carbohydrates during exercise appears to be important to maintain performance.

When working with endurance athletes or team sports athletes, coaches should consider using the heart rate response as an indicator of intensity. Heart rate increases linearly as both workload and oxygen consumption increase (50, 61). Because of this tight relationship, heart rate has become a popular way of quantifying exercise intensity in aerobic exercise. To maximize the effectiveness of heart rate–based training, a graded exercise test should be used to determine the athlete's maximal heart rate, anaerobic or lactate threshold, and $\dot{V}O_2$max. Although not as accurate as a graded exercise test, an age-predicted maximum can be used to estimate the athlete's maximal heart rate (61):

$$\text{Maximal heart rate} = 220 - \text{Age}$$

Once the maximal heart rate is determined, heart rate training zones can be established, and training can be based on those zones (tables 4.3 and 4.4). Faria and colleagues (22) suggested that the individual anaerobic threshold (IAT) is a crucial marker that can be used

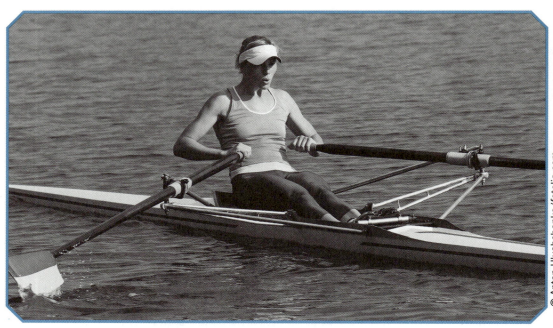

Knowing what intensity zone your activity falls in can help you better understand what systems your body uses to provide energy for competition.

TABLE 4.3 — Australian Institute of Sport Heart Rate Training Zones for Male Cyclists

Training zones	Heart rate (% heart rate maximum)	Perceived exertion
Endurance 1	<75	Recovery (easy)
Endurance 2	75-85	Comfortable
Endurance 3	85-92	Uncomfortable
Endurance 4	>92	Stressful

Adapted, by permission, from N. Craig et al., 2000, Protocols for the physiological assessment of high-performance track, road, and mountain cyclists. In *Physiological tests for elite athletes*, edited by C.J. Gore (Champaign, IL: Human Kinetics), 258-277.

TABLE 4.4 — USA Cycling Heart Rate Training Zones for Cyclists

Training zones	Heart rate (% heart rate maximum)	Description of training
1	<65	Recovery ride (easy)
2	66-72	Basic endurance training
3	73-80	Tempo training
4	84-90	Anaerobic threshold training
5	91-100	Maximal efforts

Courtesy of USA Cycling.

TABLE 4.5 — Heart Rate Training Zones Based on Individual Anaerobic Threshold

Training zones	Low end	High end	
Basic training zone	HR (IAT) − 50	HR (IAT) − 30	
Evolution training zone	HR (IAT) − 5	HR (IAT) + 5	
Example			
Basic training zone	120	140	HR (IAT) = 170
Evolution training zone	165	175	

HR = heart rate; IAT = individual anaerobic threshold.
Adapted from Faria, Parker, and Faria 2005 (22).

to determine basic and evolution heart rate training ranges (table 4.5). The basic training zone is used to stimulate increases in aerobic fitness, whereas the evolution zone is used to improve lactate tolerance (22). The basic training zone is calculated as the IAT − 50 beats per min, through the IAT − 30 beats per min. Thus for an athlete with an IAT of 170, the basic zone would be 120 to 140 beats per min. The evolution training zone is calculated as the IAT − 5 beats per min, through the IAT + 5 beats per min. For example, an athlete with an IAT of 170 would have an evolution training zone of 165 to 175 beats per min. Faria and colleagues (22) suggested that the evolution zone should be used after a period of basic training and closer to competition.

In the sport of cycling, you can also quantify intensity based on the measurement of power output (9, 36). When using a power-based training plan, the athlete must first determine her functional threshold, which is calculated by subtracting 5% from the average power achieved during a 20 min time trial performed on a flat surface (9). Once this is accomplished, seven distinct training zones can be established and used to develop a training plan (table 4.6).

High intensities of training result in rapid progress but lead to less stable adaptation, a lower degree of consistency, a greater incidence of high-intensity overtraining, and a plateau in performance. Conversely, low-level training loads result in slower development and minimal stimulus for physiological adaptation, which correspond to a lower but more consistent performance. The training plan should systematically alter volume and intensity to maximize the physiological and performance adaptations stimulated by training.

There are two types of intensities: absolute intensity, which corresponds to the percentage of maximum necessary to perform the exercise, and relative intensity, which measures the intensity of a training session or microcycle, given the absolute intensity and the total volume of work performed in that period.

TABLE 4.6 Power-Based Training Zones for Cycling

Training zone	Zone name	Percentages		Example calculations[b]	
		Average power[a]	Average heart rate[a]	Average power	Average heart rate
1	Active recovery	<55%	<68%	<124	<121
2	Endurance	56%-75%	69-83%	126-129	123-148
3	Tempo	76%-90%	84-94%	171-203	150-167
4	Lactate threshold	91%-105%	95-105%	205-236	169-187
5	$\dot{V}O_2$max	106%-120%	>106%	239-270	>187
6	Anaerobic capacity	121%-150%	N/A	272-337	N/A
7	Neuromuscular power	N/A	N/A	N/A	N/A

[a]Based off of the functional threshold (average power for a 20-minute time trial—5%).
[b]Based off of a functional threshold average power of 225 and threshold heart rate of 178.
Based on Allen and Coggan 2006 (9).

Relationship Between Volume and Intensity

Fundamental to the training process is the trade-off between volume and intensity. The interaction of these variables is the foundation for periodized training plans because of their specific effects on physiological and performance adaptations. Periodization of training attempts to target performance outcomes by manipulating both volume and intensity of training in a fluctuating fashion (74). The volume and intensity of training are inversely related in most instances. For example, when the intensity of training is the highest, the volume is generally low. Different physiological and performance adaptations can be stimulated by shifting the relative emphasis on these components in training. However, because training entails both a quantity and a quality, it is impractical to consider volume and intensity separately because the work accomplished is considered a good indicator of training stress (74). The greater the workload (e.g., the higher the intensity of training and the longer it is maintained), the greater the physiological stress as indicated by decreases in energetic substrates (e.g., muscle glycogen and PCr), increases in hormonal disturbances (e.g., cortisol release), and increases in neuromuscular fatigue.

High workloads develop endurance, create a work capacity base, establish the duration and stability of corresponding training effects, and serve as a foundation for intense efforts that are involved in special and technical preparation (74). Many strategies can be used to increase workload: (a) increasing the number of repetitions per set or increasing the distance with a corresponding decrease in intensity; (b) increasing the number of **sets**, exercises, or both; and (c) manipulating the frequency (e.g., density of training within the microcycle or training day). A good example of using these methods to increase workload can be seen in long-distance swimming. In the preparatory phase of training, the swimmer can increase the training volume by increasing the number, length, or distance of intervals used in training or by increasing the load density (e.g., increasing the frequency of high-volume training) (56). To increase training volume, a decrease in training intensity will most likely occur. However, this low-intensity, high-volume training will serve as the base on which higher-intensity work will be built (56, 74).

The relationship between volume and intensity of training varies throughout a training year depending on the focus of the phase of the annual plan (figures 4.2 and 4.3). With many sporting activities, these fluctuations in training can include alterations in time or alterations in the emphasis on technical, tactical, and physical training. Typically, in the preparatory phase of training, the emphasis in the early portion of the phase is on developing a physical training base with the use of high workloads. High workloads are accomplished via an increase in training volume with a concomitant decrease in **training intensity**. As the athlete progresses through this phase of training, the volume of physical training will progressively decrease as the training intensity increases. When the workload is very high, the athlete's readiness decreases as a result of cumulative fatigue (60, 74, 76, 77). If the athlete continually undergoes high volumes of training, performance will not be optimized even though preparedness increases. However, if training intensity is not increased, the athlete will continually train at intensities below those needed for competition. Thus, to elevate and ultimately increase performance the workload has to be decreased while intensity is increased. Therefore, it is important to consider the relationship between training volume and intensity in the context of the emphasis of each phase of the annual training plan.

Determining the optimal workload, which entails combinations of training volume and intensity, is a complex task that depends on many factors including the specifics of the sport, the phase of the annual training plan, and the athlete's level of development. It is much easier to quantify volume and intensity with sports that can be assessed objectively. In weightlifting, for example, it is relatively easy to determine the volume of training (e.g., multiply the sets by repetitions and resistance) and training intensity (e.g., tonnage divided by total repetitions, or percentage of maximum capacity). In many team sports and sports like gymnastics, it is much more difficult to quantify these variables. One strategy is to use the total number of actions, elements, repetitions, and distances covered to determine volume. Another possibility is to quantify the duration of a training session or the number of repetitions of a skill to determine volume. In these sports, the velocity or speed at which the athlete performs the activities of training or the average heart rate may be used to quantify the intensity of training.

Dynamics of Increasing Volume and Intensity

The amount of work that international-class athletes perform has increased markedly over the past 3 to 5 decades (6, 24). This marked increase in workload has been accomplished via an increase in training frequency, individual training session volume, and microcycle volume, all of which contribute to markedly greater training loads for the yearly training plan. Contemporary athletes often increase their training load by increasing training frequency, where training is undertaken frequently during the microcycle (8 to 12 sessions per week), typically with multiple training sessions being used in the same day. Although distinct physiological and performance benefits can occur from increasing the frequency of training (31, 58, 77, 78), these increases in training load (volume and intensity) and frequency (density) must be implemented in a progressive and systematic fashion (as described in chapter 2).

As the athlete becomes more trained, a workload that previously was considered a stimulating load (a training load high enough to induce physiological changes) is now a retaining load (a load that maintains physiological adaptations) or a detraining load (a load that is not high enough to maintain physiological adaptations and a loss of physiological adaptations occurs) (77, 78). For example, a novice athlete may optimize strength gains from a strength program with 3 days of training per week (58, 62); on the other hand, a more advanced athlete may require more frequent (e.g., four to eight sessions per week) strength training sessions to maximize the training stimulus. As the athlete becomes more developed she will need greater training variation, which comes from manipulating the training load (volume and intensity), frequency of training, and periodic changes in exercises or activities. These alterations in the training load should not be sudden, unless one is using planned overreaching or concentrated loading strategies (60, 64, 74). As the athlete becomes more trained and her work capacity increases, she should periodically increase the training load progressively, yet in a nonlinear fashion. Coaches need to be extremely careful when attempting to increase training load because most training plans entail a delay in training adaptations.

When attempting to increase training load via alterations of volume and intensity, the coach can consider several example strategies.

Strategies for Altering the Volume of Training

- Increase the duration of the training session. This can be a useful strategy when working with endurance athletes. For example, if the athlete is performing three sessions of 60 min duration, an increase in volume could be accomplished by increasing some of the training sessions to 75 min. In this way the athlete's training volume progressively increases over time.
- Increase the frequency of training (i.e., density, or number of training sessions) per week. If, for example, the athlete is performing 3 sessions per week, an increase to 5 days per week would increase the training frequency. Another possibility is to increase the number of sessions in the training day. For example, if the athlete is training 3 days per week, he could maintain a 3-day-a-week training plan but now include two sessions per day, for a total of six training sessions per week. When the frequency of weekly training is increased, the weekly training volume must be distributed over the new number of sessions and then gradually raised to the previous sessions' volume, if necessary.
- Increase the number of repetitions, sets, drills, or technical elements per training session.
- Increase the distance traveled or the duration per repetition or drill.

Strategies for Altering the Intensity of Training

- Increase the velocity of movement over a given distance or the quickness or tempo of performing tactical drills.
- Increase the load (i.e., resistance or weight) in strength training.
- Increase the power output of the training activity.
- Decrease the rest interval between repetitions or tactical drills.
- Require the athlete to perform endurance, interval, or tactical work at a higher percentage of maximal heart rate.
- Increase the number of competitions in the training phase, but only if this fits into the training plan for the athlete and does not impede the athlete's development.

Many factors are involved in the dynamics of intensity used in training. Three factors are often discussed: the characteristics of the sport, the training or competitive environment, and the athlete's performance level.

- *Characteristics of the sport:* Each sporting activity stimulates distinct physiological adaptations. In sports where maximal speed or power (e.g., sprinting, throwing, weightlifting) is of primary importance, the resultant physiological stress is considered to be high in response to the activity's reliance on anaerobic energy supply. Conversely, in endurance sports (e.g., running, distance cycling, triathlon), the intensity is considered to be low as a result of the lower power outputs encountered and the reliance on aerobic energy supply (19, 74). The intensity of sporting activities that rely on technical mastery (e.g., gymnastics, diving, synchronized swimming) is determined by looking at the degree of difficulty of the individual skills performed and the predominant energy supply system. In most instances, these activities rely heavily on the anaerobic energy systems and require high power outputs or quick movements. Therefore, most of these activities fall on the high end of the intensity spectrum. The classification of team sports is often difficult because of the fluid changes in intensity that can occur. Most team sports should be considered high intensity as a result of their reliance on anaerobic energy supply (see table 1.2 for a summary of sporting activities and their primary energy suppliers). For any activity, the periodized training plan should include a variety of intensities because systematic variations of intensity result in superior physiological adaptations, which ultimately elevate the athlete's performance ability.

- *Training or competitive environment:* The training or competitive environment significantly affects the intensity of a training session. For example, running in sand or uphill can significantly increase intensity, which can be seen in an increase in the heart rate response to the training session. Using drafting strategies in cycling, running, and skating to decrease drag can significantly affect intensity. In cycling, for example, drafting behind another cyclist while riding at 24.5 m/h (39.5 km/h) has been shown to result in an approximately 7.5% reduction in average heart rate and an

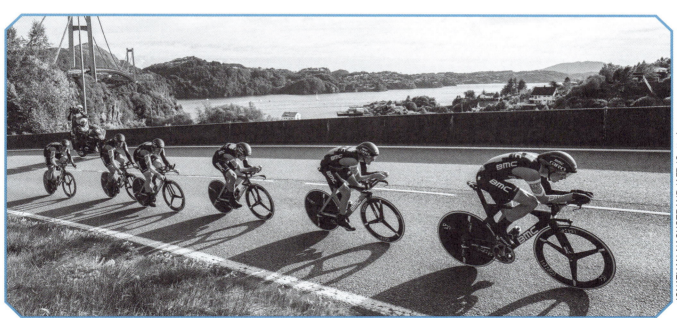

Drafting during training can modify the heart rate response to the training session; this is an example of the training environment affecting performance.

approximately 14% reduction in oxygen consumption ($\dot{V}O_2$) compared with cycling alone (35). Thus drafting has the potential to decrease the intensity of the activity while maintaining a very high speed of movement. Using aerodynamic devices (e.g., aero-handlebars, disc wheels, skin suits) can reduce the drag forces encountered in cycling and thus decrease the intensity of cycling at the same absolute speed (23).

- *Preparation of the athlete's performance level:* The athlete's physical development appears to play a very large role in determining the content of the athlete's training program. When athletes of different training levels are introduced to the same training content (e.g., workload), differing physiological responses will most likely occur because the load represents different intensities of training for different athletes. For example, a training load that is of medium intensity for an elite athlete may be a supermaximal load for a novice athlete. Conversely, a medium load for a novice athlete may be a detraining load for an elite athlete. These contentions support the importance of using individualized training plans to optimize each athlete's physiological adaptations and ultimately his performance.

As suggested previously in this chapter, the heart rate response to training can be a useful tool for prescribing and evaluating training intensities. Heart rate may be used to compute the intensity of training as an expression of the total demand experienced during a training session. The intensity of a training session can be calculated by using the following series of equations proposed by Iliuta and Dumitrescu (37). The first step of this process is to calculate the partial intensity with the following equation:

$$\text{Partial intensity} = \frac{HR_p \times 100}{HR_{max}}$$

In this equation, HR_p is the heart rate that results from performing the exercise for which the partial intensity is being calculated, and HR_{max} is the maximum heart rate achieved in performing the activity of that individual. Once the partial intensity is established, the intensity can be calculated with the following equations:

$$\text{Overall intensity} = \frac{\sum(\text{Partial intensity} \times \text{Volume of exercises})}{\sum(\text{Volume of exercises})}$$

Another possible use for monitoring heart rate is the concept of training impulse (TRIMP) (52, 67). TRIMP is the product of training duration and intensity, where heart rate is multiplied by a nonlinear metabolic adjustment based on the lactate curve and the training session duration (52). Although the TRIMP method of determining training stress is useful, its application is limited to aerobic training intensities that result in heart rates below maximum.

Rating the Volume and Intensity

Because the human body has the ability to adapt to a given training stimulus, actual performance can be changed in response to the training program. Additionally, the type of training undertaken can result in very distinct genetic and molecular adaptations that underlie these performance outcomes (17). To achieve the primary goal in the development of athletes, which is to maximize performance outcomes via an appropriate training stimulus, all elements of the training plan must be in line with the concept of training specificity. Coaches must consider the bioenergetic, mechanical, and movement characteristics of the sport and target these areas in the training plan. Furthermore, individualization of the training program is essential to the success of the plan. The workload should be based on the individual athlete's level of development or ability to tolerate training, the phase of the annual plan, and the ratio between the volume and intensity of training. If the appropriate workload dosage is implemented, the correct physiological responses will be stimulated and performance will improve.

In training, two classifications of load have been established: external and internal (34, 59). The external load, or dosage, is a function of training volume and intensity. The external load is based on the interrelationships of the volume, intensity, and frequency of the training stimuli. These factors are easily monitored, and the coach and athlete should keep detailed records of what has been accomplished. The external load elicits the physiological and psychological adaptations that occur as a result of the training program. These individual responses are at the same time affected by and specific to the internal load, or dosage, which is expressed in degree and magnitude of fatigue experienced by the athlete. The magnitude and intensity of the internal load are direct results of the external dosage that is applied during the training plan.

Application of the same external load does not always result in the same physiological or psychological responses between athletes or for the same athlete (because of, for instance, accumulated fatigue). Internal responses to training are a function of the individual athlete's response to the applied external load. Therefore, the internal response can only be estimated in general terms. The internal response is best tracked by using training logs or diaries and periodic physiological testing, including heart rate variability (HRV) monitoring, dynamometers and accelerometers data, and psychological testing (74).

Relationship Between Volume and Adaptation

The implementation of a well-structured training plan results in very specific physiological and psychological adaptations that alter the athlete's performance capacity (60, 67, 74). These adaptations are related to many factors, including the genetic endowment, health status, and training history of the athlete (67). The training plan is a key factor in determining performance outcomes because training intensity, volume, and frequency all play a significant role in modulating the physiological adaptations that are central to performance (17, 67, 75).

Of particular interest is the relationship between the dosage of training and these adaptations. The physiological systems must be progressively overloaded to induce the adaptations necessary to improve performance. For example, a high volume of work performed by highly trained endurance athletes at a low intensity does not appear to significantly improve performance or related physiological adaptations (42). A higher work volume or intensity of work is necessary for continued adaptations to occur (14, 34, 42, 59). In another example, the tonnage (i.e., Tonnage = Sets × Repetitions × Resistance in kg) of training encountered in a strength training plan is strongly related to the muscular adaptations that occur in response to training. Froböse and colleagues (26) offer evidence that the greater the tonnage of training, the greater the stimulus for muscular growth and adaptation, which ultimately could have a profound effect on performance for some athletes.

If the work volume, training volume, or training intensity is elevated too sharply or exceeds the athlete's work capacity, a maladaptive response can occur that can result in overtraining (see chapter 5) (27, 28, 72). If this situation occurs, performance can stagnate or even decline in response to the overtraining syndrome induced by the misapplied training stimulus. The training program must include variations in intensity, volume, and frequency so that the athlete alternates between stimulation and regeneration (i.e., work and rest); this usually happens at the macrocycle level (by placing an unloading week at the end of it) and microcycle level (alternating workloads within it).

The positive adaptation to a training stimulus increases the training stimulus required by the athlete in training. This increased demand for training stimulus occurs as a result of physiological adaptations that allow the athlete to tolerate greater training loads. Therefore, if the same training load is encountered again, significantly less physiological disturbance occurs, resulting in significantly less physiological adaptation. To continue to stimulate appropriate physiological adaptations, the external dosage or workload must be progressively increased, as suggested by the theory of progressive overload (25, 74). Furthermore, if the training load is substantially reduced, the training effect is diminished and an involution phase results. Although a reduction in workload is necessary when the athlete is attempting to dissipate fatigue, recover, or peak for a competition, remaining in periods of subthreshold training for too long will result in a loss of physiological adaptations and ultimately performance capacity as a result of detraining (53, 54). For instance, during the annual plan if the transition phase is too long and contains passive recovery instead of active recovery, many of the adaptations stimulated by the preparatory and competitive phases of training could be lost.

Frequency

The frequency (i.e., **density**) of training can be defined as the distribution of training sessions (74). The frequency of training can be thought of as a relationship that is expressed in units of time between working and recovery phases of training. Thus the greater the frequency of training, the shorter the recovery time between working phases of training. When increasing the frequency of training, the athlete and coach must establish a balance between work and recovery to avoid inducing excessive levels of fatigue or exhaustion, which can lead to overtraining.

It is very difficult to calculate the optimal amount of time needed between multiple training sessions (e.g., within the training day or microcycle) because many factors can contribute to the athlete's rate of recovery. The intensity and volume of training encountered within the training session plays a major role in determining the amount of time needed before another training session is undertaken (74, 77). The greater the workload (i.e., intensity and volume) of the training session, the greater the amount of time needed to recover before readiness or performance capacity is restored (77, 78). Additionally, the training status of the athlete (77, 78), chronological age of the athlete (20, 41, 66), nutritional interventions used by the athlete (16), and use of recovery interventions (10, 51) can all affect the ability to recover from training bouts. Complete recovery from a training session is not needed before the next training session. A common strategy is to increase the frequency of training and promote recovery by using training sessions of differing workloads within the training day or microcycle.

Two methods are commonly used to optimize the work-to-rest interval during endurance or interval-based training: (a) fixed work-to-recovery ratios (12, 43, 44, 68, 70) and (b) recovery durations that require heart rate to return to a predetermined percentage of maximum (7, 43, 44, 65). In these cases, it is the training frequency that is manipulated. Training density can be defined as the frequency at which an athlete performs a series of repetitions of work per unit of time (13).

- *Fixed work-to-recovery ratios:* Several researchers have used fixed work-to-rest ratios when studying interval-based training (12, 43, 68, 70). By manipulating the work-to-rest interval, the coach and athlete can design a training program that targets specific bioenergetic adaptations (18). Work-to-rest ratios of 3:1 to 1:4 target the development of endurance characteristics, whereas ratios of 1:5 to 1:100 target strength- and power-generating characteristics (table 4.7).

TABLE 4.7 Work-to-Rest Intervals for Sprinting

Training objective	Average work time (s)	Work-to-rest ratio	Intensity
Acceleration (10-40 m)	2-5	1:30-1:45	Maximal
Maximum speed (50-60 m)	6-7	1:35-1:60	Maximal
Speed endurance (80-200 m)	9-24	1:40-1:110	Maximal
Special endurance (250-400 m)	30-60	1:4-1:24	Submaximal

- *Predetermined heart rate:* Another method for determining the length of the recovery period is to establish a heart rate that must be achieved prior to performing another work bout (7, 43, 65). One method of using this technique is to set a heart rate range of 120 to 130 beats per min as the cutoff for the initiation of the next work bout (7, 65). A second method is to set the recovery period as the time it takes the athlete's heart rate to return to 65% of maximum (43, 44).

Computing the density of a training session can be accomplished by calculating what is termed the **relative density**. The relative density is the percentage of work volume the athlete performs compared with the total volume within the training session. The relative density equation is as follows:

$$\text{Relative density} = \frac{\text{Absolute volume} \times 100}{\text{Relative volume}}$$

The absolute volume is represented by the total volume of work that the individual performs, whereas the relative volume represents the total amount of time (duration) for a training session. For example, if the absolute volume of training is 102 min and the relative volume is 120 min, then the relative density of the training session would be calculated as follows:

$$\text{Relative density} = \frac{102 \times 100}{120} = 85\%$$

This calculated percentage suggests that the athlete worked 85% of the time. Although the relative density has some value to the athlete and coach, the **absolute density** of training is more important. The absolute density can be defined as the ratio between the effective work an athlete performs and the absolute volume. The absolute density or effective work is calculated by subtracting the volume of rest intervals from the absolute volume using the following equation:

$$\text{Absolute density} = \frac{(\text{Absolute volume} - \text{Volume of rest intervals}) \times 100}{\text{Absolute volume}}$$

For example, if the volume of rest intervals is 26 min and the absolute load is 102 min, then the absolute density would be calculated as follows:

$$\text{Absolute density} = \frac{(102 - 26) \times 100}{102} = 74.5\%$$

These calculations indicate that the absolute density of training was 74.5%. Because training frequency is a factor of intensity, the index of absolute density could be considered medium-heavy intensity (see table 4.1). Determining the relative and absolute density of training can be useful for establishing effective training sessions.

Complexity

Complexity refers to the degree of sophistication and biomechanical difficulty of a skill. The performance of more complex skills in training can increase training intensity. Learning a complex skill may require extra work, in comparison to basic skills, especially if the athlete possesses inferior neuromuscular coordination or is not fully concentrating on the acquisition of the skill. Assigning complex skills to several individuals who have no previous experience with those skills discriminates quickly between well-conditioned and poorly conditioned athletes. Therefore, the more complex an exercise or skill, the greater the athlete's individual differences and mechanical efficiencies.

The complexity of previously learned skills may impose physiological stress, even though the skills have been mastered. For example, Eniseler (21) demonstrated that heart rate and lactate accumulation are higher with tactical training compared with technical training in soccer players. In that study, the technical portion of the training session centered on skill practice without the presence of an opponent. The addition of an opponent during tactical training significantly increased the complexity of the drills and thus increased heart rate and lactate production. Additionally, when simulated games were undertaken, the complexity of the activities increased again, resulting in a concomitant increase in heart rate and lactate production. The highest heart rates and lactate levels were seen in actual games. In light of this information, the coach should consider the physiological stress of the different portions of the training session in the context of the complexity of the skills or activities used.

Index of Overall Demand

Volume, intensity, frequency, and complexity all affect the overall demand (i.e., workload) an athlete encounters in training. Although these factors may complement each other, an increased emphasis on one factor may cause an increased demand on the athlete if the emphasis on the other factors is not adjusted. For instance, if the coach intends to maintain the same demand in training, and the needs of the sport require developing high-intensity endurance, the volume of training must increase. When increasing the volume, the coach must consider how this increase will affect the frequency of training and how much the intensity of training must be decreased.

The planning and direction of training are the primary functions of manipulations of volume, intensity, and complexity. The coach must guide the evolution of the curve of these components, especially volume and intensity, in direct relationship with the athlete's index of adaptation, phase of training, and competition schedule. The appropriate integration of these factors in the annual training plan will enhance the athlete's ability to peak at the appropriate times, thus resulting in optimal performances at these times.

The overall demand of a training program can be calculated with the **index of overall demand (IOD)** (37). The IOD can be calculated with the equation proposed by Iliuta and Dumitrescu (37):

$$\text{Index of overall demand} = \frac{OI \times AD \times AV}{10{,}000}$$

For example, if the OI (overall intensity) is 63.8%, the AD (absolute density) is 74.5%, and the AV (absolute volume) is 102 min, then the OI, AD, and AV can be substituted into the IOD equation as follows:

$$\text{Index of overall demand} = \frac{63.8\% \times 74.5\% \times 102}{10{,}000}$$

In this example, the IOD of training is very low (48.5%), slightly less than 50%.

Summary of Major Concepts

The amount of work encountered in training is a key variable in the success of a training plan. A large amount of work that encompasses and integrates physical, technical, and tactical training is essential to stimulate the physiological adaptations that serve as the foundation for improvements in athletic performance. The application of workload should be individualized because each athlete has a tolerance to the volume, intensity, and frequency of training.

The workload encountered in training has progressively increased over the past 50 years, with athletes now undertaking multiple training sessions per day and accumulating many hours of training within the microcycle. Athletes must progressively increase their training volume, intensity, and frequency across their athletic careers. If these factors are increased too sharply or too soon, overtraining likely will occur. Thus, an athlete's increase in workload should be individualized and progressive.

The coach must monitor training loads and performance measures to determine the effectiveness of the training plan. The coach should quantify the frequency of a training session or complexity of the skills practiced to account for the workload in tactical and technical training. One useful tool that has gained popularity in many sports (e.g., soccer, rugby) is the tri-axial accelerometer with gyroscope and GPS, which is used to quantify training and competitive intensities and has replaced quantification using the heart rate monitor. The coach should monitor factors that increase the workload or training stress and coordinate them with recovery and restoration. The coach also should consider restoration techniques and the time needed to restore energy stores.

PART II
PLANNING AND PERIODIZATION

Periodization of Biomotor Abilities

The periodization of biomotor abilities and the annual plan are the tools that guide training over a year. They are the essential components of periodization because they help the coach divide the training year into distinct phases with very specific training objectives. Periodization of biomotor abilities and the annual training plan are the necessary methodological tools to maximize physiological adaptations, as they are the intrinsic foundation necessary to improve performance. It is equally important to also acknowledge that technical, tactical training, psychological, and nutrition plans also rely on the concept of periodization and should be integrated into the annual plan in order to bring adaptations and performance to the highest possible levels. In other words, the same phases defined in the annual plan are also used for the periodization of all the activities used in an athlete's training.

Periodization represents the basis for the compilation of any athlete's training plan. The term *periodization* originates from the word *period*, which is a way of describing a division of time. Periodization of training is a method by which the training process is divided into smaller, easy-to-manage segments, which are typically referred to as phases of training. Periodization of training has evolved over the centuries, with many sport scientists and authors contributing to its development.

Matveyev (25) borrowed the term of periodization from other fields of human activities, specifically from history. For instance human history is divided into specific phases (not blocks) or periods, such as the Stone Age, Bronze Age, Iron Age, Middle Ages, and the Renaissance. Periodization is also applicable to English literature (Shakespearean, Victorian), architecture (Ionian, Dorian, Roman, Gothic, Baroque), and economics (Pre-commerce, Commerce, Industrial Revolution, Capitalism, Socialism).

Perhaps without periodization, athletes' training would still be in the guessing stages of pre-world War II!

Brief History of Periodization

Periodization is not a new concept, but many people are not familiar with it or do not understand its history. The origins of periodization are unknown, but an unrefined form of the concept has existed for a long time. Evidence suggests that a simplified form of periodization was used to train athletes for the ancient Olympic Games (776 BC to 393 AD). Greek physician Flavius Philostratus (AD 170-245) included simple forms of planning in his writings and is considered one of the early proponents of periodization. Philostratus referred to the simple annual plans used by the Greek Olympians, where a preparatory phase preceded the ancient Olympic Games with a few informal competitions before and a rest period after the Games.

Roman physician Claudius Galenus (Galen, AD 129-217) expressed concerns regarding the intensity of training for the Greek Olympians. He made a distinction between mind and body, the need to relax after training (a bath and psychological relaxation), and how to treat psychological problems via "talk therapy" (psychotherapy) to reveal his patients' secrets and passions. In his book, *De Sanitate Tuenda* (Preservation of Health), Galen suggested that after training an athlete has to bathe to relax and then have good nutrition. Finally, Galen suggested a simple (periodized?) 10-month training program for the Olympic Games, with a month-long specific program prior to the games. We can assume that the 12th month was for relaxation/recovery, a phase we now call the transition period.

A similar approach was used by both American and European athletes to prepare for the modern Olympic Games (1896). Athletes planning for the European competitions at the beginning of the 20th century also followed a similar pattern. However, planned periodization became more sophisticated, culminating with the Finnish runners from 1910-20 and the very methodic German program for the 1936 Olympic Games. Finnish long-distance runner Paavo Nurmi followed Galen's structure of annual planning but greatly emphasizing the preparatory phase, with lots of over-distance aerobic work. The German specialists created the first long-term plan for the 1936 Olympic Games in Berlin. Beginning in 1932, coaches created a 4-year plan composed of four annual training plans. Not surprisingly, the German athletes were very successful in the Berlin Olympic Games.

In 1964, Tudor Bompa had the incredible chance to meet with one of the original German planners for the 1936 Olympics. The planner explained a few elements of the German system, specifying that after World War II, the Soviets captured most of the German planning documents as spoils of war. A great admirer of the ancient precursors of theory of training and that of the pre-1936 training plans created by the German specialists for the Berlin Olympics, Tudor Bompa has never used the Soviets' terminology in planning where the macrocycle refers to an annual plan and mesocycle to a monthly training program.

After WWII, Soviet Russia started a state-funded sport program, using athletics as a means to demonstrate the superiority of their Communist political system. In 1965, Leonid P. Matveyev, a Russian sport scientist, published a model of an annual plan based on a questionnaire that asked Russian athletes how they were trained before the 1952 Olympic Games in Helsinki, Finland. Matveyev analyzed the data collected on the Russian athletes and produced a model of an annual training plan that was divided into phases, subphases, and training cycles, similar to the plans produced by the Germans. Some refer to Matveyev's plan as the "classic" model of periodization. However, the true classical model should be considered the works of Galen, Philostratus, and the Germans before Matveyev.

Even before Matveyev's publication, Tudor Bompa created and applied a periodized annual plan starting in 1961 for 1964 Olympic javelin champion Mihaela Penes of Romania. During that time, Bompa also created the concepts of periodization of biomotor abilities, particularly the periodization of strength and power. This training approach, novel at the time, made an unknown athlete (Mihaela Penes) an Olympic champion just in 5 years! This concept has been refined during the years into a determinant training methodology, a tool utilized to improve sport-specific abilities that has maximized athletic performance (please refer to the Periodization of Biomotor Abilities section later in this chapter). Thus, Bompa has developed several aspects of periodization of dominant biomotor abilities: periodization of strength and power (5, 7); periodization of endurance and muscle endurance (8); and periodization of agility (9).

Matveyev's structured training referred only to an annual plan with only one competitive phase, or **monocycle** (25). However, this practice did not meet the needs of all sports; therefore, as the theory of periodization evolved, training plans were adapted to meet the competitive needs of athletes who participated in more than one major competition per year. Thus, two main competitions per year (**bi-cycle** plans), three main competitions per year (**tri-cycle** plans), and multiple peak plans were developed (9). During the mid- to late 1900s, several Russian (e.g., Matveyev, Ozolin, and Verkhoshansky), German (D. Harre), Hungarian (Nádori), Ukrainian (V. Platonov), American (e.g., Stone, Kraemer, Fleck, O'Brian), and Romanian/Canadian (Bompa) sport scientists published books about the evolution of periodization from ancient times to the present (1-10, 18-20, 23-25, 27-30, 32-43, 46-49).

Periodization Terminology

Periodization can be examined in the context of two important aspects of training:

1. **Periodization of the annual plan**, which divides the annual training plan into smaller training phases, making it easier to plan and manage the training program and ensure that peak performance occurs at the main competitions
2. **Periodization of biomotor abilities**, which allows the athlete to develop the highest levels of speed, strength, power, agility, and endurance possible for the main competitions of the year

Many are unaware of the difference between periodization as a division of the annual plan and periodization of biomotor abilities. In most sports, the annual training plan is divided into three main phases: preparatory, competitive, and transition. The preparatory phase is divided into two subphases, which are classified as general and specific because of their differing tasks. The focus of the general subphase is to develop a physiological base by using many nonspecific and specific training methods. The specific subphase is used to develop characteristics needed for a sport by using mainly sport-specific modalities. The competitive phase of training is subdivided into precompetitive and competitive phases. Each phase of the annual plan contains macrocycles and microcycles. Each of these subunits has objectives that contribute to objectives of the annual training plan. Figure 5.1 illustrates the division of the annual training plan into phases and cycles.

Athletic performance depends on the athlete's physiological adaptations and psychological adjustments to training, combined with the ability to develop and master the skills and abilities required of the sport. The duration of each subphase of the annual plan depends on the time necessary to increase the athlete's training status (preparedness) and express her physiological potential (readiness) at the main competitions of the year. The main determinant of the duration of each phase of training is the competitive schedule. To optimize performance at the appropriate time (i.e., for major competitions), athletes undergo several months of training. The training plan must be well organized, sequentially develop physiological adaptations, and manage fatigue so that it does not compromise the athlete's performance capabilities. The optimal periodization model for each sport, and the time required for an optimal increase in training status and readiness, have yet to be elucidated. Confounding the coach's ability to optimally dose training is the individual athlete's ability to tolerate and adapt to a training plan, which is influenced by many factors including genetic endowment,

Phases of training	Annual Training Plan					
	Preparatory		Competitive		Transition	
Subphases	General preparation	Specific preparation	Precompetitive	Competitive	Transition	
Macrocycles						
Microcycles						

FIGURE 5.1 Divisions of an annual plan into phases and cycles of training.

psychological traits, training status, nutrition, social stressors, and recovery methods used. Because of this individuality of response to training, programs must be tailored to meet the individual's needs as well as the demands of the sporting activity.

A note of caution: In the past several years, some authors have adopted different terms to replace the terminology commonly used in training theory and methodology. It seems that training has become like fashion: This is modern, that is not! Often these changes only reflect the author's desire to be perceived as trendy. For example, the usual physiological term of *training effect* is often replaced by Russian terms of *long-lasting residual effect; preparedness* is used in the wrong context, instead of being used as *readiness* (see chapter 9). In the same way, each period, with a certain training direction emphasis within a sequential training process, has been defined as a *phase;* but in the last few years, some authors and coaches have replaced the term *phase* with the term *block*. The term "block" was introduced to training theory by Prof. Yuri Verkhoshansky to define a period of concentrated load of one biomotor ability at the expense of the others (for instance, strength). This term contrasted with the complex or concurrent models commonly employed by his colleagues; thus in complex or concurrent models, there is no appropriate use of the term "block."

Needs of Periodization

The phases of training are structured to stimulate physiological and psychological adaptations and are sequenced to develop specific components of performance (physical, technical, and tactical) while elevating the athlete's performance capacity. In the context of periodization, training follows a sequential approach to developing the athlete's skills and motor potential. This approach is undertaken for three reasons: (1) It takes time to bring to an optimal level each component of the athlete's performance capacity; (2) such process requires an escalation of specificity of training methods and training means, eliciting morphofunctional adaptations that potentiate the training methods and training means of the next phase and ultimately the performance capacity of the athlete (figure 5.2); and (3) it is not possible to maintain the athlete's physiological and psychological abilities for a prolonged period of time. The athlete's readiness to perform will vary depending on the phase and type of training, as well as the psychological and social stress encountered. Therefore, the annual training plan must be subdivided into phases that sequentially and simultaneously develop specific aspects required to maximize performance.

The preparatory phase is the time when the physiological foundation for performance is established, whereas the competitive phase is the time when performance capacity is maximized. If the preparatory phase is inadequate, performance will not be maximized during the competitive phase because the physiological adaptations necessary for optimum performance have not been developed. After the competitive phase is completed, a transition phase is necessary to remove fatigue developed across the competitive season and enable the athlete to recover from the physiological and psychological stresses of competition. Additionally, the transition phase allows the athlete to relax and prepare psychologically for the next annual training plan, which will commence shortly. This phase of training is a transition, not an off-season. The term *off-season* is inappropriate because serious athletes do not have an off-season; rather, they

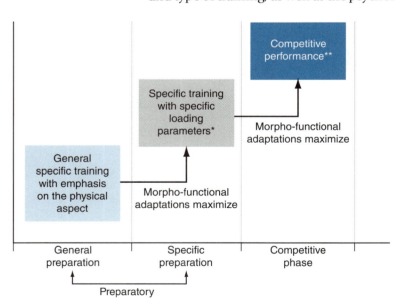

FIGURE 5.2 Enhancing of the training effect and performance potential from one phase to the next.

* While maintaining and supporting general biomotor abilities
** While maintaining and supporting general and specific biomotor abilities

transition from one annual training plan to another. Therefore, the transition is an important link between annual training plans.

The development of skills, strategic maneuvers, and biomotor abilities requires a special approach that is unique to each phase of training. Technical skill sets and tactical maneuvers are learned over time in a sequential fashion across the phases of training. The athlete attempts to perfect her technical capabilities, and as her skill level increases the complexity of tactical training can also increase. The sequential approach is also essential for the development and perfection of biomotor abilities. When attempting to improve biomotor abilities and stimulate physiological adaptations, the coach must alternate the volume and intensity of training, as proposed in the principle of load progression. Training should not occur in a linear fashion, and periodization is truly a nonlinear approach to training.

Climatic conditions and the seasons sometimes influence the duration of training phases within a periodized training plan. For example, seasonal sports such as skiing and rowing are restricted by climate. In a periodized plan, the phases of training are tailored to meet the needs of the sport and will account for climatic conditions. In cycling, rowing, canoeing, and rugby, the preparatory phase of training occurs during the winter, and the competitive phase typically occurs in the spring, summer, or fall. The reverse is true for winter sports such as speed skating, ice hockey, and Alpine and Nordic skiing.

Competition and intense training create a large amount of physiological stress and cumulative fatigue. If this stress is applied for too long, overtraining can occur and performance capacity will decrease. Therefore, stressful training or competition phases should be alternated with periods of recovery and regeneration. These types of phases are transition phases that will remove fatigue and allow the athlete to prepare for the next phase of training.

Misapplication of the Term "Periodization"

As previously stated, periodization is a term used in several scientific fields and borrowed by training science to indicate a phase-based process of training management. Since the first Eastern European publications of the 1960s, the concept of training periodization has evolved, especially in its practical application by coaches; it has been enriched by the unique characteristics in each sport to which it was applied with undeniable success. Nevertheless, its rigid misapplication by some coaches led to a misunderstanding of the concept of periodization as rigid and mechanistic. Nothing is further from the truth! The only somewhat rigid part of periodization is the competitive phase within the annual plan, since the competition calendar is determined by each sport federation. Yet, the coach can still choose when to initiate the competitive phase, what competitions to attend, when to peak, and when to end the competitive phase.

When it comes to the actual training program, periodization is even more flexible. It is recommended that the coach design the detailed training program only one macrocycle at a time, so that the program of the next macrocycle can be based on the actual progress of each athlete, in each aspect of the physical, technical, and tactical preparation. Finally, the daily training program can and should be adjusted according to objective and subjective data on the athlete's readiness to perform the planned session.

Because of the misunderstanding of the concept of training periodization, some have misused the term and employed foreign meanings of periodization, such as traditional, linear, undulatory, and flexible. In our opinion these new terms betray the spirit of the scientific thought. Here is a very brief explanation of discrepancies among some of the new terms:

- *Linear periodization:* Since periodization has originated from the term *period* (of time), its meaning is only in this regard. In sports training the term linear has been used for a certain loading methodology, when training load is constantly increased (e.g., 50%, 60%, 70%, etc.). The only activity that employs such linear loading is **bodybuilding**. This is why bodybuilders are either overtrained or need to train quite infrequently.
- *Undulatory periodization:* This term does not belong to periodization; rather it is a method of managing the load in training (figure 5.3). Load undulation within the

microcycle is an old methodological concept that, for instance, was already used by weightlifters in the late 1950s. Furthermore, periodization already implies an undulation of the load at microcycle level, at macrocycle level, and between macrocycles (figures 5.3, 5.4, and 5.5)

- *Flexible periodization:* As stated previously, the concept of program flexibility is implied by the concept of periodization, as objective and subjective data is collected to direct

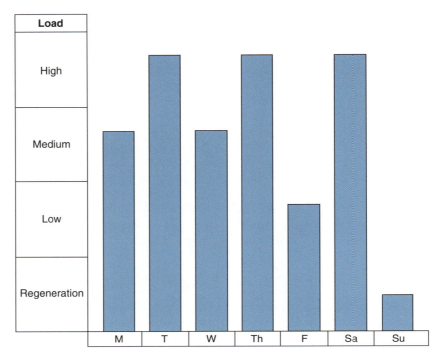

FIGURE 5.3 Load undulation within a preparatory microcycle.

Reprinted, by permission, from T.O Bompa and C. Buzzichelli, 2015, *Periodization training for sports,* 3rd ed. (Champaign, IL: Human Kinetics), 166.

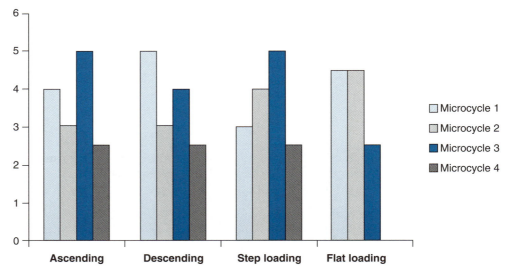

FIGURE 5.4 Four ways to design an undulating macrocycle.

Reprinted, by permission, from T.O Bompa and C. Buzzichelli, 2015, *Periodization training for sports,* 3rd ed. (Champaign, IL: Human Kinetics), 96.

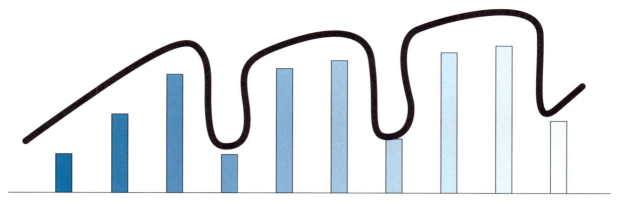

FIGURE 5.5 Placing an unloading microcycle between macrocycles undulates the load.

Reprinted, by permission, from T.O Bompa and C. Buzzichelli, 2015, *Periodization training for sports*, 3rd ed. (Champaign, IL: Human Kinetics), 97.

the training process. It is not the fault of periodization of training if some coaches applied the same program to all the athletes, regardless of their actual progress.

- *Block periodization:* As stated previously, the term "phase" cannot be substituted with the term "block," unless it is referring to a phase with a concentrated load of just one biomotor ability (strength, speed, or endurance) at the expense of the others. In this model, general preparation is composed through a strength **block,** and specific preparation is composed through the sport-specific biomotor ability (speed or endurance), with no maintenance training for strength. It would seem that few elite athletes have been trained with the block periodization model in its pure form.
- *A.T.R. (Accumulation-Transmutation-Realization):* A.T.R. is a periodization model for multiple peaks, with very short phases (general preparation-specific preparation-competition) repeated multiple times during the year. Despite being a necessity for some professional athletes who compete often, this model never really maximizes the motor potential of athletes.

Confusion Between Periodization and Loading

Periodization is sometimes confused with loading patterns. As noted earlier in the chapter, some refer to linear and undulatory (or wavelike) periodization. However, periodization strictly refers to phase-based training; thus periodization cannot be linear or undulatory. In fact, periodization is nothing other than a sequence of training periods (hence the term periodization), or phases. Each of these phases has specific training goals with the final goal of helping athletes reach their highest-possible potentials prior to and during the competitive phase.

As a flexible concept of planning, periodization also has several variations from the main model, depending on the specifics of sports, the schedule of competitions an athlete participates in per year, and the characteristics of the athlete. There is no linear or undulatory periodization—these two terms refer only to the methodology of loading within the training program for an athlete or team.

While periodization has been briefly defined here, the methodology of loading has several variations. De Lorme and Watkins (11) were among the first to refer to progressive loading, which has since been referred to as the linear method of load progression, or the method of constantly increasing the load of training. Linear loading is specifically visible in bodybuilding training; this loading pattern is one of the reasons that athletes in this sport are constantly overtrained. The physiological principle of progressive adaptation to stress of a biological system is often disregarded by individuals who promote linear periodization and still believe more is better from a mathematical perspective.

The undulatory loading method was promoted by Bompa in 1956 in Romania (5), used by Soviet weightlifters in those same years, and also published in the United States in 1983 (9).

Selective Periodization

Far too often the annual training plans developed for elite athletes are also used for young athletes who lack the training experience and physiological maturity to tolerate intensive competitive schedules. This is one reason why periodization of training should be individualized. The coach should consider the athlete's readiness for intensive competitive schedules, using the following guidelines:

- A monocycle is strongly suggested as the basic annual training model for novice and junior athletes. Such a plan has a long preparatory phase during which the athlete can develop foundational technical, tactical, and physical elements without the major stress of competitions. The monocycle is the typical annual plan for seasonal sports and sports for which endurance is the dominant biomotor ability (e.g., Nordic skiing, rowing, cycling, long-distance running).
- The bi-cycle annual training plan is typically used for advanced or elite athletes who can qualify for national championships. Even in this scenario, the preparatory phase should be as long as possible to allow for the development of fundamental skills and physiological potential.
- The tri-cycle annual training plan is recommended for advanced or international-level athletes. Presumably, these athletes have a solid foundation that allows them to handle an annual plan that contains three or more peaks. The usual scheme in individual sports is as follows: First peak for winter championships, second peak for summer Nationals, and third peak for Worlds or Olympics. The time lapse between Nationals and Worlds or Olympics should be enough to recover from the physiological and psychological stress of the Nationals, resume training, and then unload again to return to peak for the most important competition of the year.
- The multiple-peak training plan is characterized by a reduced number of weeks per cycle, and clearly shorter preparatory phases. This is why multiple-peak annual plans are suggested only for athletes with a very good training background (4-6 years), a high level of athleticism, and the capacity to tolerate many and stressful competitions. A typical example of a sport for this type of annual plan is tennis: it features many tournaments, short recovery times between tournaments, and an equally short number of weeks to prepare for the next tournament.

The duration of the training phases depends largely on the competitive schedule. Table 5.1 provides guidelines for distributing the training weeks contained in each training phase of four examples of annual plan.

TABLE 5.1 Guidelines for the Distribution of Weeks for Each Training Phase Contained in the Classic Types of Annual Training Plans

Annual plan structure	Total weeks per cycle	Number of weeks per phase		
		Preparatory	Competitive	Transition
Monocycle	52	≥28	12-22	4
Bi-cycle	26	12-16	6-12	1-4
Tri-cycle	20-24 (winter) 16-18 (spring/summer) 4-6 (summer)	12-20 (winter) 10-12 (spring/summer) 2-4 (summer)	4-6 (winter) 8-12 (spring/summer) 2-4 (summer)	1-2 (winter) 1-2 (spring/summer) 3-6 (summer)
Multiple-peak	11-16	9-12	1-2	1-2

Applying Periodization to the Development of Biomotor Abilities

The concept of periodization is not limited to the structure of the annual plan. Periodization also applies to the development of dominant biomotor abilities for a chosen sport, which ultimately affects the type of training included in each training phase. The outcome of applying periodization principles to the development of dominant biomotor abilities assists the athlete to fully develop his motor potential and reach peak performance during the competitive phase. If the dominant abilities do not reach high levels of development prior to and during major competitions, the achievement of high performance is unlikely. Because an in-depth discussion about the development of biomotor abilities is provided in later chapters (chapters 10-12), the present discussion centers on topics related to the periodization of biomotor abilities within the annual training plan.

Some sports, mostly individual, have a loose structure of periodization, especially regarding endurance. However, in most team sports the periodization of dominant abilities allows room for improvement. In many sports, the dominant biomotor ability is power. Recognizing this, some coaches focus only on exercises and drills aimed specifically at developing power throughout the year, from the early preparatory phase to the beginning of the competitive phase. This type of approach stems from a misunderstanding of exercise physiology and the concept of adaptation, as well as methodological concepts such as periodization and the principles of specificity. A high power output is deeply dependent on a high level of maximum strength. Therefore it is physiologically essential to first develop maximum strength (training the nervous system to voluntarily recruit a high number of motor units, including the fast-twitch muscle fibers) during the early part of the preparatory phase, and then convert strength gains into power-generating capacity prior to and during the competitive phase (figure 5.6).

Figure 5.6 refers to a monocycle; the approach for a bi-cycle or tri-cycle is similar, but far more condensed. Time constraints for these types of annual plans require the coach to shorten the time necessary for the development of each biomotor ability, often at the expense of reaching the highest possible level. In the case of a multiple-peak plan, the time to develop the necessary abilities is even shorter, creating some problems for athletes and coaches. The only sport disciplines that seem to be less affected by frequent competitions,

	Preparatory		Competitive			Transition
	General preparatory	Specific preparatory	Precompetitive	Main competition		Transition
Strength	Anatomical adaptation	Maximum strength	Conversion • Power • Muscular endurance • Both	Maintenance • Maximum strength • Power	Cessation	Compensation
Endurance	Aerobic endurance	• Aerobic endurance • Specific endurance (ergogenesis)	Sport- or event-specific endurance (ergogenesis)			Aerobic endurance
Speed	Aerobic and anaerobic endurance	HIT • Anaerobic power • Anaerobic endurance • Lactate tolerance	Specific speed Agility Reaction time Speed endurance			

FIGURE 5.6 Periodization of main biomotor abilities.

HIT= high-intensity training, typically interval-based training that models the sport or activity targeted by the training plan.

In this figure, the training phases are not limited to a specific duration. Rather, the focus is on the sequence and the proportions between the training phases.

are the alactic ones (such as the jumps and throws in track and field). Because of the lower residual fatigue, alactic events allow athletes to easily train through some of the planned competitions. For all the other sports, multiple-peak training plans have to be reserved for top class athletes who have many years of experience in training. The application of multiple-peak training programs among junior athletes is not advisable because it may result in multiple injuries (particularly for sports such as soccer and tennis). Several examples of periodization of dominant abilities are presented in figures 5.7 through 5.11.

Dates	Sept.	Oct.	Nov.	Dec.	Jan.	Feb.	Mar.	Apr.	May	June	July	Aug.
Competitions					Detroit	L.A.	Toronto	Prov. Orillia	Nat. championships Vancouver			
Periodization	Preparatory				Competitive						Transition	
	General prep.		Specific prep.		Precomp.		Main competition				Transition	
Period. of strength	Anat. adapt.		Maximum strength		Conversion to power		Maintain maximum strength and power				Regeneration	

FIGURE 5.7 Monocycle periodization model of strength training for gymnastics.

Period. = periodization; prep. = preparation; precomp. = precompetition; anat. adapt. = anatomical adaptation.

Dates	June	July	Aug.	Sept.	Oct.	Nov.	Dec.	Jan.	Feb.	Mar.	Apr.	May
Competitions								Division champ.	Nat. champ.	World champ.		
Periodization	Preparatory						Competitive				Transition	
	General prep.		Specific prep.		Precomp.		Main competition				Transition	
Period. of endurance	General end. (run, bicycle)		Specific endurance (run, skate)				Specific endurance				General endurance	
Period. of strength	Anat. adapt.		Maximum strength		Conversion to power		Maintain maximum strength and power				Regeneration	

FIGURE 5.8 Monocycle periodization model for dominant abilities for figure skating.

Period. = periodization; prep. = preparation; precomp. = precompetition; end. = endurance; anat. adapt. = anatomical adaptation.

Dates	July	Aug.	Sept.	Oct.	Nov.	Dec.	Jan.	Feb.	Mar.	Apr.	May	June
Training phases	Preparatory	League games				R/R	League games and international matches				Transition	
Period. of strength/ power/ agility	AA MxS Power Agility	Maintain strength, power, and agility				R/R	Maintain strength, power, and agility				Transition	
Period. of speed	Anaerobic and speed	Maintain specific speed				R/R	Maintain specific speed				Transition	
Period. of endurance	Aerobic endurance	Maintain specific endurance				R/R	Maintain specific endurance				Transition	

FIGURE 5.9 Monocycle periodization model for a European professional soccer team.

Period. = periodization; AA = anatomical adaptation; MxS = maximum strength; R/R = recovery and regeneration (a low intensity maintenance program).

Dates	Nov.	Dec.	Jan.	Feb.	Mar.	Apr.	May	June	July	Aug.	Sept.	Oct.
Competitions								League games				
Periodization	Preparatory						Competitive				Transition	
	Gen. prep.		Specific prep.			Precomp.	League games				Transition	
Period. of strength	Anatomical adaptation		Maximum strength			Conversion: –Musc. end. –Power		Maintain: –Power -Muscular endurance			Regeneration	
Period. of speed	Aerobic endurance	Anaerobic endurance	Specific speed				Specific speed, reaction time, and agility					
Period. of endurance	Specific endurance						Perfect specific endurance				Aerobic endurance	

FIGURE 5.10 Monocycle periodization model for dominant abilities for a baseball team.

Period. = periodization; prep. = preparation; precomp. = precompetition; musc. end. = muscular endurance.

Dates	Nov.	Dec.	Jan.	Feb.	Mar.	Apr.	May	June	July	Aug.	Sept.	Oct.
Competitions					Winter champ.						Summer champ.	
Periodization	Preparatory 1			Comp. 1		T	Preparatory 2			Comp. 2		Trans.
	General prep.	Specific prep.	Precomp.	Main. comp.		T	Gen. prep.	Spec. prep.		Pre-comp.	Main. comp.	Trans.
Period. of strength	Anatomical adaptation	Maximum strength	Conv.: –Power –Musc. end.	Maintain: –Power –Musc. end.		Anat. adapt.	Max strength		Conv.: –Power –Musc. end.	Maintain: –Power –Musc. end.		Regen.
Period. of speed	Aerobic endurance	Anaero. end. and ergogenesis	Specific speed and ergogenesis			Aerobic and anaerobic endurance			Anaer. end. and ergogenesis	Specific speed and ergogenesis		Games

FIGURE 5.11 Bi-cycle periodization model for dominant abilities in swimming (200 m) with winter and summer national championships.

Comp. = competitive; T or trans. = transition; prep. = preparation; precomp. = precompetition; conv. = conversion; anat. adapt. = anatomical adaptation; musc. end. = muscular endurance; regen. = regeneration; anaer. end. = anaerobic endurance.

Simultaneous Versus Sequential Integration of Biomotor Abilities

The concept of integrating the development of biomotor abilities is not a new one (5, 6, 9, 10). Both types of integration have been successfully used. In fact, both types represent a training (physiological) necessity, depending on the type of plan and physiological profile of a sport. It is our firm opinion that they are not mutually exclusive—one type of integration cannot be used at the exclusion of the other.

However, Issurin (17) has proposed that the integration of biomotor abilities (and skills) has to be sequential rather than simultaneous; further, Issurin has postulated that modern sports with very long competitive phases (e.g., soccer and other team sports, or even tennis) require a sequential integration approach.

Examination of the examples of periodization of biomotor abilities shown in figures 5.6-5.11 reveals that the development of each biomotor ability is sequential, but integration of these abilities is simultaneous. In addition, the development of one ability positively

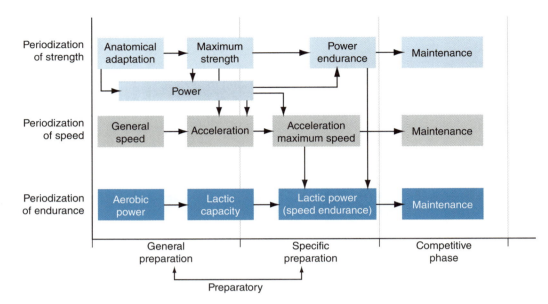

FIGURE 5.12 Sequential development and simultaneous integration of biomotor abilities for a sprinter in track and field.

influences the others (figure 5.12). For instance, high levels of speed cannot be achieved before maximum strength and power are highly developed. A swimmer will be faster only by increasing the application of force against the water resistance. Therefore, the higher the force application to the ground or water, the higher the velocity.

Consider just one biomotor ability, such as strength. Periodization of strength follows a sequential approach dictated by physiology (and not because it is in fashion now). In order to increase the level of power prior to the main competitive phase, the sequence of periodization must be the following: Start with anatomical adaptation (3 weeks or longer) to adapt the muscles and ligaments to the sport or activity and to train an injury-free athlete. Next, move into the maximum strength phase (4 weeks or longer), which involves training the nervous system to voluntarily recruit the highest number of motor units of the prime movers (muscles that perform a technical skill) and thereby overcome an external resistance. Finally, in order to maximize power development, a conversion phase (4 weeks or longer) has to be planned, in which dynamic exercises of low-medium loads are performed explosively. These exercises allow for quick application of force against resistance, which results in an increase in the **discharge rate** of fast-twitch muscle fibers. At the end of these 11 or more weeks of training, power will reach superior levels, resulting in maximized performance.

The development of speed, agility, and endurance has to follow a physiologically and methodologically sound sequence of periodization, too. Furthermore, the periodized development of each biomotor ability has to integrate each ability with the others to maximize the motor potential of the athlete and ultimately, her performance (figure 5.12).

Issurin (17) asserts that because modern training has a very long competitive phase, training has to follow a sequential integration approach. For example, in professional soccer, the competitive phase is 10 to 10.5 months long, and it is followed by a short holiday. When does the coach have the time to apply sequential integration of biomotor abilities and skills when the preparatory phase is just 3 to 4 weeks? What is the performance of the team going to be like during the strength block? What happens to the injury rate and performance level when the accumulation block is performed multiple times during the competitive season?

Periodization of biomotor abilities must also follow the simultaneous approach when other biomotor abilities have to be developed (e.g., speed, agility, and endurance). If these abilities are not trained simultaneously, it will be almost impossible to reach the level of expected development. Distributing the load of each biomotor ability instead of concentrating it allows for a rational progression over time without abrupt overloads of the physiological systems of the athlete. Such sudden increases of load for one or more components of the training program normally leads to maladaptation, decreased performance, or injury.

Issurin's sequential development of biomotor abilities and skills doesn't devote enough time to each component of performance to fully develop the athlete's motor potential or retain her technical-tactical proficiency; on the other hand, such a short exposition avoids the potential for a lasting "residual effect." Sequential integration with bigger blocks probably has worked in seasonal sports such as kayaking or canoeing, or for certain events in track and field, where long preparations of 5 to 6 months are the norm. But to suggest that sequential integration has to be used for all sports is quite unrealistic and certainly will not lead to the maximization of performance. In fact, Platonov found that sequential integration lowered the probability of peaking at the most important competition of the year to just 5% to 15% (30).

Periodization of Strength

The objectives, content, and methods of a strength training program will change throughout the phases of an annual training plan. These changes aim to maximize the developent of the specific type of strength required in a sport while considering the individual characteristics of the athlete in order to achieve optimum performance. These changes also depend on the phase of the annual training program and the targeted physiological adaptations for that phase.

Anatomical Adaptation

After the transition phase, when most athletes do very little strength training, it is advisable to begin a strength program to build a foundation from which future training practices are developed. This is typically accomplished during the anatomical adaptation phase of a strength training program. In this early preparatory phase, several key objectives are targeted:

- Stimulate involvement of most muscle groups, including the stabilizer muscles.
- Increase short-term work capacity, which will reduce fatigue in the later stages of training when intensity of training and the volume of technique-oriented work are high.
- Begin to work on the technical aspects of the fundamental lifts that will represent the core of the strength training program.
- Prepare the muscles, ligaments, and tendons for the stressful activities to come and, consequently, produce an injury-free athlete. When the preparatory phase, specifically the anatomical adaptation subphase, is inadequate, the risk of injury increases.

This phase of a strength training program is a crucial part of the general preparation subphase of the preparatory phase. The anatomical adaptation phase is marked by a high volume of work (e.g., two or three sets of 8-20 repetitions) performed at low intensities (40%-65% of one-repetition maximum, or 1RM). The number of exercises performed will depend on the training experience of the athlete: Usually beginners will perform more exercises than experienced athletes. This subphase should last up to 12 weeks for beginners and 2 to 4 weeks for experienced athletes, in order to achieve the physiological adaptations targeted. For junior athletes or athletes who do not possess a strength training background, a longer anatomical adaptation phase (9-12 weeks) may be warranted; for professional team sports, 2 to 4 weeks could be sufficient.

Maximum Strength Phase

All sports require power (e.g., long jump), muscular endurance (e.g., 400-800 m swimming), or some combination of both (e.g., rowing, Nordic skiing). Both muscular power and endurance depend directly on maximum strength. In support of this contention, it has been shown that stronger athletes generally produce higher power outputs (38) and express higher levels of muscular endurance (26). It appears that maximum strength must be elevated before power-generating capacity can be increased because power is the product of both force and velocity.

The maximum strength phase is a critical component of the preparation phase because it builds on the general adaptations stimulated in the anatomical adaptation phase and develops the neuromuscular attributes necessary for the development of muscular power (10, 43). The maximum strength phase can range from 1 to 3 months depending on the sport, the athlete's needs, and the annual training plan. For athletes whose sports depend heavily on maximum strength, such as American football or shot put, this phase can be on the longer end of the spectrum (3 months). In a sport for which muscular endurance is the determinant of final performance, such as cycling, triathlon, or marathon canoeing, this phase can be shorter (1 month). The development of maximum strength is best accomplished by working first on the development of the **intermuscular coordination** component of strength (2 to 6 repetitions with a load between 70% and 80% of 1RM), and then on the intramuscular component of strength (1 to 3 reps with a load between 80% and 90% of 1RM).

Conversion to Specific Strength Phase

The conversion phase transforms maximum strength into power or muscle endurance (chapter 10). It also provides a transition between the preparatory phase and competitive phase and equips athletes with the neuromuscular abilities vital for the achievement of the highest performance.

The athlete will gradually convert the strength developed in the maximum strength phase into the type of power needed for the targeted sport. This is accomplished by using

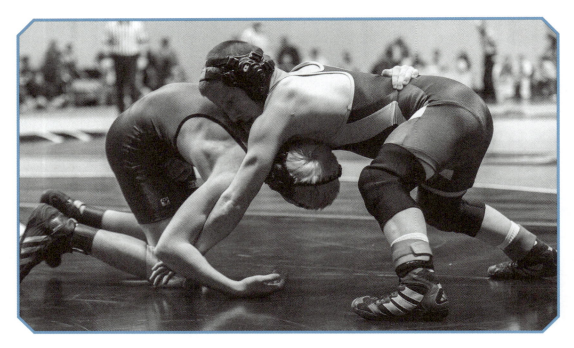

The characteristics of the sport dictate the type of power or endurance that needs to be developed during the specific strength phase of training. This ratio may be almost equal for a wrestler.

the appropriate power training methods (e.g., medicine balls, speed training, plyometrics). Maximum strength levels must be maintained during this phase; if they decline, the ability to maximize power-generating capacity will also decline. If this occurs during the competitive phase, speed and agility will also decrease.

The physiological characteristics of the sport dictate the type of power or endurance that needs to be developed during this phase of training. Because most sports require some combination of power and endurance, the ratio between these two characteristics must match the demands of the sport. For example, the ratio may be almost equal for a wrestler, while power or endurance would dominate for a canoeist (200 m and 500 m). Muscular endurance should prevail for rowing (race duration 6-8 min), swimming events of longer duration (400-1,500 m), Nordic skiing, and the triathlon.

Maintenance Phase

This phase of the annual training plan is designed to maintain the physiological and performance standards achieved during previous phases. It is very difficult to maintain these gains, and strength has been shown to decrease across the competitive season, especially when inappropriate training methods are used (18). The maintenance phase must contain a high enough strength training volume to maintain strength gains while avoiding the development of high levels of fatigue.

The maintenance program depends largely on the physiological requirements of the targeted sport. Thus the ratio of strength, power, agility, and muscular endurance must reflect these needs. For example, an American football player or shot putter would focus his strength training on maximum strength maintenance and power development, whereas an endurance athlete would focus on power and endurance development. The breakdown of training sessions that target these attributes is difficult to recommend because it depends on the competitive season. Generally, the maintenance phase contains training units with a small number of exercises (two to five exercises) that are performed for two to four sets of one to six repetitions, with a wide range of training intensities (60%-80% of 1RM for maximum strength, 30%-80% for power, 30%-60% for muscular endurance). For instance, a top soccer player will maintain strength and power by using three essential exercises: half squats, back hyperextensions, and toe raises. One may also add hip thrusts (glutes). The frequency of strength training during this phase can be 2 days per week, for a duration of 30 minutes. In individual power sports, a common approach is planning two power sessions, on Mondays and Fridays, and a strength maintenance session on Wednesdays, during the weeks that do not have a competition in the weekend. For the competition week, on the other hand, one or two low-volume power sessions are planned.

Cessation Phase

It is usually recommended, mostly for individual sports, that the strength training program end 5 to 7 days prior to the main competition. This reduces the athlete's level of cumulative fatigue, decreases levels of stress, and facilitates physiological and psychological supercompensation. However, this recommendation may not be adequate for all sports. Athletes in sports with a high strength-and power requirement (field events in track and field, wrestling) may benefit from simply reducing the number of sessions during the week prior to the major competition. Such a program would contain a very low volume and a medium intensity, but the program should be performed explosively.

Compensation Phase

The compensation phase completes the annual training plan and coincides with the transition phase. The main objective of the transition phase is to remove fatigue and allow the athlete to recover (via the use of active rest) before initiating the next annual training plan, without a significant degradation of his biomotor level of development. Additionally, this phase is designed to induce regeneration, which is a very complex undertaking. For injured athletes, this phase is used for rehabilitation and restoration of movement capacity. When this is necessary, the athletic trainer, physical therapist, or physiotherapist should work in conjunction with the coach to treat the athlete.

During this phase, regardless of injury or rehabilitation status, all athletes should consider an active rest training plan that includes some strength training. This training should address the stabilizing musculature and target areas of weakness that could increase the athlete's potential risk for injury. This is also the time to work on compensation of other muscle groups that are not primarily used during the competitive phase.

Periodization of Power, Agility, and Movement Time

Power and agility training are discussed in details in chapters 10 and 12, so this short section covers only the elements that pertain to the periodization of power, agility and movement time. As a determinant ability in many sports, **power** refers to the quick application of force against resistance. **Agility** is perceived as an athlete's ability to swiftly accelerate and decelerate and quickly change directions during a game or other sports contests. **Movement time**, on the other hand, refers to an athlete's ability to quickly move a limb in the desired direction, such as in boxing, racquet sports, and Martial arts.

According to many authors, agility evolves from speed. In other words, an athlete will never be agile before being fast. This isn't completely true because the athlete will never be fast before first gaining strength. When an athlete develops a higher level of **relative strength** (i.e., the ratio between his maximum strength and his body weight), he is capable of moving his body more quickly with less effort. The training methods required to produce a high level of maximum strength normally aim to develop the ability of the nervous system to recruit a high number of fast-twitch muscle fibers; these methods also expose the nervous system to training with low angular velocities. Thus, in order to maximize the power capability and, consequently, the agility of the athlete, it is necessary to follow the maximum strength phase with a conversion to a power and agility phase. In other words, one has to:

1. increase maximum strength first, with the ability to recruit fast twitch muscle fibers, and then
2. increase the ability to increase the discharge rate of the same muscles (figure 5.13).

Simply put, agility does not evolve from speed. Agility improves visibly only after maximum strength is developed. In fact, as is evident in sprinting, speed will never increase without increasing maximum strength first.

Because athletes are exposed to heavy loads during the maximum strength phase, at 70%-90% of 1RM, fast-twitch muscle fibers are fully **recruited** into action in higher amounts. This physiological adaptation ensures that the athlete will successfully overcome high resistance. During the next phase, when maximum strength is converted into power and agility, the athlete is exposed to training methods that result in quick application of force and quick

		Preparatory Phase		**Competitive Phase**
Periodization	AA	MxS	Power and agility	Maintain MxS, power, and agility
Scope of training	AA	Increase the recruitment of FT	Increase the discharge rate of FT	Maintain MxS, power, and agility

FIGURE 5.13 Periodization of agility and movement time.

AA = anatomical adaptation; MxS = maximum strength; FT = fast-twitch muscle fibers.

changes of directions (acceleration–deceleration), which increases the **discharge rate** to fast-twitch muscle fibers. After 4 to 8 weeks of power and agility training (depending on the duration of the maximum strength phase), the athlete has maximized her abilities which increases her readiness for competitions.

Both power and agility training have a positive effect on movement time, or the capacity of the athlete to move a limb in the desired direction. As the arms and legs become stronger and react faster to a given signal, the speed of movement increases. In many cases athletes are just exposed to agility drills. Moreover, some of these drills, such as the speed ladder, are trained from childhood to athletic maturation. This training methodology may be challenged by asking why athletes have reached a plateau. To bring about change, organize a periodization of agility plan based on figure 5.13, which will use this method to induce results.

Another component of agility is perceptual decision making, which is related to reaction and movement time (e.g., visual scanning, anticipation, pattern recognition, and knowledge of situations) (50). This component has been termed **reactive agility** and is marked by the ability to react to a situation; reactive agility appears to differentiate players of different levels in various sports (12).

Periodization of Speed

The periodization of speed depends on the characteristics of the sport, including the performance level and the competitive schedule. The development of speed for a team sport athlete is very different from that of a sprinter. Team sport athletes usually follow a monocycle annual plan, whereas sprinters usually undergo a bi-cycle annual training plan as a result of having both indoor and outdoor championship competitions. Regardless of the type of individual or team sport, the periodization of speed training may follow several distinct subphases: a general speed phase; an acceleration phase; a maximum speed phase; and an anaerobic endurance phase. For team sports, there is also a specific speed, agility, and reactive agility phase, which directly follows the acceleration phase.

General Speed and Acceleration Phases

The first step in developing speed is to establish a physiological and technical base that provides the athlete with the skills needed for moving fast. This type of training is typical of the general preparation phase of the annual training plan and is designed to increase the technical proficiency of the athletes during the first part of the expression of speed (i.e., the acceleration phase).

Technical improvement is achieved by incorporating coordination drills (such as skipping or dribbling) with speed training at various intensities: moderate intensity technical runs over step-hurdles (15-30 m), high-intensity uphill accelerations (5-30 m) with full or partial rest intervals, and heavy sled towing (20-30 m) with full recovery. For track and field athletes, this is the time to train on the grass several times a week, always with flats. According to the complex integration approach, the general speed phase (speed) is planned simultaneously with the anatomical adaptation phase (strength) and the aerobic endurance phase (endurance).

The general speed phase is followed by the acceleration phase. During the acceleration phase, short-distance sprints (5-30 m) are performed at high intensities (95%-100% of maximum), with long rest intervals between repetitions (1 to 4 min). Track athletes begin using spikes at this phase. Uphill short sprints or medium- to light-load sled towing can still be used. This type of training relies on the anaerobic alactic system.

During these phases, the previous training means are used simultaneously with tempo training. Tempo training progresses from extensive to intensive, in order to elevate the general and anaerobic endurance capacity of the athlete, thereby progressively creating the metabolic adaptations necessary for the maximization of specific endurance (15).

It is important to note that for sports where aerobic endurance is not part of its ergogenesis (proportions of the systems that supply the energy for the duration of activity), such as sprinting in track and field, the traditional type of aerobic endurance with long steady runs or longer repetitions on the track (500 m or more) is not a physiological necessity. In fact, because speed of movement or sprinting ability depends largely on the rate of energy supply, it is not recommended to use methods that compromise anaerobic function (31).

The metabolic adaptations induced by tempo training have a great degree of sport specificity and translate into a physiological improvement for many individual and team sports. The use of interval-based training methods has been reported to enhance both anaerobic and aerobic metabolism (21).

As training progresses from the general preparatory to specific preparatory phase of training, additional sport-specific activities are incorporated. For team sports training, tactical drills of 2 to 5 min can be performed nonstop to develop sport-specific endurance (22). In soccer this may be accomplished via the use of small-sided games in which fewer players participate in a game simulation (i.e., 2 versus 2; 3 versus 3; 5 versus 5); it may also be accomplished by use of a soccer-specific dribble track, as recent research suggests that this practice effectively develops soccer-specific endurance capacity (16).

Maximum Speed Phase

As the competitive phase approaches, training becomes more intensive, event-specific, refined, and specialized. Training will include work designed to maximize speed, mostly via specific technical and tactical drills.

Speed can be developed with short-distance sprints (40-80 m) performed at high intensities (90%-100% of maximum), with longer rest intervals between repetitions (3 to 8 min) and sets (6 to 20 min). This type of training will stress the anaerobic systems, especially the phosphagen system. It is paramount that the athlete develops speed before he starts training speed endurance. Speed is the neural prerequisite for speed endurance, in the same way that aerobic power precedes lactic capacity (anaerobic endurance) and it is important to lay the metabolic adaptations foundation necessary to maximize this biomotor ability.

For team sport athletes, maximum speed training will also have an injury prevention function, especially for the hamstrings. Having maximum speed repetitions in training will ensure that the neuromuscular system will be ready if called upon for a long lasting maximum sprint during a game. Despite not being frequent, such long sprints can make the difference between winning and losing, so it is better to be prepared for them!

Anaerobic Endurance Phase

Speed endurance training, as noted previously, uses various distances and rest intervals. These different interval structures can be used to target physiological adaptations. For example, the lactic system power and lactate tolerance can be targeted via the use of high-intensity (95%-100% of maximum) short-distance sprints (<80 m), performed with short rest intervals between repetitions (1 to 2 min) and longer rest between sets (6 to 20 min). They can also be targeted via the use of high intensity (95%-100% of maximum) moderate-distance sprints (120-200 m) with long rest intervals between repetitions (lactic power: 12-20 min, depending on the performance level, the targeted event, and the level of intensity; lactate tolerance: 3-6 min, depending on the performance level, the targeted event, and the level of intensity).

Specific Speed, Agility, and Reactive Agility Phase

For most team sports, the specific speed can be described as acceleration with changes of direction. This must be reflected in the training program of the athletes engaged in such sports. After a previous phase dominated by linear accelerations (at sport-specific distance and slightly longer), strength and conditioning coaches should plan acceleration drills with cuts and changes of direction. Because accelerations in team sports are brief (usually less than 3 s or 20 m), followed by a short rest before another acceleration is performed, rest intervals in this phase will be short between repetitions (30 sec to 1 min) and longer between sets (3 to 5 min). One way to measure and progress the muscular load of agility drills is to calculate the total degrees of change of direction in a session.

Reactive agility can be trained by using visual and auditory stimuli (external cues) applied during complex agility drills. For this purpose, multicolored cones can be laid down after an agility course (e.g., slalom runs), with the coach giving the directional cue by calling out a color. Another drill can be performed by placing four hoops at the start of the agility course, assigning a number to each, and then calling a random sequence of the four numbers, which the players have to reproduce by rapidly stepping inside the hoop with alternating feet. Various starting positions can be utilized for agility drills: facing the other way, lying down, sitting, etc.

Periodization of Endurance

Endurance is developed in several distinct phases across the annual plan. Within an annual training plan that constrains one peak, endurance would be developed in three phases: (1) aerobic (oxidative) endurance, (2) aerobic and specific endurance, and (3) specific endurance (ergogenesis).

Aerobic Endurance

Aerobic (oxidative) endurance is developed throughout the transition phase and the early preparatory phase (1 to 3 months). Each sport requires slight alterations, as the aerobic endurance developed throughout during this phase can be aerobic capacity, aerobic power, or both, depending on the specific endurance to be developed at later stages. Aerobic capacity can be achieved via the use of a uniform and steady method with moderate intensities, whereas aerobic power can be achieved via moderate- to high-intensity interval training (see chapter 11). Individual sports that require medium or long endurance might start this phase by incorporating long, steady runs, followed by long, moderate-intensity intervals; for team sports, combat sports, racket sports, and individual sports that require only short endurance, it is appropriate to start with moderate-intensity, medium to short intervals and progress to high-intensity, short intervals at later stages. The aerobic power developed in this phase is useful for power sports, as it allows the athlete to resynthesize phosphocreatine more rapidly between bouts of anaerobic efforts (45).

The development of aerobic endurance provides the following benefits (21, 44):

Enhanced Cardiorespiratory Function

- Increased **capillarization**, which allows for an increase in oxygen and nutrient delivery
- Increased hemoglobin concentration, red blood cell number, and blood volume
- Decreased submaximal heart rate and resting blood pressure
- Increased maximal aerobic power ($\dot{V}O_2$max)
- Increased cardiac output
- Increased stroke volume
- Increased blood flow to working muscles
- Increased oxygen exchange at the lungs
- Decreased submaximal respiratory rate

Enhanced Musculoskeletal System Function
- Increased type I fiber content
- Increased oxidative **enzyme** capacity
- Increased mitochondrial density and size
- Increased myoglobin concentration
- Increased muscular endurance capacity

These adaptations improve endurance capacity as a result of more efficient use of fuel substrates (carbohydrate and fat). The adaptations are stimulated in response to the workload, especially the training volume.

Aerobic and Specific Endurance

Aerobic endurance and specific endurance are components of the endurance capacity of the athlete. After building an endurance base to maximize the development of specific endurance, training plans should introduce endurance elements that target the dominant energy systems used in the sport (see table 1.2). Endurance is developed in this phase of training through the use of uniform, alternative, and interval training (short, medium, and long duration). During the early part of this phase, the emphasis is on aerobic endurance; in the later portion of this phase, the emphasis shifts to the development of specific endurance with the use of high-intensity interval training or sport-specific, interval-based training methods (16). The shift to specific endurance development allows for a transfer of training effects, which enhances performance gains during the competitive phase of the annual training plan.

Specific Endurance Training

The development of event- or sport-specific endurance training coincides with the late preparatory and competitive phases of the annual training plan. The sport-specific activity is the preferred training mean during this phase. The appropriate training parameters depend on the bioenergetic characteristics of the sport and the needs of the individual athlete. For many sports, the coach must emphasize training intensity so that it often exceeds competition or game intensity. One tool, which may be useful for team sports like soccer, is the use of small-sided games and a soccer-specific "dribbling track" (figure 5.14) that can be used to couple tactical and conditioning activities in one training session (16). For combat sports, sparring can be performed alternating "under time" days, during which the regular duration of rounds is fractioned, with short intra-round rest intervals, and long inter-rounds rest intervals; this allows for a higher mean power output and overtime days, during which the duration of rounds is longer than the duration used in official competitions. Both undertime and overtime session parameters can be progressed over time to match the specific requirements of the event. Of course, not all sessions should be high intensity and sport-specific; alternating intensities facilitates recovery between training sessions, leading to lower fatigue levels and an optimal peak for competitions.

Integrated Periodization

An athlete is a complex being who requires not only physical, technical, and tactical training, but also an integrated periodization, in which psychological training and nutrition plans are integrated with other activities.

To maximize the coach's ability to construct and deliver appropriately designed training plans, an interdisciplinary team of experts may be needed, including sport scientists, sport psychologists, nutritionists, biomechanics, and sports medicine professionals. Given the rapidly evolving nature of sport science, the team approach may be necessary to most effec-

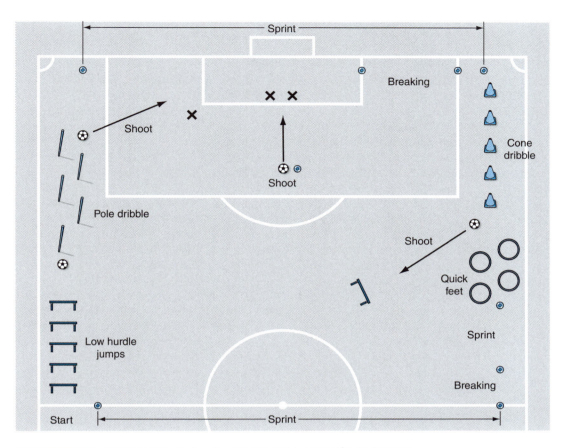

FIGURE 5.14 Dribbling track for developing soccer-specific endurance.

The dribble track requires the athlete to dribble a ball around the course. The athlete should gradually increase intensity until achieving a heart rate between 90% and 95% of maximum and hold that heart rate for 4 min. After the 4 min time period is completed, the athlete performs 4 min of exercise at 70% of maximal heart rate. The circuit can be completed two to four times depending on the phase of the periodized training plan. Athletes must dribble around cones and sticks, jump over the hurdles, accelerate and break between discs, and shoot at pre-determined points.

tively interpret, develop, and integrate new training methods in the context of a periodized training plan.

The integration of all training components into a comprehensive annual training plan (10) requires the coach and sports enhancement team to evaluate the athlete and the training goals, which will allow them to appropriately sequence training factors. Depending on the phase of the periodization plan, the training emphasis will shift to develop specific characteristics and manage fatigue. A truly comprehensive plan includes dietary recommendations and psychological training. Sport psychologists and nutritionists work with athletes, analyzing their activities and proposing techniques and nutrition plans; without their feedback, high performance would be very difficult to achieve. The knowledge and enthusiasm of these sport scientists is present, but each professional tends to work in isolation from the others. The missing element in training is the close collaboration of athletes, coaches, and experts in nutrition and sport psychology.

The foundation of integrated periodization has to be the training program produced by the coach. Psychologists and nutritionists, therefore, have to analyze a coach's programs, discuss its difficulties, and propose solutions and techniques to assist the athletes in maximizing performance.

Figure 5.15 illustrates an example of integrated periodization for a speed and power sport, where periodization of nutrition and mental training are integrated according to the

Months	1	2	3	4	5	6	7	8	9	10	11	12
Training phases	Preparatory						Competitive					Transition
Subphases	Preparatory	Specific		Precompetitive		Official and league competitions					Unloading	Transition
Speed	Anaerobic and aerobic endurance	• Maximum speed • Anaerobic endurance		• Maximum speed • Specific speed • Agility • Reactive agility	• Sport-specific preparations • Specific speed • Agility • Reactive agility						Unloading	Play, fun
Strength	Anatomical adaptation	Maximal strength	Power	Maximal strength	Conversion of power		Maintenance of power or maximal strength					Compensation
Mental training	• Evaluate mental skills • Learn new mental skills • Practice relaxation	• Mental training • Visualization • Imagery • Relaxation • Energy management			• Mental rehearsal • Energizing • Positive self-talk • Visualization • Focus plans • Simulation • Coping		• Mental skills to cope with opponents • Stress management • Relaxation • Focus plans • Mental rehearsal • Motivation • Positive self-talk				• Mental skills to aid regeneration, relaxation, stress management • Positive self-talk • Visualization	• Active rest • De-stress
Nutrition	• High carbohydrate • Moderate protein	• High protein • Moderate carbohydrate	• High carbohydrate	• High carbohydrate • Moderate protein	• High carbohydrate • Moderate protein		Fluctuates according to the competitive schedule				High carbohydrate	Balanced diet

FIGURE 5.15 Integrated periodization plan for a speed and power sport.

athlete's plan. Since this is just a hypothetical example, the interested parties have to make the necessary changes and additions, so that their solutions will consider the training plan, athlete's level of development and training objectives of a given training phase. If the training plan is not completely integrated, the likelihood that the athlete will achieve successful results is significantly decreased.

Summary of Major Concepts

Periodization, or the division of an annual plan into smaller phases, along with the periodization of the biomotor abilities, are determinant elements of planning and programming the training process. Without these intrinsic elements of structuring the training program, peak performance might be a very questionable reality.

Essential to achieving training goals is the comprehension, skills, and knowledge of periodization of biomotor abilities. A peak performance will never be realized if the athlete or the team are not at the highest standards of physical development. The higher the physical attributes, the easier it will be for the athlete to achieve high performance.

Planning the Training Session 6

Workout planning has existed since the ancient Olympic Games. As mentioned in chapter 5, evidence for this can be found in several manuals on planning and training written by Flavius Philostratus (AD 170-245) for Greek Olympic athletes. Although most of his work has been destroyed, his surviving manuals, the *Handbook for the Athletic Coach* and *Gymnasticus*, teach the reader how to train for competition and the importance of recovery. He suggests that the coach "should be a psychiatrist with considerable knowledge in anatomy and heritage." Even in ancient times, science was the foundation for the development of the training plan.

The earliest evidence of an organized training session plan is mentioned in *The Aeneid*, the great work of the Roman poet Virgil (Publius Vergilius Maro, 70-19 BC). In this poem, Virgil refers to the journey of Aeneas, a Trojan hero, who decided to emigrate to Italy after the destruction of Troy (about 1100 BC). During the trip Aeneas and his crew had to stop at several Mediterranean islands, where they were challenged by the locals to rowing races. Virgil described how Aeneas organized a training session in which the rowers did some exercises, which might be considered a warm-up, and then proceeded to row for a while. After they had completed the rowing portion of their training session, they lifted stones to improve their strength, and then concluded the training session with a bath and massage.

What is interesting about this passage is that the organization of the training session that Virgil describes is very similar to the composition of a modern training session. Even more interesting is that Aeneas integrated strength training into the training session, which in modern times is still a topic of debate. It is clear that training is an evolutionary process that spans back to ancient times and is in continual flux. This evolution continues as a result of the tireless work of sport scientists, who develop the scientific foundations of training, and the training theorists and coaches, who use this knowledge to continually improve the training process.

Importance of Planning

Planning is probably the most important tool a coach has. By using a methodical and scientifically based procedure, the coach can structure the training process in a way that will allow the athlete to optimize performance at appropriate times. The coach's ability to effectively guide the training process is dictated by her knowledge of the physiological responses of the body to training stimuli and her planning and programming skills.

The planning of training should be based on science and perfected through practice. The implementation of a well-organized and scientifically based training plan eliminates random and aimless training practices, which are sometimes still practiced by ill-informed coaches. A well-devised training plan removes poor training concepts or philosophies such as "intensity all the way" and "no pain, no gain" and replaces them with the principles of sport science and training methodology, resulting in practices that are logically devised and planned. The goal of the training plan is to stimulate specific physiological responses according to a planned design so that certain performance outcomes are achieved at the appropriate time. Nothing that occurs during training should happen by accident; responses should occur as a result of the design of the training plan. The old adage that "if you fail to plan, you plan to fail" is true of the training process.

Training consists of introducing a training stimulus, which causes a specific physiological response, and inducing recovery, which allows the athlete to adapt to the training stimulus (56). One might consider the training process as an adaptations management system in which intense periods of training, stimulating morphofunctional adaptations, are interspersed with periods of easier training or rest, designed to allow the athlete to recover and adapt. The coach must try to predict the athlete's physiological and psychological responses to the training stimuli and the fatigue induced by each stimulus; to put it another way, the coach must consider how much fatigue a certain training intervention may elicit, how the athlete will respond to that fatigue, and how that training stimulus adds to the training demand as a whole.

Central to this prediction is an understanding of the physiological responses to training and how different actions affect recovery and adaptation. This line of reasoning suggests that it may be best to consider the planning of training as a process in which the training stimulus is systematically and logically manipulated to optimize the physiological adaptations to training. This process should be undertaken in accordance with the demands of the targeted sport, with the express goal of maximizing performance outcomes.

The effectiveness of the training plan is largely dictated by the coach's expertise and experience. The coach must understand many factors related to exercise physiology and its relationship to training theory and methodology, as well as the practical aspects of an athlete's development. A coach should understand the physiological and psychological responses of the body and mind to training and exercise, the recovery process and techniques necessary to induce restoration, nutrition and its importance in training, and motor learning and its application to skill development. The greater the coach's knowledge base, the better prepared he will be to manage the training plan.

Because training is planned in accordance with the athlete's potential and rate of development, the training plan not only reflects the coach's knowledge base, but is adjusted according to the objective and subjective data collected by the coach during each training session (especially during testing days). To optimize an athlete's training plan, the coach must examine the athlete's test results, competitive results, progress in all training factors, and competition schedule. The training plan must evolve in accordance with the athlete's rate of progress and the coach's continually expanding knowledge.

Planning Requirements

To create an effective training plan, the coach must establish a long-term path of development that optimizes the athlete's potential. To help the athlete achieve long-term training goals, the coach must monitor the athlete during training, at competitions, and periodically with specialized tests that can be interpreted and used to adjust the training stimuli.

A coach must have a thorough knowledge of training theory and athlete development to successfully help an athlete reach her potential.

Develop a Long-Term Plan

Depending on the specifics of the sport, it can take 8 to 14 years of dedicated training to maximize an athlete's competitive performance. A long-term training plan is an essential component of the training process because it guides the athlete's development over many years of athletic activities. A major goal of long-term planning is to facilitate the progressive and continual development of the athlete's motor potential, skills, and performance. To accomplish this goal, the coach must consider the athlete's rate of improvement and the athlete's potential to achieve training and performance goals. The long-term training plan is at best a prognostication; the ultimate success of the plan depends on the coach's ability to forecast future developments and implement appropriate training objectives at the correct times.

Central to the athlete's sporting success is the ability of the coach to design and implement **annual training plans** that can be extracted from a long-term training structure (9).

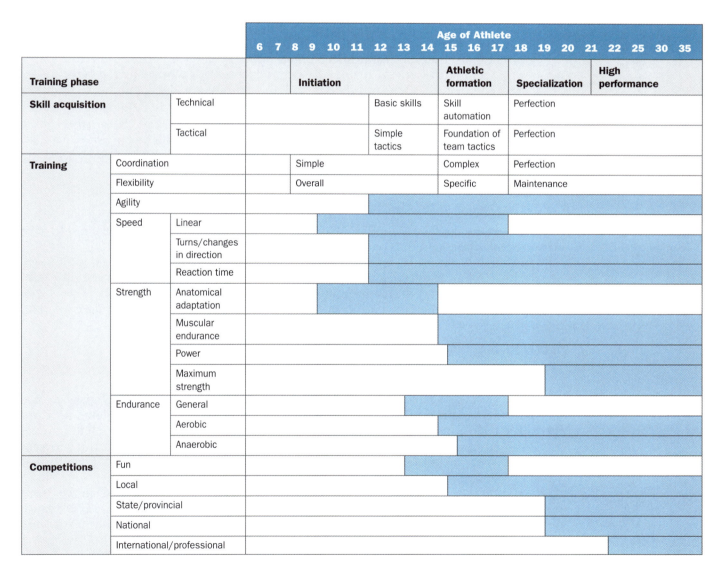

FIGURE 6.1 Long-term training model for volleyball.

Note: Shaded area shows the ages to start or end work on that ability.

Reprinted, by permission, from T.O. Bompa and M. Carrera, 2015, *Conditioning young athletes* (Champaign, IL: Human Kinetics), 260.

A specific guide of training for a long-term training plan should start from early years of athletic involvement through all of the stages illustrated in figure 6.1 (Initiation, Athletic Formation, Specialization, and High Performance).

Figure 6.1 exemplifies a hypothetical, long-term training plan for volleyball. The top of the chart lists the duration of the plan (here, from ages 8 to 35). The chart then lists the four phases of training: initiation (8 to 15 years), athletic formation (15 to 18 years), specialization (18 to 21 years) and high performance (21 to 35 years). Following is a brief analysis of each phase:

- *Initiation:* The main scope of training for the Initiation phase is skill acquisition. Since technical skill is the factor that limits performance for young athletes, and prevents the young athlete from progressing and enjoying a sporting activity, the main objective of the Initiation phase is to learn both technical and tactical skills.
- *Athletic formation:* After the first few years of primarily transforming a beginner into a player (ages 15 to 18, and sometimes 1 to 2 years earlier), the coach should try to transform a player into an athlete. Following the end of this phase, performance is affected by refinement of technical and tactical skills and the ability to improve sport-specific physical attributes. Transforming a player into a top athlete (strong, powerful, faster, more agile and reactive) capable of playing effectively for a longer period of time (specific endurance) is accomplished by utilizing training methods and means that start as multilateral and gradually increase in specificity throughout the phase.
- *Specialization.* Specialization could be considered the road to High Performance, or the stage of refining the position-specific technical and tactical skills and physical qualities.
- *High performance.* During Specialization and High Performance, the limiting factors for performance are technical and tactical excellence, maximum strength, power, and agility (reaction) time. The more effective the coach's training methodology, the higher the chances of the athletes reaching objectives of high performance.

Following the High Performance phase, the determinant scope of training is not to have six volleyball players on the court, but to have six athletes playing volleyball!

Note that the suggested long-term plan in figure 6.1 refers to all elements of training: skill acquisition (technical and tactical), training (coordination, flexibility, agility, speed, strength, and endurance training), and the progression of competition. Take a close look at every type of training and the progression proposed for the duration of the suggested long-term plan.

Integrate Periodic Testing and Monitoring Programs

An often-overlooked but highly important part of the long-term plan is a comprehensive monitoring program in which periodic testing is conducted to track the athlete's development. The inclusion of a monitoring program eliminates the random approach to training that is sometimes present in modern athlete development. An inclusive monitoring program allows the coach to examine the effects of the training program and quantify factors that scientific literature has shown to be related to performance.

The testing program should be completely integrated into the training plan, contain tests that target the athlete's development, and focus on the athlete's objectives (i.e., performance outcomes). The testing battery for any sport should include tests that reveal the athlete's progress toward her performance goals. Monitoring should occur continuously and at periodic intervals throughout the training year. For example, testing should be conducted at the beginning of each new training phase; on the other hand, certain factors (e.g., resting heart rate, heart rate variability, mood status, sleep patterns, and force capability measured with a hand-grip dynamometer or accelerometer) should be monitored daily as they can yield information about the athlete's recovery status and readiness for the planned training stimuli. An often-overlooked tool that can shed substantial light on the athlete's progress is the **training log**. The training log is a very simple tool to track daily responses to training stimuli; it yields a large amount of information, which can give the coach great insight into the athlete's response to the training plan. The analysis of daily training logs, coupled with data collected from specialized tests and performance results, will allow the coach to help the athlete maximize her performance gains.

Establish and Emphasize the Main Training Factor

When establishing the training plan, the coach must carefully examine the results of the monitoring program to determine the athlete's weaknesses. Performance results and test data will reveal which training factors have not improved or have deteriorated as a result of the training plan. Training factors that fall behind the athlete's mean development rate are the weakest links in training and must be addressed via a redistribution of training efforts. The coach and athlete must determine the underlying reason for a lack of development. For example, in gymnastics, technical improvement depends on strength development. Thus, if a gymnast is not strong enough to perform a technical skill, the coach should increase training activities designed to improve muscular strength. Once the athlete's areas of weakness are determined, the training program should be designed to target training factors that address the athlete's weaknesses. This change in program focus must be implemented in conjunction with adjustments in volume and intensity of training dictated by the training plan.

Types of Training Plans

The coach's ability to organize and use appropriate planning tools will dictate the success of the training programs. Many planning tools are available, including the individual training session, microcycle, macrocycle, annual training plan, and long-term training plan. Long-term plans (4 to 8 years) are essential for the multi-year development of young athletes and Olympic athletes.

The terms used to describe the planning of training are not consistent throughout the world. For example, Russian (Matveyev, 36-38; Zatsiorsky, 63-64) and many American authors refer to the annual plan as the macrocycle. Tudor Bompa, on the other hand, out of respect for the work of Philostratus, Galen, and the German specialists of the early 1930s (chapter 5), uses the term **annual training plan**.

Annual plans are used as guides or training projections for the year to come. Especially in individual sports and for youth athletes, they are constructed in the context of the long-term training goals and plans established by the coach. The annual plan is divided into smaller phases, described by Russian scientists as mesocycles (Matveyev, 38). Bompa describes the phases as grosse or macrocycles, terminology employed by the Germans in their preparation for the 1936 Olympic Games. The macrocycle content (training direction) is based on the phase of the annual plan and is designed in concert with the development of the **microcycle** (small cycle, or kleine in German), which is the most important functional tool for planning. The fluctuation of the load within the macrocycle determines its structure. The microcycle is a short training cycle that can range from 3 to 7 days depending on the phase of training. Finally, an equally functional type of plan for a coach is the daily training session, where all the athletic activities are programmed.

Training Session

During an individual training session or lesson, the coach explains the scope and methods used in the daily program and then attempts to apply them in training. The training session can be classified in several different fashions depending on the tasks and structure of the session.

Training Sessions Classified by Task

The training session can be classified based on the tasks within the session. There are four basic classifications of training sessions: learning, repetition, skill perfection, and assessment.

Learning Session

The athlete's main task in a learning session is to acquire new skills or tactical maneuvers. The coach uses a basic structure to organize this type of session. For example, the coach begins the session by explaining the objectives of the session and then directing the athlete through a warm-up. After the warm-up, the athlete focuses on acquiring a specific skill set. After completing the main portion of the session, the athlete cools down, and the coach gives the athlete pertinent feedback regarding his progress toward developing the skill. It is very important that the athlete is fully recovered from previous training sessions when learning new skills or tactical maneuvers because any residual fatigue could impair cognitive functions and learning.

Repetition Session

A repetition session is very similar to a learning session, in that a specific skill set or tactical maneuver is practiced. The major difference is that during the repetition session, the athlete continues to learn the skill and attempts to improve the skill set.

Skill Perfection Session

The skill perfection session is an extension of the repetition session, in that the athlete attempts to improve the overall skill set. The major difference is that, at this point, the skill has been learned and the athlete now attempts to perfect the skill to maximize performance.

Assessment Session

Assessment sessions should be conducted periodically. These sessions can include tests that evaluate the athlete's physiological responses to training and performance, or the sessions can include exhibition or practice competitions to gauge the athlete's preparedness. The results of these sessions can be used to fine-tune an athlete's training or as a tool for selecting athletes for competitions.

Training Sessions Classified by Structure

The coach may organize training sessions in several forms to accommodate individuals and groups of athletes.

- *Group sessions:* The group session is organized for several athletes, although not necessarily an entire team. For example, the coach may work with the offensive linemen from an American-style football team or a group of athletes who compete in an individual sport. Although group sessions are not optimal for the individualization of training, they can be an effective tool for developing team spirit (especially before an important competition) and psychological qualities.
- *Individual sessions:* Individual sessions allow the coach to focus attention on one athlete to address physical or psychological problems. This session provides the coach the opportunity to precisely evaluate the individual athlete and adjust her skill development. These sessions are most appropriate during the preparatory phase of the annual plan. Other types of sessions may be more appropriate during the competitive phase.
- *Mixed sessions:* A mixed session is a combination of group and individual sessions. In this type of session, the whole team may warm up together and then divide into individualized training sessions. After completing the individualized portion of the training session, the athletes come back together to either practice as a team or cool

down together. During the cool-down, the coach discusses pertinent issues to reinforce certain aspects of the training session.

- *Free sessions:* Free sessions minimize a coach's control over the athlete's training and can promote trust and confidence between the athlete and coach. This type of session develops the athlete's conscientious participation in training, stimulates his independence, and may increase his level of maturity. Free sessions can help the athlete develop problem-solving skills that can translate to the competitive arena, where the coach may not always be available. Although this type of session can greatly benefit the athlete, it should be used mostly with advanced and elite athletes; less developed athletes may not possess the physical and psychological skills to handle such a session.

Sessions generally last approximately 2 h, although they can be prolonged up to over 3 h, depending on the sport and the phase of the annual training plan. Of course, there is an inverted relationship between intensity and duration. Training sessions for team sports are usually consistent in duration, whereas training sessions for individual sports tend to vary in duration. Training sessions fall into three categories of duration: (a) short sessions, which last between 30 and 60 min;

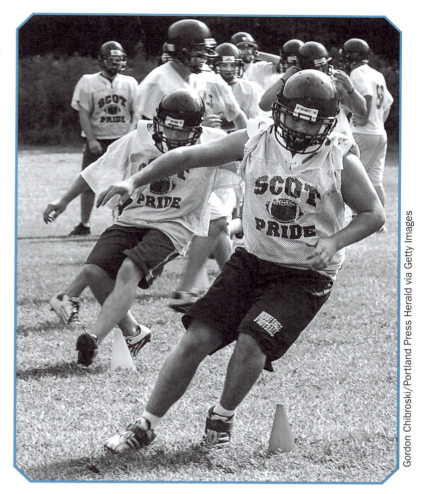

Incorporating different types of training sessions in a training plan can foster team unity as well as individual growth.

(b) medium sessions, which last 90 min to 2 h; and (c) long sessions, which last longer than 2 h. The duration of the training session depends on the tasks that are required during the session, the activities being performed, and the athlete's physical potential. A sprinter may perform a training session that lasts only 1 to 1.5 h during the competitive phase, whereas a marathon runner may undertake a session that lasts 2 to 2.5 h. Training can also be broken into smaller subunits throughout the training day. When a training session is broken into smaller subunits, the total time spent training may be slightly longer, about 2 to 2.5 h. Integral to the length of the training session are the number of repetitions being performed and the rest intervals between repetitions and sets.

Structure of Training Sessions

A training session consists of several parts that are sequenced in a way that allows the coach and athlete to follow the principle of a progressive increase and decrease in work across the training session. The training session consists of three or four main structural components. A three-part training session contains a warm-up (preparation), a workout, and a cool-down (conclusion); a four-part training session consists of an introduction, a warm-up, a workout, and a cool-down.

The selection of which structure to use in a training session depends on the training task and content, the phase of training, and the athlete's training level. The four-part structure is used during the preparatory phase of training for most athletes, especially beginners or novice athletes. Advanced athletes generally use the three-part model, especially during the competitive period of the annual training plan, because these athletes require less explanation and motivation and prefer to dedicate more time to the main body of the training session. The only substantial difference between the two structures is the inclusion of an introduction.

Introduction

The introduction of a training session is initiated by gathering the athletes into a group to facilitate communication. Several managerial tasks can be undertaken during this time, such as taking attendance (especially in team sports), relaying any information that is pertinent to the athletes' training or competitive schedules, and explaining the objectives of the training session. When discussing training objectives, the coach should explain the methods that will be used to accomplish these objectives. At this time the coach must attempt to increase the athletes' motivation and focus on the day's training tasks. After the general objectives are explained, the group should be broken into smaller subgroups according to individual or position-based goals.

The length of the introduction depends on the extent of the explanation and the level of the athlete. Beginner and novice athletes will require a 5 to 10 min introduction; as the athletes become more developed the length of the introduction can be reduced.

The coach must always be prepared and organized when explaining the training objectives. Some coaches find it useful to use audiovisual aids or handouts explaining parts of the session. Handouts may cover specific goals or objectives that need to be highlighted in the session and may be considered an expansion of the overall training plan. Athletes should receive the training program well in advance of the training session so they can familiarize themselves with and mentally prepare for the session. If this is done, the coach will only need to emphasize the important parts of the training session. The training program should also be posted so that athletes can easily refer to it prior to and during the training session. Allowing the athletes to become familiar with the organization of the training session gives them a sense of shared responsibility and increases the likelihood that they will give a focused effort during training. It is also likely that this process will allow the athletes to develop dependability and willpower.

Warm-Up

It is widely accepted by athletes and coaches that a warm-up is essential for optimal performance during either training or competition. The contemporary scientific literature supports this contention and suggests that the composition of the warm-up can affect the degree of performance improvement (4, 5, 33, 51, 60). It is well documented that an appropriate warm-up will improve muscle function and prepare the athlete for the demands of exercise or competition (60).

Types of Warm-Up Warm-ups can be broadly classified as either passive or active (4, 5, 60). A passive warm-up uses external means (e.g., saunas, hot showers, hot baths, heating pads, or diathermy) to elevate the muscle and core temperature without depleting energy substrates (4, 5). An active warm-up uses some form of physical activity to elevate muscle and core temperature (52, 60). The active warm-up can be further divided into general and specific components. General warm-up procedures include activities such as jogging, calisthenics, or cycling, whereas the specific warm-up component uses activities specific to the sport. For most athletes it is impractical to use passive warm-up procedures; therefore, athletes who are preparing for training or competition typically use active warm-ups.

Structure of a Warm-Up The composition of a warm-up depends on factors such as the activity being prepared for, the athlete's physical capacity, the environmental conditions, and the restrictions of the sporting activity. During the general warm-up, the athlete should participate in activities that will elevate muscle and core temperature, such as light jogging, calisthenics, or cycling. For most athletes the general warm-up should be performed at low intensity (40%-60% of $\dot{V}O_2max$) and for 5 to 10 min (4, 5). A low intensity is recommended because this level of activity will increase temperature while limiting the reduction in phosphate degradation (4, 5). Additionally, temperature begins to elevate within 3 to 5 min of the initiation of the warm-up and plateaus at about 10 to 20 min (52). The coach may need to tailor the warm-up to the individual athlete, because poorly conditioned athletes can achieve the same degree of temperature elevation with less warm-up time. Conversely, highly trained athletes may need to increase the duration and intensity of the warm-up to achieve the appropriate elevation of temperature (60). A good guide to determine whether the athlete is adequately warmed up is the presence of perspiration.

After completing the general warm-up, the athlete should shift to a specific warm-up. A specific warm-up is designed to prepare the athlete for a certain activity. The warm-up features progressively increasing intensities and may involve **postactivation potentiation** activities in some instances. For example, the inclusion of short, intense sprint activities has been shown to improve running and kayak performance (4, 5), provided sufficient recovery time is available between the cessation of the warm-up and the competition or training bout. It appears that at least 5 min of recovery is necessary when transitioning from the warm-up to training or competition (4, 5).

The specific warm-up is important when preparing for competition because it includes specific skill sets. For example, a gymnast may include certain technical elements in the warm-up in order to prepare physically and mentally for the competition. It has been recommended that an athlete spend 10 to 15 min undergoing specific activities during the warm-up period (29). However, as the complexity of the sport increases, the athlete may need to spend more time on the specific warm-up. An example of a warm-up that contains all of these elements is presented in table 6.1.

The total warm-up should take between 20 and 50 min and include a general warm-up designed to increase body temperature and a specific warm-up designed to prepare the athlete for his chosen sporting activity. The duration of the warm-up can be increased or

TABLE 6.1 Warm-Up Protocol for a Power Athlete

Type of warm-up	Activities contained in warm-up	Duration (min)
General	Jogging	5
	Static stretching (if external temperature allows)	5-10
Dynamic stretches/ movement assessment/ technical components	Glutei activation exercises	2.5
	A skipping → lateral walking → B skipping → lateral cross-over walking → back skipping → backward lunging → rear kicking → straight-knee running → carioca → backward running 2 × 20m, walk back recovery	10
	Ballistic leg stretches 2 × 20 per leg (frontal and sagittal)	2.5
Specific	Easy alternate bounding	5
	Jumps over medium height hurdles	5
	Short accelerations	5
Transition to competition or training	Passive recovery	5
Total warm-up time		45-50

decreased depending on the needs of the particular athlete. An athlete who participates in high-intensity activities such as sprinting may require up to 45 min to effectively warm up, although most of the activities will be interspersed with adequate rest intervals. Conversely, an endurance athlete will have a shorter, yet denser warm-up because her metabolic systems are highly trained and her neuromuscular system does not need to be prepared for high-intensity activities. An athlete who is in poor shape will probably have to decrease the duration of the warm-up or use a lower frequency (longer rest intervals). An interesting application of the warm-up is to use longer warm-ups as conditioning tools during the preparatory phase of training.

Physiological Effects   A wide variety of physiological factors are altered by an active warm-up. The primary improvement associated with a warm-up is the elevation of muscle and core temperature (4, 5, 60). Some authors claim that the elevation in temperature likely increases the nerve conduction rate and speed metabolic reactions, which can then increase the speed and force of muscle contractions (4, 5, 60). Additionally, as temperature elevates, the amount of oxygen that is delivered to the muscle increases (2) as a result of increased vasodilation and blood flow (60). The release of oxygen from both **hemoglobin (Hb)** and **myoglobin** increases as well, thus increasing oxygen delivery to the working muscle (3, 4, 5).

Although most of the effects of a warm-up are related to increases in temperature, other factors have been suggested to be major contributors to performance improvement. Of particular interest is a postactivation potentiating effect created by the warm-up protocol (40, 55, 61). Postactivation potentiation has been defined as the increased contractile ability of a muscle after a contraction (40). Potentiation effects are most likely related to phosphorylation of myosin regulatory chains (22, 28) or an elevation of calcium (Ca^{2+}) in the cytosol (1). The effects of postactivation potentiation appear to be most prevalent in strength and power performance (55, 61), and some investigators have found that these effects are limited to highly trained athletes (12).

Psychological Effects   Another warm-up–induced response involves the athlete's psychological state (4, 5). Investigators reported a lack of performance improvements when athletes were hypnotized to forget they had gone through a warm-up (35). Other investigators have shown that athletes who used mental imagery as a warm-up tool demonstrated enhanced physiological performance characteristics (34). It appears that the warm-up prepares the athlete not only physiologically but also psychologically.

Possible Effects of an Active Warm-Up

- Increased resistance of muscle and joints
- Increased release of oxygen from hemoglobin and myoglobin
- Increased rate of metabolic reactions
- Increased nerve conduction rate
- Increased thermoregulatory strain
- Increased vasodilation and blood flow to the muscle
- Decreased internal viscosity
- Increased speed and force of muscle contractions
- Increased baseline oxygen consumption
- Increased preparedness for competition or training

Injury It has been well documented that an appropriate warm-up will reduce rates of injury (60). It is likely that the increased temperature that occurs during a warm-up reduces the potential for injury. Support for this contention can be seen in animal studies demonstrating that a 1 °C (33.8 °F) increase in temperature reduces the occurrence of skeletal muscle injury.

Stretching Contemporary scientific literature has demonstrated that dynamic stretching is superior to static stretching during the warm-up period (53, 58). Performance decrements associated with static stretching are most noted in strength and power sports, but static stretching decreases performance in all activities (53). The force production inhibitory effect of static stretching can be avoided if it is placed at the end of the general component of the warm-up. The progressively increasing intensity of the following exercises will dissipate the inhibition. Such structure has been used successfully for years by the world's best sprinting groups. To this end, the warm-up should include dynamic stretching activities that involve sport-specific movements, whereas attempts to increase flexibility should be reserved for the cool-down.

Glutei Activation Exercises The gluteus maximus, a powerful monoarticular muscle, is the primary hip extensor that operates in conjunction with the semimembranosus muscle, the semitendinosus muscle, and long head of the biceps femoris, as synergistic movers. As stated by Stuart McGill (42), world-renowned expert in spine biomechanics, an increasing number of people suffer from what he called "gluteal amnesia," which can be found in several populations of athletes (differentiated by geographical region and sport). This dysfunction can be defined as the inability to engage the glutei in the extension of the hip, thus transferring a higher workload to the hamstrings and low back. This could be one of the main reasons for the high incidence of hamstring injuries in sporting activities, especially in the presence of high eccentric loads.

For this reason, we suggest the implementation of glutei activation exercises within the warm-up, possibly before the athletic drills, in the form of a straight-knee supine march, one or two leg bridges, and quadruped hip extensions with bent knee.

Athletic Drills A variety of athletic drills should be considered and used as dynamic stretches, technical refinement drills, and movement assessment tools. This includes skipping (As, Bs); shuffling; lateral walking, crossover, and backward walks; backpedaling; rear kicks; straight-knee runs; and cariocas. The use of these drills as movement assessment tools is often overlooked by coaches who rely on static exercises for testing batteries, which are implemented every few months in order to assess posture and balance of athletes. The athletes then perform dynamically, with coaches assessing movement quality at every training session via athletic drills, speed training, or technical-tactical training.

Main Body of the Session

Specific training objectives are addressed in the main body of the training session. This is when the athlete learns new skills and tactical maneuvers, develops specific biomotor abilities, and enhances psychological qualities.

The content of this part of the training session depends on many factors including the athlete's training status, gender, and age; the sporting activity; and the phase of training. The main body of the training session may stress technique while simultaneously focusing on biomotor abilities and psychological traits. For less advanced athletes, the following succession is a general recommendation:

1. Learn and perfect a technical or tactical element.
2. Develop speed and agility.
3. Develop strength.
4. Develop endurance.

The athlete should be well rested when learning new skills, and technical and tactical elements should be addressed early in the main body of the training session. This is particularly important because fatigue will impede the athlete's ability to master motor skills (46). When the athlete is attempting to sequence learning or perfect technical and tactical elements, she should consolidate elements or skills acquired in previous lessons. She should work on perfecting the most important technical elements or skills and then conclude by applying those skills in simulated competitions.

If perfecting a technique requires heavy, fatiguing work, the athlete should perform these activities later in the main body of the training session. It is advisable to precede these activities with speed exercises. This approach may be appropriate for weightlifters or track and field athletes.

Activities that are designed to improve speed and agility are usually of a high intensity and are undertaken for relatively short durations. These types of exercise are extremely taxing, and the athlete should perform them when well rested. For this reason, these activities usually are performed in the early part of the session (when the athlete is still fresh) and precede both strength and endurance training. However, the focus of the training session will change the relative order of activities. For example, if speed development is the primary focus of the session, then speed-based exercises should immediately follow the warm-up. If coordination or agility is the major focus, it should be addressed early in the training session because fatigue can significantly affect motor skills (46).

Strength-developing exercises usually are placed after technique development and speed exercises. Although this is appropriate for most athletes, it may not be advisable in some cases. For example, several studies suggest that performing a heavy-load strength exercise (70%-90% of one-repetition maximum) prior to sprint activities results in a postactivation potentiation response that manifests itself as an increase in running velocity (40, 61). This technique appears to be very effective at increasing sprint performance if the volume of the strength activity is low. This method of sequencing strength training only appears to be effective with highly trained athletes (12).

Exercises for developing general or specific endurance should be placed in the last portion of the main body of the training session. These activities generate large amounts of fatigue, which will impede the athlete's ability to acquire or perfect movement or tactical skills, develop speed and agility, and maximize strength development. This sequencing should not be confused with the strategy of practicing certain drills under fatigue to prepare the athlete for a specific game scenario.

If learning (which requires a high level of concentration) is the dominant objective for beginning athletes, the training sequence should be technique, speed, strength, and endurance. However, a single training session should rarely include all four of these elements. This same general sequence for training can be used with elite athletes; however, advanced athletes may benefit from altering the order of training depending on the objectives of the individual training session and the objectives of the microcycle.

The structure of the main body of training will be dictated by the objectives established for the individual training session. Each training session should focus on only two or three objectives, because it is very difficult to effectively target more than three training objectives. Trying to target too many objectives will likely impair the athlete's rate of improvement and may result in the occurrence of overtraining. The individual training session objectives should be linked to the microcycle and macrocycle objectives, the athlete's performance level, and the athlete's potential. Although it may be advisable to plan objectives derived from different training factors (e.g., technical, tactical, physical, or psychological), these factors should be chosen based on the needs of the sport and the abilities of the athlete.

The coach can plan 15 to 20 min of supplementary physical development, or what is sometimes referred to as a conditioning program, to take place after the athlete has achieved the objectives of a given training session. This addition should be considered for less demanding training sessions that do not challenge the athlete. This supplementary development should be specific to the dominant biomotor abilities of the sport and should address factors that are limiting the athlete's rate of improvement.

Cool-Down

After the conclusion of the main portion of the training session, the athlete should undergo a cool-down period. The cool-down begins the recovery process and facilitates the body's return to homeostasis. The postexercise recovery period is a time when the body must remove waste products, replenish energy stores, and initiate tissue repair (30). The body usually does not return to a resting state immediately after a training bout or competition. Depending on the intensity and volume of the session, recovery can require up to 48 h (32, 41). To initiate and speed up the posttraining or postcompetition recovery, the athlete needs to undergo a structured cool-down session that is designed to stimulate recovery. This portion of the training session is often overlooked, but when implemented correctly it is a very valuable tool for maximizing the recovery from and adaptation to a session.

The cool-down should last for 20 to 40 min and consist of two major parts: The first part entails active recovery exercise and lasts for 10 to 20 min. This active recovery exercise should be of a low intensity (<50% of the athlete's maximum heart rate). Although limited data are available in the scientific literature, it appears that active recovery is much more effective in inducing postexercise recovery than is passive recovery (7, 44, 45). The activities included in the active recovery will depend on the athlete's sport. A cyclist may use a continuous bout of very low-intensity cycling for 20 min as the active exercise portion of the cool-down, whereas a soccer player might use very light jogging. A shot putter may use an interval series that contains low-intensity and short-duration jogging after a training session. Regardless of the sport, this portion of the cool-down should be low intensity and should not overly tax the athlete.

The second part of the cool-down should contain 10 to 20 min of stretching. Although static stretching is not usually recommended during the warm-up, the cool-down is an excellent

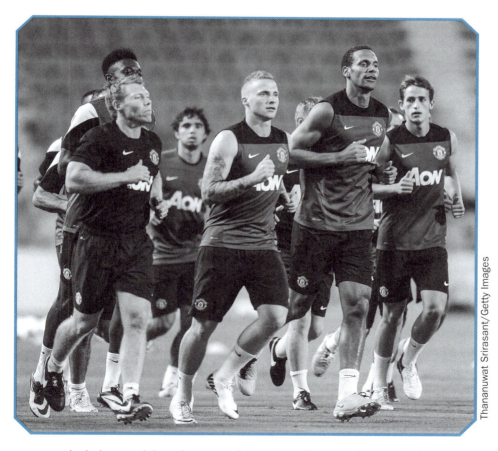

Include a cool-down in your training plans. The cool-down period is an important part of a training workout.

time for this activity (29). There are several reasons to include stretching in the postexercise period. First, stretching brings the muscles back to their anatomical length progressively, facilitates metabolic exchanges, and speeds up recovery processes. Furthermore, stretching can improve flexibility without compromising performance. It appears that the stretching portion of a cool-down can improve range of motion (flexibility) as a result of increased muscle temperature (29). Second, the inclusion of a postexercise stretching protocol has been demonstrated to reduce the onset of muscle soreness that can be stimulated by a training session (11). Third, it has been reported that the combination of active recovery followed by a period of stretching significantly increases the rate of recovery from training and competitive stress (50).

While the athletes are stretching during the cool-down, the coach can ask them whether they achieved the training session's objectives and how they felt about the session; the coach also can use this time to further the athletes' understanding of training.

Duration of Each Part of the Session

The length of a training session depends on many factors, but sessions usually last about 2 h (table 6.2). The duration of each component of the session will depend on the type of session; the athlete's age, gender, stage of development, and athletic experience; the characteristics of the sport; and the phase of training in which the session occurs. For example, a novice athlete may not have the fitness to tolerate a training session for 2 h, and so the session will be modified to accommodate the athlete's training status. The coach can use either the three- or four-component structure discussed previously to modulate the time commitment to each element of the training session. Examples of the three- and four-component models are provided in table 6.2.

TABLE 6.2 Average Durations for Each Part of a Two-Hour Training Session

Training session parts	Four-part training session	Three-part training session
Introduction	5 min	—
Preparation	30 min	30 min
Main body	65 min	70 min
Conclusion	20 min	20 min
Total time	120 min	120 min

Fatigue and Methodological Guidelines for Sessions

From a holistic perspective, fatigue is a multifactorial response to some sort of exercise, training, or competitive stress (30). Conceptually fatigue is defined as an acute impairment in exercise performance, which ultimately can impair the ability to produce maximal force or control motor function (30, 54). Fatigue can occur in response to an exercise bout or competition when one or more of the following situations arise: a reduction in energy substrate availability, an accumulation of metabolic by-products, neuromuscular transmission failure, impairments in Ca^{2+} handling by the sarcoplasmic reticulum, central disruption, and a response to conscious perception (18, 47). Although there are numerous potential causes of fatigue, the two broad categories of peripheral and central fatigue are often discussed.

Peripheral fatigue has received the most attention in the scientific literature and generally is related to factors in the muscles themselves (18, 19). These factors can include impairments in neuromuscular transmission (including beta-2 adrenergic receptors down-regulation (20), impulse propagation, sarcoplasmic reticulum failure, substrate depletion, and various other metabolic factors that can disrupt energy production and muscular contraction (16). Research exploring peripheral fatigue has centered on the availability of fuel substrates during a bout of exercise or competition (13). When exercise bouts are intense or undertaken for long durations, the availability of fuel substrates such as carbohydrates can become compromised. This can substantially reduce the athlete's ability to maintain high levels of performance (26).

The second type of fatigue that is discussed in the literature, central fatigue, is related to the brain (16). Central fatigue is often associated with a failure of the central nervous system to recruit skeletal muscle (47). It appears that fatigue-induced alterations in neurotransmitters such as dopamine, serotonin, and possibly acetylcholine have the potential to alter the ability of neural impulses to reach the muscle (15, 47). For example, it has been suggested that exercise-induced increases in serotonin (5-HT) can lead to central fatigue and possibly mental fatigue, which could impair performance (14). Along these lines, it appears that the conscious perception of body functions such as breathing, increased cardiac output (pounding of the heart), body temperature, and sweating can affect fatigue. These cognitive sensations also are believed to affect motivation, which appears to be linked to previous exposure to similar situations (54).

It is clear that both central and peripheral fatigue can accumulate in response to a training or competitive bout. Gandelsman and Smirnov (21) suggested there are two major phases of fatigue: latent and evident. In the early portions of a competition or training bout, physiological changes occur in order to meet the demands of the exercise bout. During this phase, latent fatigue can result, in response to the increased neuromuscular activity and metabolic stress stimulated by the bout of exercise. If the exercise bout is prolonged at the same intensity, fatigue will accumulate, resulting in the occurrence of evident fatigue. Consequently, the athlete's ability to maintain maximal work capacity will progressively decrease.

Many strategies can be used to deal with fatigue, ranging from modifying the structure of the training session to including dietary supplements to offset reductions in energy substrates (26). For example, increasing the length of the rest interval can decrease the occurrence of latent fatigue, which may facilitate the development of specific biomotor abilities such as power. Under some circumstances, training under conditions of latent fatigue can help prepare the athlete for the end of competitions, when fatigue is high. Such training also may enable the athlete to develop the psychological tools to deal with an accumulation of training-induced latent fatigue, which may improve her performance in the later stages of a competition (54). Strategies to deal with evident fatigue can include a structured cool-down period, as outlined previously in this chapter. Recovery techniques such as massage and contrast baths may alleviate this form of fatigue as well.

The intensity of the training session will affect the amount of fatigue that is developed, and the session should be structured to address this. A session that contains high-intensity activities should have only a few objectives and be of short duration. Conversely, a session containing lower-intensity bouts of exercise could have multiple training objectives and last longer. For example, the session may focus on perfecting a technical element, incorporating those elements into the team's tactical scheme, and doing tactical drills with a high endurance component. Even with this format, athletes can experience latent fatigue as a result of the metabolic disturbances stimulated by the volume of work.

The athlete's ability to dissipate fatigue and recover from a training session or microcycle of intense training depends on many factors. The athlete's physical preparedness and training age may dictate his ability to tolerate training. For example, an athlete who lacks the appropriate physical development will experience greater levels of fatigue, which may result in an inability to tolerate training stress. Therefore, the coach must modify the training lesson to accommodate this athlete's deficiencies. This process may require more variations in the training plan with greater fluctuations in training intensity and volume in an attempt to dissipate fatigue and stimulate restoration. In the end, the recovery rate is proportional to the degree of physiological disturbance stimulated by the training session. The greater the training intensity and volume (which constitute the training load), the greater the accumulated fatigue and the more time needed before readiness is elevated.

Supplementary Training Sessions

Most athletes want to maximize the time that they spend training while minimizing the occurrence of overtraining. One way to maximize training time and increase training volume is to use supplementary training sessions, which can consist of individual training sessions or special group sessions, such as training camps. These training sessions can be performed during the early morning, before school or work. Sometimes they are performed before breakfast, but it is probably advisable that the athlete consume a small amount of food before training, especially when the session lasts longer than 30 min (10). The time spent in these sessions depends on the athlete's schedule. Even though each session may be short in duration (30-60 min), over the course of the training year these small increases in training volume can result in a substantial increase in yearly training volume. For example, an athlete who trains an extra 30 to 60 min each day will accumulate an additional 150 to 300 training h per year, which could significantly improve her potential.

Although these sessions are considered supplemental, they must fit into the structure of the training plan designed by the coach. The coach will prescribe the content and dosage of these sessions in accordance with the athlete's objectives, weaknesses, and phase of training. These sessions, 20 to 40 min in duration, can be structured to improve the athlete's general endurance, general or specific flexibility, and even general or specific strength. One use for supplemental training sessions might be to improve an area of weakness to enhance certain abilities. For example, an athlete who lacks flexibility can undertake a supplemental training session that directly targets flexibility. Any resulting improvement in flexibility could transfer to improve a technical aspect that the athlete is attempting to perfect.

A supplemental training session lends itself best to a three-part structure (table 6.3). Because these training sessions may be undertaken independently of the coach, an introduction phase is not included. Therefore, these sessions contain the major components of a three-part training session: warm-up, main body, and cool-down. The goal and format of each session are no different than those of a regular training session. The main body of these sessions should have no more than two objectives; one objective is optimal.

TABLE 6.3 Three-Part Supplemental Training Session

Training session part	Duration (min)
Warm-up	5-10
Main body	20-40
Cool-down	5-10
Total session time	30-60

Sample Training Plan

The training plan is a tool utilized by the coach to structure and guide the training session. The written version of the training plan should contain all pertinent information and be easy to follow. It is advisable to give the athlete a copy of the training plan well in advance of the training session, allowing the athlete to prepare for the training session mentally and physically. The coach should briefly introduce the plan during the introduction portion of the session and, if space is available, post the day's training plan so that the athletes can refer to it during the session.

There are many formats by which the training plan can be presented, but it should contain some basic elements. One of the most important items to include in a training plan for an individual session is the objective of that session. The session's objective guides the training session, allowing the athlete to understand what happens during the training session. The plan should include the date and location of the training session as well as the equipment needed. The training plan should specify the exercise, drills, and activities that the athlete must complete during each portion of the session. The plan should provide a detailed explanation of the dosage (repetitions, sets, duration) and intensity (percentage maximum strength, heart rate range, time, and power) of the training session. Another item to include, especially when working with team sports, is a section detailing the most difficult drills an athlete can perform during the lesson. Finally, the training plan should note items that the athlete needs to focus on while performing the drills and exercises. These notes can be very specific to the individual athlete or address global needs of a group of athletes. A sample training session plan is presented in figure 6.2.

The length of a session plan will depend on the sport and the coach's experience. Inexperienced coaches need to be as specific as possible and include as much information as possible in the training plan. This provides a blueprint to work from during the training session and decreases the chance they will forget an important aspect of the training session. More experienced coaches may be able to get away with a more generalized training plan, but it may still be worthwhile to present a detailed plan to the athletes so they can prepare mentally and physically for the training session.

Training Lesson Plan 148
Date: June 14
Place: York Stadium
Equipment: Starting blocks
          Barbells

Coach: _____
Objectives: Perfect start
           Specific endurance
           Power training

Part	Exercises	Dosage	Formations	Notes
Introduction	1. Describe the lesson's objectives.	3 min		
	2. Stress what the athletes should focus on during training.			John: Pay attention to arm work.
Warm-up	1. Warm-up duration	20 min		Rita: Put on two warm-up suits.
	2. Jogging	1,200 m		
	3. Calisthenics	8×		
	Arm rotations	8×		
	Upper-body rotations	12×		
	4. Hip flexibility	8-10×		Stress hip flexibility.
	5. Ankle flexibility	8-10×		
	6. Bounding exercises	4 × 20 m		Stress weak leg.
	7. Wind sprints	4 × 40-60 m		
Main body	1. Starts	6 × 30 m Rest 1-2 min		Stress arm work.
	2. Specific endurance	3 × 120 m 3/4 (16 s)		Maintain a constant velocity throughout all repetitions.
	3. Power training	60 kg ——— 4 sets 8–10 reps		Between exercises, relax arms and legs.
Cool down	1. Jogging	800 m		Stay light and relaxed.
	2. Stretching	10-15 min		Focus on hip flexors.
	3. Massage	5-10 min		Work with partner.
Session notes	Remember that 8× = 8 times; 8-10× = 8-10 times			

FIGURE 6.2 Training session plan for a sprinter.

Daily Cycle of Training

An important aspect of implementing a training plan is to organize the athlete's daily schedule to make optimum use of her time, especially at professional level. It is important to strike a balance between training, personal free time, work schedules, and relaxation. This is best accomplished by organizing the training day into time allotments. The best organizational strategy appears to be multiple training lessons that occur on the same training day. Research by Häkkinen and Kallinen (27) suggests that splitting the day's training volume into two shorter sessions results in a greater improvement in performance, compared with performing one long training session. This finding supports the practical observations of European coaches who have noted that long training sessions decrease the quality of training because they elicit large amounts of fatigue. This increase in fatigue appears to decrease the athlete's ability to develop biomotor abilities and perfect technical and tactical skills. Therefore, when possible, the daily training volume should be broken into smaller subunits to maximally develop the athlete's capabilities.

The actual structure of the training day depends on many factors, including the time available for training, the developmental status of the athlete, and the availability of training facilities. If the athlete is attending a training camp, the frequency of training sessions may be substantially greater. It appears that the training day can be broken into two training sessions, one in the morning and one in late afternoon or evening. An example of how training might be structured for an athlete who is working full time and also training two times per day is shown in the sidebar. When athletes attend training camps, they will most likely undergo a greater frequency of training, such as three to four sessions per day or more, as shown.

Structure for Multiple Training Sessions Per Day of Training

Time	Activity
Two training sessions per day	
5:30 a.m.–6:00 a.m.	Wake up, eat snack, prepare for training
6:00 a.m.–7:30 a.m.	**First training session**
7:30 a.m.–8:00 a.m.	Eat breakfast
8:00 a.m.–8:30 a.m.	Prepare for work
8:30 a.m.–9:00 a.m.	Travel to work
9:00 a.m.–10:30 a.m.	Work
10:30 a.m.–10:45 a.m.	Eat snack
10:45 a.m.–12:30 p.m.	Work
12:30 p.m.–1:00 p.m.	Eat lunch
1:00 p.m.–5:00 p.m.	Work
5:00 p.m.–5:30 p.m.	Travel to training
5:30 p.m.–6:00 p.m.	Eat pretraining snack and prepare for training
6:00 p.m.–7:30 p.m.	**Second training session**

Time	Activity
Two training sessions per day (continued)	
7:30 p.m.–8:00 p.m.	Travel home
8:00 p.m.–8:30 p.m.	Eat dinner
8:30 p.m.–10:00 p.m.	Have free time
10:00 p.m.–5:30 a.m.	Sleep
Three training sessions per day	
6:30 a.m.	Wake up
7:00 a.m.–8:00 a.m.	**First training session**
8:30 a.m.–9:00 a.m.	Eat breakfast
9:00 a.m.–10:00 a.m.	Rest
10:00 a.m.–noon	**Second training session**
12:00 p.m.–1:00 p.m.	Rest and recovery session
1:00 p.m.–2:00 p.m.	Eat lunch
2:00 p.m.–4:00 p.m.	Rest
4:00 p.m.–6:00 p.m.	**Third training session**
6:00 p.m.–7:00 p.m.	Rest and recovery session
7:00 p.m.–7:30 p.m.	Eat dinner
7:30 p.m.–10:00 p.m.	Have free time
10:00 p.m.–6:30 a.m.	Sleep
Four training sessions per day	
6:30 a.m.	Wake up
7:00 a.m.–8:00 a.m.	**First training session**
8:30 a.m.–9:00 a.m.	Eat breakfast
9:00 a.m.–10:00 a.m.	Rest
10:00 a.m.–noon	**Second training session**
Noon–1:00 p.m.	Rest and recovery session
1:00 p.m.–2:00 p.m.	Eat lunch
2:00 p.m.–4:00 p.m.	Rest
4:00 p.m.–5:30 p.m.	**Third training session**
5:30 p.m.–6:30 p.m.	Rest and recovery session
6:30 p.m.–7:30 p.m.	**Fourth training session**
7:30 p.m.–8:00 p.m.	Recovery techniques
8:00 p.m.–8:30 p.m.	Eat dinner
8:30 p.m.–10:00 p.m.	Have free time
10:00 p.m.–6:30 a.m.	Sleep

Modeling the Training Session Plan

A training model is a simulation of a competition, the goal of which is to increase certain training adaptations and translate those adaptations to competitive performance. The modeling process can be thought of as a method for creating a training session that mimics the physiological, technical, tactical, and psychological elements encountered during a competition. Any training session can be designed to coincide with the objectives of a given phase of training while modeling competitive performance (8).

The coach must avoid the temptation to structure the training session the same way all of the time. Variation of the training stimulus is very important for inducing physiological and performance gains. The model approach is one method for inserting a new or novel training stimulus into the training plan. This method can be used to increase the athlete's motivation, induce a new physiological challenge, and present him with novel tasks that prepare him for competition. There are many ways to use the model approach, and coaches should modify the following examples to best suit their training objectives.

Model Training Session for Skill Acquisition

A model can be developed to enhance skill acquisition and refinement. New skills are best learned when athletes are rested, when they are capable of concentrating on the task, and when fatigue will not impede learning. Additionally, cumulative fatigue makes it more difficult to retain skills that have recently been acquired. Thus drills that are used to teach and develop skills should take place immediately after the warm-up. Table 6.4 presents an example of this type of model. This model can be used to develop speed, agility, and power.

TABLE 6.4 Model Training Session for Skill Acquisition

Training component	Time (min)	Goals
Warm-up	20-30	Get the athlete ready to train.
Technical and tactical drills	45-60	Improve and refine a specific skill set.
Physical training	30-45	Develop a specific biomotor ability in accordance with the daily plan.
Cool-down	10-20	Initiate the recovery.

Note: This basic model structure can be modified for agility, speed, and power training.

Model Training for Skill Refinement Under Conditions of Fatigue

This type of model may be used to mimic the conditions that are encountered at the end of a game, match, or race, where the athlete may be required to perform certain skills under fatigue. Although mastery of skills is best addressed when the athlete is fresh, athletes must also practice skills under the influence of fatigue. The objective in using this type of model is to create a situation of fatigue similar to that seen in the later part of a competition. To accomplish this objective, the coach should create technical and tactical drills that stress the glycolytic and oxidative energy systems in a way similar to that seen in competition (see chapter 1). This situation challenges the athlete's ability to cope with and overcome fatigue, both physically and psychologically (i.e., via determination, motivation, and willpower). An example of how this model may be incorporated into a training session is presented in table 6.5.

TABLE 6.5 — Model Training Session for Skill Refinement Under the Condition of Fatigue

Training component	Time (min)	Goals
Warm-up	20-30	Get the athlete ready to train.
Fatigue-inducing technical and tactical drills	45-60	Stress the athlete's glycolytic and oxidative system. Induce a situation of fatigue under which the athlete must perform specific skills.
Technical and tactical drills	20-30	Improve the accuracy of passing and shooting. Develop precision and accuracy of shooting. Work on quickness and power under conditions of fatigue.
Cool-down	10-20	Initiate the recovery.

Note: This model can be adapted to challenge the athlete's ability to perform fast, agile, and precise movements under the condition of fatigue.

This model can also be adapted to challenge the abilities of the athlete to perform fast, agile, and powerful athletic movements under the condition of fatigue. For this reason, its utilization is suggested when preparing martial artists, racket sport players, athletes in contact sports, or any athlete working to perform technical and tactical skills effectively during the last part of a sporting contest. The goal of this model is to improve performance at the end of the game, match, or competition when fatigue is at its highest, thus allowing the athlete to physiologically and psychologically adapt to this scenario.

Model Training for Controlling Precontest Arousal

To achieve maximum effectiveness during an afternoon or evening competition, the athlete must be in a state of arousal and psychological alertness. A short morning (e.g., 10:00 a.m.) session may facilitate optimal arousal for the afternoon contest, reduce anxiety, and help the athlete overcome feelings of excitability, nervousness, and restlessness. This type of session should be used to promote calmness and controlled confidence. The session should be relatively short and contain a brief series of short, explosive movements (table 6.6). These short actions, which should not induce fatigue, can arouse the athlete for the contest and improve later performance by increasing the contractility of the major skeletal muscles used in the sporting movements (17). These activities must be of short duration, include longer rest intervals, and not induce fatigue, since fatigue will decrease performance capacity. An additional strategy is to use long rest intervals between each activity bout to ensure recovery (39).

TABLE 6.6 — Model Training Session for Controlling Precontest Arousal

Training component	Time (min)	Goals
Warm-up	10-20	Start with a short, light warm-up to prepare the athlete.
Technical, tactical, or speed drills	10-15	Perform short technical, tactical, or speed drills, separated by long rest intervals; this is designed to prepare the athlete for an afternoon competition.
Cool-down	10-20	Initiate the recovery.

Summary of Major Concepts

This chapter emphasizes the benefits of organization and planning. Training effectiveness depends on the coach's and athlete's ability to organize and plan training from a single workout to a long-term plan. A workout plan is not difficult to construct, and it is a powerful tool that can maximize performance outcomes. The objectives and goals of the individual training sessions must be clearly outlined for the athlete. The athlete must receive feedback about her progress toward attaining these objectives.

The workout plan includes several key components. The warm-up is an often overlooked but essential component. This important segment prepares the athlete for the training session and should never be compromised or removed from the training plan. The warm-up should contain general dynamic activities and progress to dynamic muscle actions that are specific to the sporting activity.

The cool-down is another often-overlooked component that can influence the effectiveness of the training session. This portion of the session allows the body to return to homeostasis and initiate recovery. This is the ideal time to include static stretching and improve flexibility. If implemented correctly, the cool-down can be a very effective part of the training session.

Planning the Training Cycles

Training cycles can be structured into long-term plans such as the **quadrennial** (4-year) plan and the individual annual plan (1 year). Based on the terminology used by the German training specialists preparing for the 1936 Olympics, the annual plan can be further subdivided into grosse (macrocycle) and kleine (microcycle) plans. Macrocycles can be structured in 2- to 6-week increments, whereas microcycles traditionally last 1 week.

Although some authors suggest that eight or nine microcycle variants exist, it is probably simpler to use four basic variants: developmental, competition, recovery–regeneration, and peaking–unloading. Although the four basic microcycle types are used most of the time, it is likely that some coaches use variations of these broad categories.

Microcycle

The term microcycle is rooted in the Greek word *micros*, which means "small," and the Latin word *ciclus*, which refers to a regular sequence of events. In training methodology, a microcycle is a weekly training program within an annual plan. The microcycle is the most important programming tool in the training process. The content of the microcycle determines the quality of the training process. The microcycle is structured according to the objectives, volume, intensity, and methods that are the focus of the training phase. The physiological and psychological demands placed on the athlete cannot be steady. The mix of general and sport-specific stimuli must change according to the phase of the annual plan; they must also take into consideration the athlete's working capacity, the athlete's need for recovery, and the competition plan. The microcycle must be flexible enough that individual training sessions can be modified to address the residual fatigue of the athlete (i.e., internal load, or degree of readiness) in relation to the training objectives of the training session. When the training unit is modified, subsequent training lessons must be modified to maintain the focus of the microcycle and ensure that the training objectives of the phase are achieved.

Constructing Microcycles

The microcycle has a strong historical precedence and can be found in the works of Philostratus, an ancient Greek scholar. Philostratus proposed a short-term plan that he called the "tetra system," a 4-day training cycle:

- *Day 1:* Undertake a short and energetic program.
- *Day 2:* Exercise intensely.
- *Day 3:* Relax to revive the activity.
- *Day 4:* Perform moderate exercise.

The tetra system structure was to be repeated continually. Such ancient training practices are the foundation of the microcycle structure.

The main criteria determining the microcycle structure are the training goal, training factors, and desired improvements in athletic performance. The appropriate microcycle structure will dictate the rate of improvement in the various training factors. The sequencing within the microcycle is of particular importance because the fatigue generated in one session can significantly affect subsequent training sessions. For example, if a session focuses on endurance development or contains a very intense stimulus, and that session precedes a technical training session, the fatigue generated by the first session might impair the development of technique in the next session. Thus, the sequencing of the training stimuli throughout the microcycle must account for accumulated fatigue in order to maximize the development of specific performance or biomotor factors. The microcycle should be structured using the same concepts suggested for the training session plan:

- Technical or tactical training
- Development of speed, agility, or power
- Development of strength
- Development of specific endurance

Constructing a Microcycle

Repetition of a training stimulus is essential for the athlete to improve a technical element or develop a biomotor ability. *Repetitia est mater studiorum* is a Roman phrase meaning "repetition is the mother of study." To maximize gains, exercises that target specific biomotor abilities must be undertaken with varying frequencies during the microcycle. Depending on the athlete's ability, targeted training sessions with similar objectives and content may need to be repeated two or three times during a microcycle to maximize the training effect and its adaptations. Of particular importance is the training stimulus used, because the amount of fatigue generated will affect the recovery required before that stimulus can be used again. For example, in strength training a load with a 20-repetition maximum requires significantly more recovery than a set that doesn't push the athlete to muscle failure. Thus a longer recovery period may be warranted before performing this type of strength training.

When the athlete and coach are targeting specific endurance with submaximal intensities, three training sessions per week will suffice. However, for specific endurance of maximum intensity during the competitive phase, the athlete should engage in endurance training twice per week and dedicate the remaining days to lower-intensity training. The athlete should use one or two training sessions per week to maintain strength, **flexibility**, and **speed**. It appears that 2 or 3 days per week are optimal for plyometric, speed, and agility training.

Various training loads should be alternated throughout the microcycle. The athlete should use maximal loads no more than twice per week, interspersed with low-intensity training days and active rest days. It is particularly important to schedule active rest and relaxation the day after a competition. Active rest or low-intensity exercise should be interspersed throughout the microcycle, especially after sessions that have high to maximal demand.

When planning the microcycles, the coach can repeat the basic structure across several microcycles, especially during the preparatory phase. Throughout a macrocycle, microcycles of similar nature (i.e., content and methods) can be repeated two or three times; this can result in qualitative improvements based on the athlete's adaptation. The types of microcycle fluctuations will vary depending on the athlete's level of development.

Structural Considerations

The annual training plan dictates the structure of the macrocycle and microcycle plans. Individual microcycle plans should be developed to meet the objectives of each phase of the annual and macrocycle training plans. This approach must permit flexibility in the training program, allowing the coach to modify the training content in response to the effects of training performed previously and the athlete's improvement. In this approach the macrocycle is considered a guideline, and the daily and weekly programs can be altered to address the athlete's response to the training stimuli. However, the microcycle should be constructed in accordance with the training objectives and the phase of training. When structuring the microcycles of the training plan, the coach should consider many factors:

- The objective of the microcycle and the dominant training factors
- The training demand (e.g., number of sessions, number of hours, volume, intensity, and complexity) targeted during the microcycle
- The intensity of the microcycle and the intensity fluctuations contained in the microcycle
- The methods that will be used to induce the training stimulus in each training session
- The days on which training and competition will occur (if applicable)
- The need to alter intensity each day (i.e., start the microcycle with a low- or medium-intensity training session and progress intensity in a undulatory fashion)
- The timing of competitions in the context of the microcycle (i.e., when the microcycle leads into a competition, the highest intensity or peak training session for that week should occur 3 to 5 days prior to the event)

The coach must determine whether the athlete should perform one or more sessions per day. If the athlete's development and work, school, or personal schedule allow for multiple training sessions, the coach should plan the timing of such sessions.

It is helpful to begin each microcycle with a meeting during which the coach and athlete discuss the objectives for each training factor contained in the microcycle and how those objectives will be achieved. The coach and athlete should discuss the volume and intensity of training, the number of training session contained in each training day, and where the most difficult training sessions will fall. The coach may want to target performance standards for the microcycle. Additional personalized information can be given to athletes at this time. Finally, if the microcycle is leading into a competition, the coach should give the athlete details about the upcoming contest and motivate the athlete to attain each competition goal.

If there is no competition at the end of microcycle, a short meeting should be held after the last training session of the microcycle to analyze whether the athlete achieved the microcycle training objectives and goals. The coach should use this meeting to critique the athlete's performance during training, making sure to highlight the positive aspects while targeting others for improvement. The coach can strengthen the evaluation of the microcycle by collecting input from the athlete. The coach should then take all information obtained from the meetings and training outcomes to formulate strategies for future microcycles with similar objectives and goals. The meeting following a microcycle is a tool with which coaches and athletes can coordinate their focus on performance outcomes.

Classifying Microcycles

Several different microcycle structures are presented in this chapter, but specific training circumstances result in an infinite number of structural variations. The dynamics of the microcycle is dictated by many factors including the phase of training, the developmental status of the athlete, and the training factor emphasis (technical, tactical, or physical preparation). One of the most important factors dictating the microcycle structure is the athlete's level of development and training capacity. For example, a highly trained athlete may be able to tolerate a greater frequency of training sessions performed at higher intensities than a novice or less-developed athlete. Athletes on the same team may have different work capacities and training needs, so individualization of microcycle content may be warranted.

To create an individualized training stimulus, the coach must eliminate standardization and rigidity when structuring the microcycle. This flexibility allows the coach to use information gathered from training, assessments, or competition to modify the training program, thereby helping the athlete meet performance and training objectives.

One method for classifying microcycles centers on the number of training sessions per week. As stated previously, the number of training sessions that the athlete can tolerate without overtraining occurring is dictated by the athlete's level of development and physical preparation. Additionally, the microcycle structure will change depending on the available time for training and whether the athlete is participating in a training camp or undergoing regular training sessions.

There are a variety of microcycle structures: 3 days per week (figure 7.1), 4 days per week (figure 7.2), and 5 days per week (figure 7.3) are common structures. Advanced athletes who have a high work tolerance and can meet the time requirements can undergo eight or nine training sessions per week (figures 7.4 and 7.5), sometimes up to 12 or 13. Microcycles with additional training session may be used during holidays or during training camps, when more time is available for training, or with more advanced athletes.

Session time	Day						
	Monday	Tuesday	Wednesday	Thursday	Friday	Saturday	Sunday
a.m.							
p.m.	Training		Training		Training		

FIGURE 7.1 Microcycle with three training sessions per week.

Session time	Day						
	Monday	Tuesday	Wednesday	Thursday	Friday	Saturday	Sunday
a.m.							
p.m.	Training	Training		Training		Training	

FIGURE 7.2 Microcycle with four training sessions per week. A variant is to have the fourth training session on Friday.

Session time	Day						
	Monday	Tuesday	Wednesday	Thursday	Friday	Saturday	Sunday
a.m.							
p.m.	Training	Training		Training	Training	Training	

FIGURE 7.3 Microcycle with five sessions per week.

Session time	Day						
	Monday	Tuesday	Wednesday	Thursday	Friday	Saturday	Sunday
a.m.	Training	Training		Training		Training	
p.m.	Training	Training		Training		Training	

FIGURE 7.4 Microcycle with eight sessions per week.

Session time	Day						
	Monday	Tuesday	Wednesday	Thursday	Friday	Saturday	Sunday
a.m.	Training		Training		Training	Training	
p.m.	Training	Training	Training	Training	Training		

FIGURE 7.5 Microcycle with nine sessions per week.

There are many ways to increase the number of training sessions. The athlete can use a 3+1 microcycle, training on 3 successive half days, followed by a half day of rest, for a total of 9 training sessions during the microcycle (figure 7.6). This model can be modified for an athlete whose training tolerance or potential is higher and can tolerate more intensive microcycles. A 5+1 microcycle (training on 5 days, followed by a half day of rest) (figure 7.7) and a 5+1+1 microcycle (training on 5 days, followed by a half day of rest, followed by a half day of work) are intensive microcycles (figure 7.8). The structure of these more intensive microcycles depends on the amount of time that is available and the type of training stimulus used during each session.

The microcycle structure can be further expanded by integrating multiple training sessions throughout the day that target different training factors. For example, a three-component microcycle may be constructed where a sprint–agility or a plyometric session is conducted in the morning and the main training session, which targets tactical or technical development followed by strength training, may be performed in the late afternoon or early evening (figure 7.9).

An additional aspect of the microcycle structure relates to the variations in training intensity and demand. The training dynamics should not be uniform across the microcycle. They

Session time	Day						
	Monday	Tuesday	Wednesday	Thursday	Friday	Saturday	Sunday
a.m.	Training	Training	Training	Training	Training	Training	
p.m.	Training		Training		Training		

FIGURE 7.6 Microcycle with a 3+1 structure.

Session time	Day						
	Monday	Tuesday	Wednesday	Thursday	Friday	Saturday	Sunday
a.m.	Training	Training	Training	Training	Training	Training	
p.m.	Training	Training		Training	Training		

FIGURE 7.7 Microcycle with a 5+1 structure.

Session time	Day						
	Monday	Tuesday	Wednesday	Thursday	Friday	Saturday	Sunday
a.m.	Training	Training	Training	Training	Training	Training	Training
p.m.	Training	Training		Training	Training		

FIGURE 7.8 Microcycle with a 5+1+1 structure.

Session time	Day						
	Monday	Tuesday	Wednesday	Thursday	Friday	Saturday	Sunday
7:00 a.m.	Plyometric training		Plyometric training		Plyometric training		
3:00 p.m.	Sprint and agility training	Aerobic training	Sprint and agility training	Aerobic training	Sprint and agility training	Aerobic training	
5:00 p.m.	Strength training		Strength training		Strength training		

FIGURE 7.9 Microcycle with the integration of multiple training factors.

should vary depending on the characteristics of the training, the type of microcycle used, the environmental conditions (e.g., climate, weather), and the phase of the annual training plan. The intensity of training can alternate between the six intensity zones, ranging from very high (90%-100% of maximum) to a recovery day where no training is undertaken (table 7.1). These alterations are dictated by the objectives of the microcycle. For example, the objectives of an intensive microcycle may require 1 (figure 7.10), 2 (figures 7.11-7.15), or occasionally 3 (figure 7.16) high-demand to very high-demand training days depending on the objective of the microcycle.

When planning the modulations of intensity or training demand within the microcycle, the coach should consider the principles of load progression. The microcycle usually should contain only one peak, which occurs during the middle 3 days of the week. In some instances, a microcycle can contain two peaks that are followed by 1 or 2 days of regeneration sessions. An exception to this rule may occur when model training is being used; in this case, two peaks can occur on adjacent days to simulate a competitive situation.

TABLE 7.1 Intensity Zones and Training Demand

Intensity zone	Training demand	Percentage of maximum performance	Intensity
1	Very high	90-100	Maximum
2	High	80-90	Heavy
3	Medium	70-80	Medium
4	Low	50-70	Low
5	Very low	<50	Very low
Recovery	Recovery	No training	Recovery

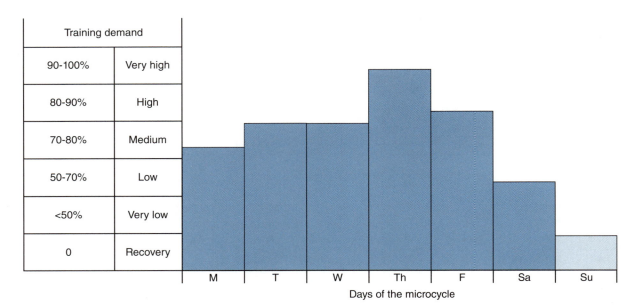

FIGURE 7.10 Microcycle with one peak.

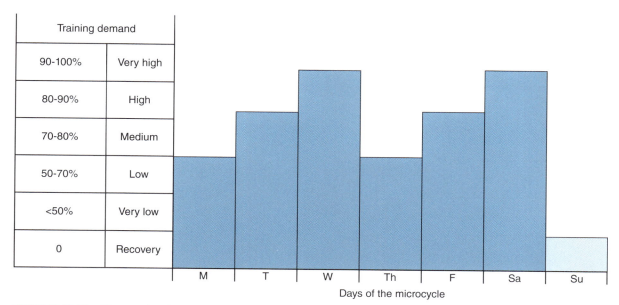

FIGURE 7.11 Two-peak microcycle.

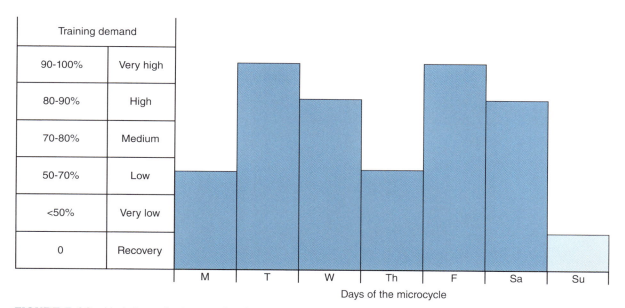

FIGURE 7.12 Variation of a two-peak microcycle.

The microcycle structure can be modified if the athlete is training at high altitude or has traveled a long distance and crossed several time zones (i.e., time difference of 5-8 h). In these situations, it may be warranted to add an adaptation microcycle that does not contain a peak. The microcycle structure also should be altered when the athlete is training in a hot and humid climate. In this situation it is recommended that the peak occur at the beginning of the week when the athlete has more vigor.

The sample microcycles in figures 7.10 through 7.16 represent **total training demand** rather than the separate variables of volume and intensities. The use of total training demand

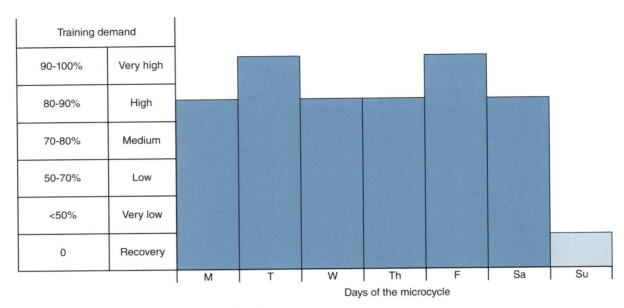

FIGURE 7.13 Two-peak microcycle with high demand.

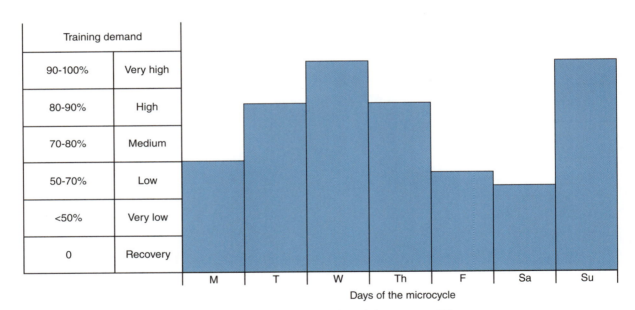

FIGURE 7.14 Two-peak microcycle in which the second peak is a competition.

allows for the microcycle structure to be used in a variety of sporting activities because sports vary in their area of emphasis, with some being dominated by speed-power, maximum strength, or endurance. Additionally, team sports contain a complex interaction of many factors that can best represented by total training demand.

A microcycle can be structured many ways; some authors speculate that there are at least 22 possible microcycle structures. This number of microcycle variants may complicate the

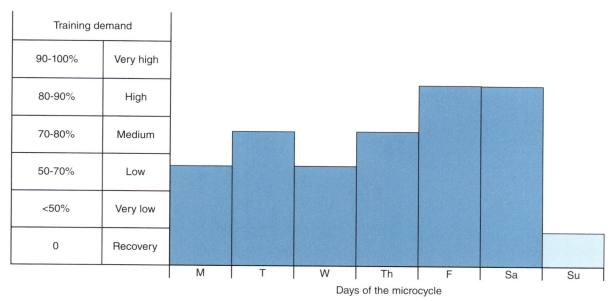

FIGURE 7.15 Microcycle model with two adjacent peaks.

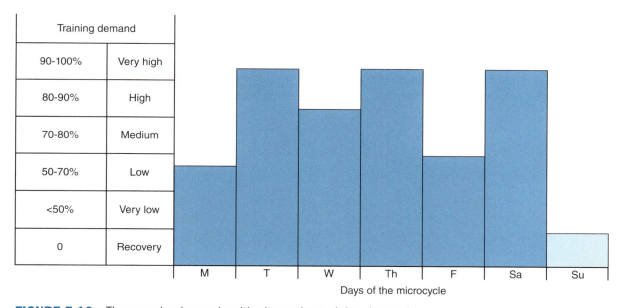

FIGURE 7.16 Three-peak microcycle with alternating training demands.

training and planning process, so it may be better for the coach to use the most common microcycle structures and adapt them to individual training needs.

The microcycle should be functional and, therefore, as simple as possible. The plan should specify the date, objectives, and content for each training session. The content should be succinct and easy to understand and should emphasize major items to target in the training session. Figure 7.17 shows a microcycle plan from the competition phase.

Sport/Event: Javelin	Microcyle # 29
Date : 20.07-27-09	**Objectives:** 1. Perform 67:00 m 2. Perfect the rhythm of the last three strides under higher velocity conditions 3. Develop the ability to concentrate for the morning competition 4. Maintain leg and arm power

Time	Mon.	Tues.	Wed.	Thurs.	Fri.	Sat.	Sun.
a.m. 10:00-11:00	• 15 min warm-up • Sprints: $\frac{20, 30, 40 \text{ m}}{\frac{2}{4}; \frac{3}{4}}$ 6	Competition warm-up: 6 throws		Same as Tuesday	Competition warm-up	Competition 10:45	
p.m. 16:00-18:00	• Warm-up: 20 min • Sprints: $\frac{30 \text{ m}}{\frac{4}{4}}$ 3 • Technique: • Last 3 strides • 30 throws with baseball • 15 medicine ball throws • 2 × 30 m bounds	• Warm-up: Competition • Throws: • 6 throws 4/4 • 15 throws, 3/4 with short approach • Warm-up: 7 min specific warm-up • Weight training: 30 min • Flexibility: 5 min	Basketball game: 2 × 15 min	Same as Monday	• Warm-up: Competition • Throws: 15 medium approach • Walk and throws: 15 min at different targets placed in the grass • Relaxation: Special exercises	Basketball game: 2 × 15 min	

FIGURE 7.17 Competition phase microcycle plan for a female javelin thrower.

Classification of Microcycles Based on Training Objectives and Phase of Training

The structure of the microcycle depends on the training objectives and thus the training phase. From this point of view, there are four general microcycle classifications: developmental, competition, recovery–regeneration, and peaking–unloading.

Developmental Microcycles

Developmental microcycles are specific to the preparatory phase of training. The objective is to increase the level of adaptation, improve skills, and develop biomotor abilities. Such cycles could have two or three peaks of medium and high demand. The microcycle uses an alternation of energy systems and loads, creating an undulatory loading dynamic. The actual structure of the microcycle depends on the athlete's classification, sport characteristics, and the preparation subphase the athlete is in. Figure 7.18 illustrates a microcycle for the early part of the preparatory phase, presenting training sessions for early adaptation and development.

Recovery–Regeneration Microcycles

The goal of a regeneration microcycle is to dissipate residual fatigue. As a consequence, it can be used to elevate the athlete's level of readiness, which will improve performance; for example, it can be used between the end of the preparatory phase and the beginning of the competitive phase for a team sport. This microcycle is marked by a significantly lower training demand, which can be created by decreasing training intensity, volume, or some combination of both. Another approach to using this type of microcycle, specific to the

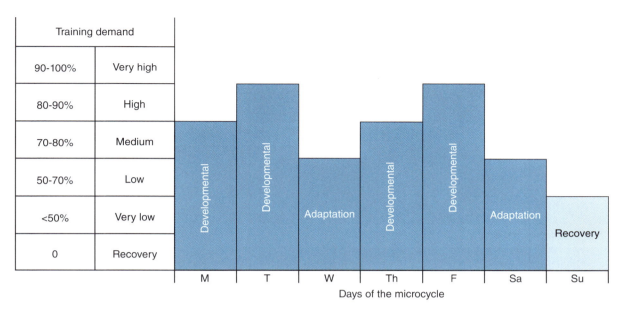

FIGURE 7.18 Developmental microcycle. The scope or focus of this microcycle is adaptation.

transitory phases, is to include activities that train physiological characteristics similar to the targeted sport but that are different than the typical training activities.

Peaking–Unloading Microcycles

Unloading microcycles are placed at the end of every macrocycle in order to dissipate fatigue and elevate the athlete's level of athletic readiness; this ultimately increases sport-specific performance. Before the most important competitions of the year, two unloading microcycles are used back to back to allow for peaking (chapter 9). This type of microcycle is created mainly by decreasing weekly training volume (by 50% or more) and by maintaining or decreasing intensity (by 5%-10%). The reduction of training demand will result in physiological responses that allow supercompensation to occur. The unloading microcycle elevates performance and decreases the potential for overtraining.

Microcycle Dynamics During the Competitive Phase

During the competitive phase, the sequencing of individual microcycles depends on the competitive schedule. Timing of competitions also affects the placement of regeneration and unloading days within the microcycle. The format used when planning a competitive microcycle will be affected by the requirements of the sport. In team sports there may be several competitions in 1 week, whereas in individual sports (figure 7.19) competitions may occur over several consecutive weeks. With one competition per week, 1 or 2 days of rest and recovery should be included each week. The bulk of training, including strength and power training, will be conducted during the middle of the microcycle. In this example, a medium to high training demand is used. After the bulk of training is completed, unloading should then be planned for the 2 days prior to the next competition.

This basic competitive microcycle can be modified when the opponent is weaker or the competition is of little importance. Such a competition will not present a high physiological challenge, and the subsequent competition-induced fatigue will be markedly less than usual. It may be warranted in these situations to replace the recovery day that is planned for Monday (in this example) with an additional technical or tactical training session. Addition-

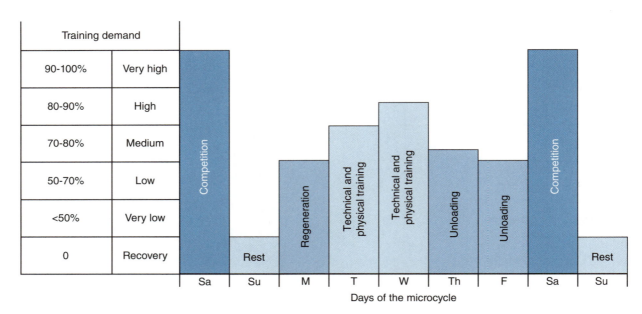

FIGURE 7.19 Microcycle with weekly competitions.

ally, it is likely that only one unloading day would be needed before a minor competition. This schedule results in a net gain of 4 training days, with at least one of those days being of a high demand. Activities for maintaining the level of physical training have to also be planned, although they should be less challenging than during a microcycle with no competitions. Emphasis should be given to the maintenance of the dominant biomotor abilities in the targeted sport.

When teams have multiple competitions or games in one microcycle (see figure 7.20), Monday is a short regeneration session that contains a very low training demand. The second session of the microcycle (Tuesday) is a tactical day that is used to elevate performance during the Wednesday competition. On Thursday a regeneration day is planned, and Friday is the only high-demand training session of the microcycle. Strength and power training is

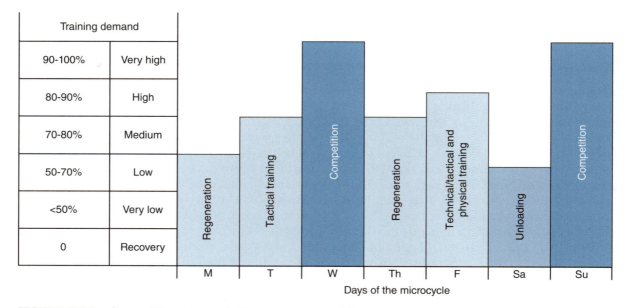

FIGURE 7.20 Competitive microcycle for a team sport with two games in 1 week.

suggested for Friday, but of medium-low demand. The number of exercises must be very low (two to four) and they should strictly address the prime movers. To facilitate a good performance for the Sunday game, an unloading day is planned for Saturday.

If the competitive schedule is organized over the 2 days of a weekend (e.g., team sports tournament or several races in track and swimming), then the microcycle can be organized as depicted in figure 7.21. Two unloading training sessions are used on the 2 days (Thursday and Friday) prior to the weekend competition so that fatigue is dissipated and supercompensation may be achieved at the time of competition. The highest training demand occurs at the beginning of the microcycle (Tuesday), thus progressively decreasing the training demand across the microcycle. On those days you can also plan a short session for the maintenance of strength and power.

If the microcycle contains a multiple-day tournament, the coach should plan regeneration activities that may include active recovery. Active recovery performed at very low intensities can facilitate lactate removal (1, 9, 11, 13, 16), dampen central nervous system activity, increase the tone of the parasympathetic nervous system, and reduce muscle soreness (14). Active recovery should include very low intensities of exercise that do not significantly affect muscle glycogen stores. Tournament play can significantly affect glycogen (8), so glycogen stores must be replenished before the next competitive match. The best method for accomplishing this is to follow a post-exercise supplementation program and to ensure adequate dietary intake of carbohydrate between matches (3, 7). A microcycle for a weeklong tournament is presented in figure 7.22. Note that the morning after every game includes a very low-intensity regeneration session that is designed to speed recovery. Additionally, a low-intensity tactical training session is planned for the late afternoon on the day prior

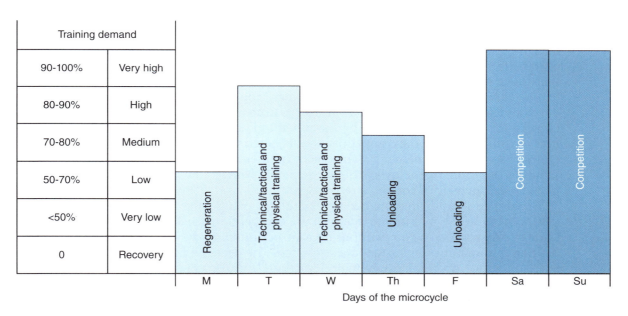

FIGURE 7.21 Competitive microcycle for a team sport with two games in one weekend.

Time	Days of the Microcycle						
	M	T	W	Th	F	Sa	Su
a.m.	Game	Regeneration	Game	Regeneration	Game	Regeneration	Game
p.m.		Tactical training		Tactical training		Tactical training	

FIGURE 7.22 Microcycle for a weeklong team sport tournament.

to each game. A microcycle formatted in this fashion will provide the athlete with the best potential to recover and maximize performance.

Model of a Microcycle for Competition

The vast majority of microcycles in the annual training plan target the development of skills and abilities required by the sport. However, during the competitive phase, the focus of the training plan shifts to maximizing performance capacity during competition. This is accomplished by modifying the microcycle structure in accordance with the demands of the sport and the athlete's physiological and psychological needs. One strategy is to develop the microcycle based on a model of the competition (model training). This model, especially in individual sports, can be used repeatedly prior to main competition. The model should contain training sessions of various intensities and should alternate between active rest and recovery. The daily cycle should be identical to the day of the competition.

Many sports (e.g., regional-level track and field and swimming, tennis, some team sports, martial arts) have qualifying rounds followed by finals in the same day (e.g., Friday at 10:00 a.m. and 6:00 p.m.). Models designed to address this competitive schedule would place the main training day on Friday, which would contain two training sessions that would occur at the same times as the targeted competition.

Other sports (e.g., some team sports, national- and international-level track and field and swimming, boxing, tennis, wrestling) may contain 2 to 4 days of consecutive competitions. This type of competitive format can also be modeled by modifying the microcycle structure to correspond to the demands of the competition. This model should be repeated several times prior to the contest. However, the model should only be used every 2 or 3 weeks, with developmental microcycles placed between each microcycle containing this competitive model.

Some tournaments such as the Olympic Games, World Championships, or international competitions are organized over 4 to 9 days. It is not feasible to model this competitive format because such a model will create a large amount of physiological stress and significantly affect the time that can be dedicated to training. To prepare for larger tournaments, the athlete should participate in smaller tournaments that last 2 or 3 days and contain four or five competitive efforts. To prepare for these tournaments, the athlete should follow developmental microcycles and daily training structures that contain characteristics of the targeted tournament. It may also be warranted to familiarize the athlete with the competitive schedule by using the competitive model, altering between competition and recovery typically seen in a tournament. It may be recommended that training days that fall on the same day of a tournament involve higher demands, whereas the day after this session should be of lower intensity or contain a recovery session.

The athlete should alternate between simulated competitive days and rest and recovery days to maximize her ability to adapt to the competition schedule. Many athletes do not favor free days between competitions because performance during the second day of competition is sometimes not as good as expected. The decrease in performance seems to be based on postcompetition psychological reactions (e.g., overconfidence, conceit) rather than an accumulation of fatigue. To facilitate the athlete's ability to tolerate the rest days between competitions, the coach can include competition-based microcycles in all macrocycles contained in the competitive phase of the annual training plan. If the competitive phase is short, the coach can introduce the competitive model during the last part of the preparatory phase.

Although the competitive model can be used to prepare for a major competition, the athlete likely will participate in several additional competitions. Such competitions may occur on a different day of the microcycle than the major competition. The microcycle model usually should not be modified in these situations, especially if the athlete is likely to qualify for the major competition.

The main goal of the microcycles preceding the major competition is to allow the athlete to completely recover from the physiological and psychological stress of training so that peak performance occurs. The athlete can peak by reducing the training load by approximately 40% to 60% across the microcycle before the major competition. Another strategy is to manipulate the training load across two microcycles. In this situation peaking can be accomplished in 8 to 14 days with gradual reductions in training load. Several examples of peaking strategies are presented in chapter 9.

Recovery and Regeneration Microcycles

Elevations in readiness and performance occur when fatigue is dissipated, and some authors claim that fatigue management is central to the actual training process (15). If fatigue is managed appropriately, a supercompensation effect will occur, elevating the athlete's readiness and performance potential.

Recovery and regeneration can be integrated into a microcycle in several fashions. For example, by including rest days, variations in training intensity, and alternative methods of training, a coach can facilitate recovery between or within training sessions (15). A regeneration microcycle should be incorporated at the end of a macrocycle. Figure 7.23 presents a classic 3:1 (loading and unloading) step structure in which week 4 is an unloading or regeneration microcycle. These microcycles can be structured the same as a training microcycle, but the intensity or frequency of training can be reduced.

Another restoration microcycle structure contains actual training sessions that are designed to stimulate recovery. These sessions can contain a slightly longer warm-up and a relatively short training session consisting of either light work applicable to the sport or complementary activities followed by a series of activities designed to facilitate recovery. Table 7.2 offers a sample regeneration session and several regeneration techniques.

Regeneration microcycles are integral parts of the annual plan and are particularly important during the competition phase. During the competition phase of training for many sports, 2 or 3 microcycles can be included that contain a series of competitions. The use of many competitions will increase the amount of fatigue experienced by the athlete. To enable the athlete to tolerate this high amount of physiological and psychological stress, regeneration and recovery microcycle structures should be used. An example of a regeneration microcycle is presented in figure 7.24. This microcycle is designed to remove physiological and psychological fatigue, aid in the replenishment of energy substrates, and supercompensate the athlete at the end of the cycle.

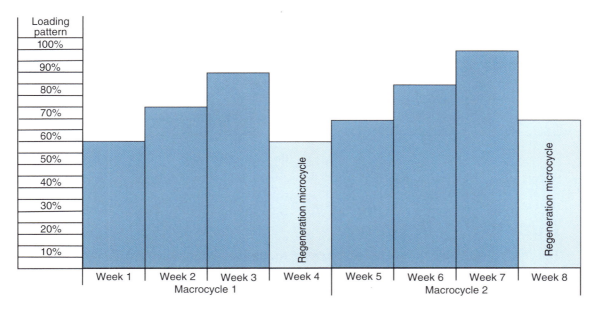

FIGURE 7.23 Placement of a recovery and regeneration microcycle.

TABLE 7.2 Regeneration Session

	Description	Duration (min)
Warm-up	General warm-up Specific warm-up	10 20
Training session	Low-intensity work from either the sport being trained for or a complementary activity	30
Cool-down	Static stretching	10
Regeneration	Warm water immersion • 37 °C-39 °C (98.6 °F-102.2 °F) for the whole body • 37 °C-40 °C (98.6 °F-104 °F) for the legs • 37 °C-45 °C (98.6 °F-113 °F) for the arms or hands	10-20
Alternative regeneration techniques	Total body massage Sauna • 60 °C-140 °C (140 °F-284 °F); 5-15% humidity Contrast therapy • Thermotherapy: 37 °C-44 °C (98.6 °F-111.2 °F) • Cryotherapy: 7 °C-20 °C (44.6 °F-68 °F) Cold water immersion • 12 °C-18 °C (53.6 °F-64.4 °F)	10-20 30 20 4 1 20

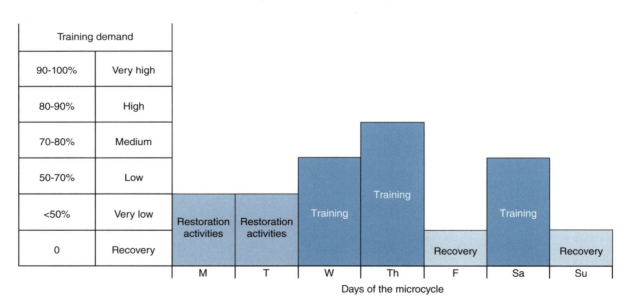

FIGURE 7.24 Regeneration microcycle.

Quantifying Training

The coach and athlete should use objective methods to plan training intensities or loads. Too often training programs are based on subjective preferences. In the best-case scenario, the plan alternates heavy training days with easy days throughout the year. In the worst-case scenario, the plan uses a "no pain, no gain" philosophy and the loading or intensity of training is constantly very high, which ultimately leads to high levels of fatigue and even to overtraining.

Although few coaches quantify the loading parameters contained in their training programs, quantifying training is one of the most important parts of developing a training program. In individual sports (track and field, swimming, rowing), volume is often quantified using mileage, as in the kilometers or miles per microcycle, macrocycle, or year of training. In throwing events volume may be quantified as the number of throws completed in the individual cycles. Intensity may be quantified as distance jumped or thrown, the percentage of maximum speed, or maximum power output or heart rate. In strength training, the volume of training is quantified as the **tonnage** (volume load) lifted, weekly repetitions per exercise, or total sets per session; intensity is determined by the athlete's maximum strength or one-repetition maximum (1RM). Training intensity and volume are rarely quantified in team sports, which makes it difficult for coaches to monitor athletes' training. Only in the last few years GPS and accelerometer devices utilized by top teams have assisted with the exact quantification of training. At best, time in minutes is used to specify duration of high-intensity drills.

The quantification of training is often a difficult undertaking, which is easier to accomplish when the training program is designed for an athlete with whom the coach is very familiar. The coach should know the athlete's training background, ability to tolerate physiological and psychological stress, strengths and weaknesses, and training environment. Because these characteristics are different for each athlete, training programs should not be shared by athletes. Understanding the athlete's needs and abilities is an essential component of designing a training plan. The intensity of training should be planned using established equations, and the volume of training should be quantified.

In all programs, the training intensity throughout the microcycle must be varied to enhance the athlete's physiological adaptation to the training load and stimulate regeneration after a training session. To quantify the training intensity, the coach may identify four to five training intensities based on the physiological demands of the sport. Each intensity must correlate with the activity's rhythm or tempo, the training type and method, and the athlete's heart rate response (plus or minus a few beats per min). The intensity zones should be determined according to the bioenergetic characteristics of the sport or the percentage contribution of the various energy systems. After gathering this information, the coach can plan the percentage of each intensity level contained in the microcycle (table 7.3). From the late specific preparation onward, the highest percentage of the training load should target the development of the dominant ability and the bioenergetic characteristics of the sport.

Table 7.3 and figure 7.25 show this concept applied in a microcycle for rowing. In table 7.3, intensity zones 3 and 4 comprise 70% of the total training load for the competitive phase of the annual training plan. The same two intensities dominate the example in figure 7.25, which shows the link between the theoretical concept and its application in the training of rowers.

If an objective means of quantifying training does not exist, the coach can subjectively divide skills and training into more difficult (pace of game, race, or match) and less difficult stratifications. The pace of the game, race, or match should be simulated with intensity zone 2; this intensity should be used for at least 50% of the training time per week.

A better quantification system contains five intensities, in which zone 5 is a low intensity to be used for compensation between other intensities or to facilitate supercompensation. An example of a five-category stratification follows:

1. Maximum intensity
2. Higher than the pace of the game, race, or match
3. Pace of the game, race, or match
4. Lower than the pace of the game, race, or match
5. Compensation

In either case, the intensity higher than the pace of the game, race, or match is dominated by anaerobic energy supply, whereas aerobic energy supply dominates intensities that are below game, race, or match pace.

TABLE 7.3 Example of Intensity Zones for Rowing

Characteristics	Intensity zones*				
	1	2	3	4	5
Characteristics	Speed endurance	Power endurance	Specific racing endurance	Aerobic endurance of medium distance	Aerobic endurance of long distance
Rhythm of activity	Maximum	Very high, greater than the racing rate and rhythm	Rapid, the optimal rhythm and ratios	Moderate, lower than the racing rhythm	Low
Stroke rate	>40	37-40	32-36	24-32	<24
Type of training	Starts and sprints up to 15 s; rest 1.5 min	Repetitions of 250-1,000 m; rest 3-10 min	Races and controlled racing; interval training of 3-4 min; rest 4-5 min	Long repetitions; variable rate and power; long-distance rowing with sprints of 30-60 s	Long-distance (steady-state) technique
Heart rate	>180 beats/min	170-180 beats/min	150-170 beats/min	120-150 beats/min	<120 beats/min
Bioenergetics Anaerobic Aerobic	80% 20%	65% 35%	25% 75%	15% 85%	5% 95%
Total training volume	10%		70%		20%

*Intensity zone 1 is the most demanding, and intensity zone 5 is the least demanding.

Time		Microcycle						
		Mon.	Tues.	Wed.	Thurs.	Fri.	Sat.	Sun.
9:30-11:30 a.m.	Intensity zone*	4	3	5	4	3	4	
	Distribution (km)	24	20	24	24	20	24	
	Training	Long repetitions: 8 × 2 km	Interval training: 10 × 3 min, work/rest ratio 1:1	Aerobic endurance, long distance	Variable rate, variable power	Interval training: 6 × 3 min, work/rest ratio 1:1.5	Aerobic endurance: 3 × 1 min	
16:00-18:00	Intensity zone	2	4		1	4	2	
	Distribution (km)	20	24		20	24	20	
	Training	Model training: 1 × 250 m, 2 × 500 m, 2 × 1,000 m, 2 × 500 m, 2 × 250 m	Variable rate, variable power		Sprints: 500 total strokes, rest 1.5 min	Long reps: 3 × 6 km, rest 5 min	Model training: 1 × 250 m, 6 × 1,000 m, 2 × 500 m, 2 × 250 m	
	Weight training	Maximum strength	Muscular endurance		Maximum strength	Muscular endurance		

FIGURE 7.25 Example of using numeric-based intensity zones to construct a microcycle for rowing.

*Intensity zone 1 is the most demanding, and intensity zone 5 is the least demanding.

Whether using objective or subjective methods to quantify training, the coach should follow the correct sequence when planning the microcycle. The first step is to plan the intensity zones for each day of the week and indicate this on the training plan (figure 7.25). Intensity zones should be chosen for each day of the week to provide variations in intensities, type of work, or energy system targeted. After this step of the planning process is completed, the training program should be developed (step 2). For the best results, the coach should include several variables of work for each intensity, irrespective of whether this refers to technical, tactical, or physical training. Each plan should include one to three intensity symbols, which means it is possible to train at least two types of work that tax the same energy system. This suggestion is mostly valid for sports of high technical and tactical complexity. A team sport example illustrates this sequence. Table 7.4 is an example of a method for quantifying training, and table 7.5 is an example of how to plan intensity zones.

TABLE 7.4 Quantification of Training for Team Sports

	Intensity zones*				
	1	2	3	4	5
Characteristics of training	T: complex; TA: lactic acid tolerance training	T/TA: suicide drills	TA: $\dot{V}O_2$max	T/TA: phosphagen	T: skills: accuracy in shooting, serving, passing
Duration	30-60 s	20-30 s	3-5 min	5-15 s	10 min (several bouts)
Rest interval (min)	3-5	3	2-3	1-2	1
Heart rate (beats/min)	>180	>180	>170	>170	120-150
Bioenergetics					
Anaerobic (%)	80	90	40	90	10
Aerobic (%)	20	10	60	10	90
Total training volume (5)	40		20	20	20

T = technical; TA = tactical.
*Intensity zone 1 is the most demanding, and intensity zone 5 is the least demanding.
Note: During the rest interval, athletes can practice technical skills of low intensity (e.g., shooting the basketball).

TABLE 7.5 Example of Alternating Intensities During a Microcycle for a Team Sport

Day						
Monday	Tuesday	Wednesday	Thursday	Friday	Saturday	Sunday
1*	2	4	2	1	5	
3	5	5	3	4		
5			5	5		

*Intensity zone 1 is the most demanding and intensity zone 5 is the least demanding.
Note: Several intensities are planned for a given day. As per the planned intensities, Wednesday and Saturday are compensation days.

Alternating Intensity and Energy System Focus During a Microcycle

Alternating training intensities during a microcycle is one of the most effective methods to prevent **exhaustion,** staleness, and overtraining. The higher the intensity or power output of the activity, the greater the reliance on anaerobic energy supply (phosphagen and fast glycolytic). A plan that modulates the intensity of training will target a specific energy system, thus facilitating recovery and regeneration or stimulating adaptation. The structure of this variation will be dictated by the phase of training (preparatory versus competitive) and the need to supercompensate a specific energy system prior to competition. This is best accomplished through creating microcycle variations based on the interaction of exercise physiology and training methodology. A plan that is appropriately varied will greatly increase the athlete's probability of reaching peak performance at the appropriate time.

For most sports, the energy demand of the activity preferentially targets at least two energy systems (10, 15). Although the primary energy system targeted can be isolated, all of the energy systems are active at the same time and the intensity of the activity (i.e., power output) will dictate which energy systems are preferentially targeted (2). Therefore, a high intensity will increase the influence of the phosphagen and fast glycolytic systems, whereas a lower intensity will increase the emphasis on the slow glycolytic and oxidative systems (15). If the competition depletes the athlete's energy reserves, training intensity during the postcompetitive training days should be reduced. Reducing the intensity of training will dissipate cumulative fatigue, thus creating a microcycle that induces recovery and regeneration and thereby prepares the athlete for subsequent training.

Although it is important to alternate work and regeneration, it is not always necessary for the athlete to be completely recovered for the next bout of training. For example, during the preparatory phase of training, when the major focus is on developing a strong physiological foundation, the athlete will not fully recover and performance will not supercompensate. When the training demand is lowered in later unloading microcycles, the athlete's level of athletic shape (i.e., readiness) will be elevated and performance will increase. Therefore, during the preparatory phase of training, the plan can include developmental microcycles without allowing the athlete enough time to remove all of the accumulated fatigue. This process will challenge the athlete's physiological systems and result in greater performance improvements after future unloading microcycles. As a competition approaches, the fatigue generated in the preparatory phase can be reduced by alternating training intensities and lowering training volume; this stimulates physiological adaptations, removes fatigue, and allows physical parameters to supercompensate.

Alternating the focus on intensity and energy systems can be very difficult with complex sports (e.g., team sports) in which multiple energy systems play a large role in performance and the technical and tactical skills rely on all of those systems. Such activities can require the athlete to maximize power, speed, and high-intensity endurance in order to be successful. Thus, planning involves a conundrum in which many tasks must be trained to meet the demands of the sport without inducing overtraining. The best approach is to vary intensities of training, thereby changing the bioenergetic targets of training, to develop multiple facets of the athlete's physiology. A two-step process can be used to vary training intensities in an attempt to target specific energy systems.

The first step is to classify all of the skills and types of training according to the energy systems that are taxed. Table 7.6 gives an example of skill classification. Although this table can be used as a guideline for classifying skills, you may still want to systematically classify the skills and biomotor abilities that are relevant to the sport. One method for planning the daily training session is to target a specific energy system with all skills and physical training activities. Conversely, the daily session can target one training option and leave the balance of the other activities for other days.

The second step is to plan a microcycle that alternates the training options from table 7.6, in order to target specific energy systems. The alterations in training loads coupled with

TABLE 7.6 — Classification of Skills and Physical Training for Alternating Energy Systems

Anaerobic alactic day	Anaerobic lactic day	Aerobic day
1. Technical skills (1-10 s)	1. Technical skills (10-60 s)	1. Long-duration technical skills (>60 s)
2. Tactical skills (5-10 s)	2. Tactical skills (10-60 s)	2. Long- and medium-duration tactical skills (>60 s)
3. Acceleration and maximum speed	3. Speed endurance (10-60 s)	3. Aerobic endurance
4. Maximum strength and power	4. Power endurance, muscle endurance short	4. Medium and long muscle endurance

Reprinted, by permission, from T.O. Bompa and C. Buzzichelli, 2015, *Periodization training for sports*, 3rd ed. (Champaign, IL: Human Kinetics), 169.

appropriate nutrition will allow the athlete to restore energy sources, facilitating physiological adaptations that will eventually increase performance.

In terms of microcycles that alternate energy systems, these types of training cycles are not planned throughout the annual plan. During some phases of training, fatigue must be dissipated to stimulate supercompensation, whereas in other phases high levels of fatigue are generated to challenge the athlete's physiology to adapt. Even though the training loads are alternated in these microcycles, it is likely that the overall training demand will create a large amount of fatigue, which will decreases preparedness and ultimately suppress the supercompensation effect.

Several examples of how to manipulate the training demand are presented in this chapter (see the figures in the sections that follow). Alternating the training demand will challenge the athlete on some training days, which will induce a high level of fatigue; on other days fatigue will be removed in response to a less challenging training bout. Each sample microcycle contains a diagram of the dynamics of fatigue or supercompensation in response to various training sessions.

Team sports are very complex, and a single training session for these sports will stress multiple energy systems as well as the neuromuscular system (technique, maximum speed, strength, and power). Figure 7.26 gives an example of how the microcycle can be varied. Monday's session taxes the neuromuscular, phosphagen, and glycolytic energy systems. Activities involving speed, power, and maximum strength training performed for short durations rely

Day	Microcycle day						
	M	T	W	Th	F	Sa	Su
Training demand	Technique	Tactical	Technique	Tactical	Technique	Technical or tactical	
	Speed	Endurance		Endurance	Speed	Endurance	
	Power or maximum strength		Power or maximum strength		Power or maximum strength		
Theoretical fatigue curve							

FIGURE 7.26 Microcycle to be used at the end of the preparatory phase of training for a team sport.

on ATP-PCr as fuel. However, a large volume of these activities, requiring inadequate rest intervals to restore creatine phosphate, can deplete glycogen stores. Depending on the volume and intensity of training, the rate of recovery from Monday's workout should be relatively quick, allowing the athlete to perform Tuesday's training session without much fatigue.

In a traditional plan in which the athlete experiences high levels of physiological stress almost every day, the demanding session occurring on Monday in figure 7.26 could nearly deplete the glycogen stores and produce a high level of accumulated fatigue. Alternating training intensities may help the athlete better manage this fatigue. For example, in figure 7.26 Monday is a training day with a high amount of physiological stress, whereas Tuesday's training session contains tactical and endurance training performed at a much lower intensity. The remainder of the microcycle alternates training stressors in order to modulate fatigue.

Another example of how one might alternate training stressors during a microcycle is presented in figure 7.27. This figure presents a hypothetical model for a sport in which speed and power are dominant. Training for speed and power occurs on the same day as power endurance training, which is marked by repeating power exercises 10 to 25 times per set. Two high-intensity training days, in which the phosphagen and glycolytic systems are taxed, precede a training day that focuses on tempo training and the development of endurance (compensation).

Figure 7.28 is a microcycle for a sport that is dominated by aerobic endurance capacity and therefore relies predominantly on **oxidative metabolism**. The plan simultaneously includes types of strength training that tax the same energy system on that particular day. Consequently, muscular endurance or high-volume (many repetitions) strength training is performed after the bout of endurance training. Higher-intensity activities (maximum strength or power endurance training) occur on the day that specifically taxes the phosphagen and glycolytic systems. Event-specific intensity training is performed on Thursday. This type of targeted training is sometimes termed **ergogenesis**.

Figure 7.29 shows a microcycle structure for an endurance sport in which competition lasts between 4 and 6 min. In this example, high-intensity endurance that stresses both the phosphagen and glycolytic systems is important for a successful performance. Days that target the development of high-intensity endurance (i.e., produce significant glycolytic stress) are followed by low-intensity aerobic work that is used as a compensation activity. The goal is to develop the ability to produce high levels of lactic acid formation, and then buffer this

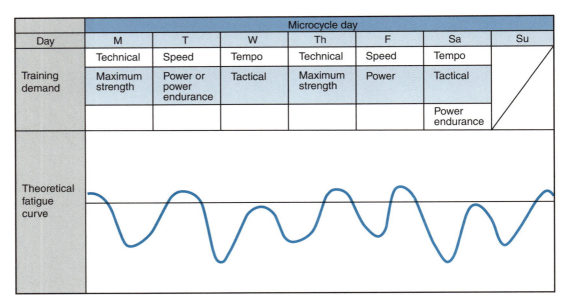

FIGURE 7.27 Alternating training stress for a sport that requires speed and power.

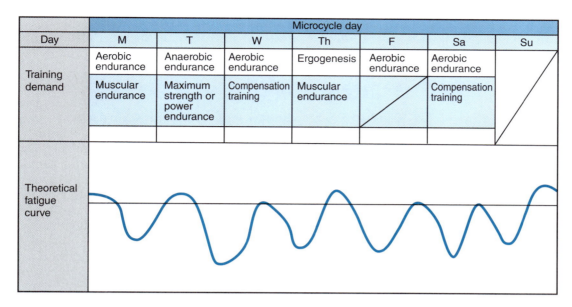

FIGURE 7.28 Alternating training stress for a sport where endurance is dominant.

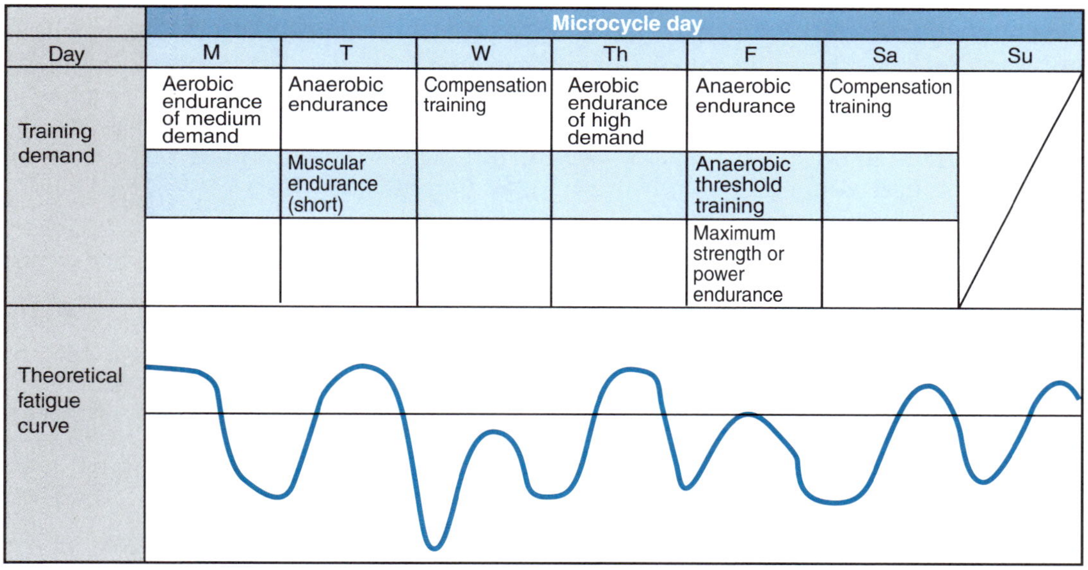

FIGURE 7.29 Alternating training stress for a sport that requires endurance for 4 to 6 min (aerobic power).

lactic acid and remove it quickly, inducing a faster recovery rate. In this example, days that follow high-intensity interval training are always followed by compensation training days designed to enhance recovery.

Macrocycle

The term *macro* is derived from the Greek word *makros,* meaning "large." A training macrocycle is a phase that lasts 2 to 6 weeks or microcycles. The microcycle is used to plan for the immediate future, whereas the macrocycle projects the structure of a training program several weeks in advance. Therefore, one could think of the macrocycle as the general structure of training and a projection for the future, whereas the microcycle is the exact plan used to accomplish the targeted goals.

Duration of a Macrocycle

Although the macrocycle plans used to prepare athletes for various sporting activities may have some similarities, it is likely that each sport will have requirements that must be addressed. These requirements will in most instances dictate the macrocycle structure. The loading structure and the duration of the macrocycles may be different depending on the sport and the phase of training. Therefore, the macrocycle must be crafted carefully to meet the individual athlete's training objectives. Table 7.7 presents a macrocycle structure for the strength training plan of an American university women's soccer team.

When establishing the length of the macrocycle, the coach must consider the phase of training. During the preparatory phase, the macrocycle is generally longer (4 to 7 weeks) than those in the competition phase to address the objectives of this portion of the annual training plan. In this context the macrocycle should be long enough to develop biomotor abilities, technical skills, or tactical elements. Therefore, one method for determining a macrocycle's length is to consider the time necessary to perfect an ability or its components.

The macrocycle structure is also influenced by the competitive schedule. During the competitive phase, macrocycles are shorter in accordance with the competitive schedule, and contain two or three 1-week microcycles. Competitions should fall at the end of the unloading microcycle, which coincides with the end of the macrocycle; this will give the coach information about the athlete's progress toward the target performance level. If the competition phase contains several competitions during the month (possibly as many as eight), as typically seen in team sports, the coach must decide which competitions are the most important. In this type of macrocycle structure, less emphasis is placed on the minor competitions because they are simply used to train through and to provide feedback on the

TABLE 7.7 Macrocycle Structures for the Strength Training of an American University Women's Soccer Team

Month	May	June	July	August	September	October	November
Phase	Preparatory	Preparatory	Precompetitive	Precompetitive	Competitive	Competitive	Competitive
Focus	Anatomical adaptation	Maximum strength (70%-85% 1RM)	Power and agility		Maintenance	Maintenance	Peaking
Number of microcycles	4	4	6	2	4	4	4
Emphasis on training objectives							
Muscular endurance	High	Moderate	Low	—	Low	Low	—
Strength	Moderate	High	Moderate	Low	Low	Low	Low
Power	Low	Moderate	High	Moderate	Moderate	Moderate	Low
Speed	—	Low	Moderate	High	Moderate	Moderate	Moderate

athlete's preparation for the major contest. Therefore, the length of the macrocycle should allow for the last microcycle to lead into the major competition.

Structural Consideration for a Macrocycle

The development of the macrocycle structure is based on the objectives, the phase of training, and the competition schedule. Therefore, the macrocycles of the annual training plan should vary according to the training objectives for each phase of the plan (i.e., preparatory, competitive, and transition phases).

Macrocycles for the Preparatory Phase

The main objective of the preparatory phase is to induce physiological, psychological, and technical adaptations that will serve as the foundation for competitive performances. A disturbing trend in some sports is the use of year-round competitive schedules. This schedule will limit the athlete's performance capacity because too little time is dedicated to the preparatory phase of training. In an appropriately constructed annual training plan, the preparatory phase is a crucial part of the plan and is the foundation for competitive success.

Developmental macrocycles are well suited for the preparatory phase of training. The training demand of developmental macrocycles usually follows the step-loading method. Figure 7.30 depicts two step-loading examples, the 4:1 and the 3:1 loading patterns. In the 4:1 loading pattern, the training load is increased across four microcycles, and unloading or regeneration is planned for the last microcycle. This loading pattern works well during the very early part of the preparatory phase when the athlete is attempting to develop a physiological base, correct technical habits, and learn new technical or tactical skills. A 3:1 loading pattern is also well suited for the preparatory phase and is probably the most common loading plan. This loading pattern fits well with the body's natural biocycles (5). The 3:1 loading pattern contains three microcycles with increasing workloads, followed by a regeneration or unloading microcycle. If the level of fatigue is very high after the third microcycle, the load used in the fourth microcycle can be decreased even further, or a second regeneration microcycle can be used to create a 3:2 loading pattern. The higher the training stress during the macrocycle, the longer the time before the athlete shows improvement in

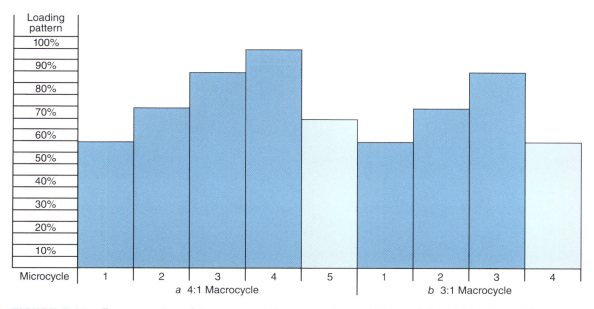

FIGURE 7.30 Two examples of developmental macrocycles: *(a)* 4:1 model and *(b)* 3:1 model.

performance or a supercompensation effect (4). Halson and colleagues reported that after 2 weeks of very high loading demands, 2 weeks of unloading are needed to return performance capacity to preloading levels.

Macrocycles for the Competitive Phase

The dynamics of the competitive macrocycles are dictated by the competition calendar. Because of this relationship, there are numerous sport-specific macrocycle structures.

A steady loading pattern should be used throughout the competitive season with team sports in which there are one or two competitions per week. Within this structure, microcycles will vary in intensity and volume, especially microcycles that contain competitions. In these microcycles, the contests will be interspersed with regeneration days and training days that fluctuate between various levels of demand (low to high). To address the unique loading demands of team sports, coaches should consider using various microcycle loading patterns.

The macrocycle loading pattern can be 4:1, 3:1, 2:1, 1:1, 2:2, or any other combination. Longer macrocycles (4:1, 3:1) are usually employed during general preparation. During specific preparation, 3:1 and 2:1 are the typical macrocycles structures, where the 2:1 is used mainly for power sports in the flat loading format. During the competitive phase, the unloading microcycles (which allow fatigue to dissipate and performance to elevate) are employed more frequently. Thus the most common macrocycle structures are 2:1, 1:1, and 2:2. Two consecutive unloading microcycles (to taper, as explained in the next section) can be planned to peak for an important competition or for when a team faces strong opponents in two consecutive weekends.

Another important consideration regarding the structure of the macrocycles is the number of peaks contained in the phase. For example, in the macrocycle presented in figure 7.31, the qualification competition occurs on July 9 and the main competition on August 14. No

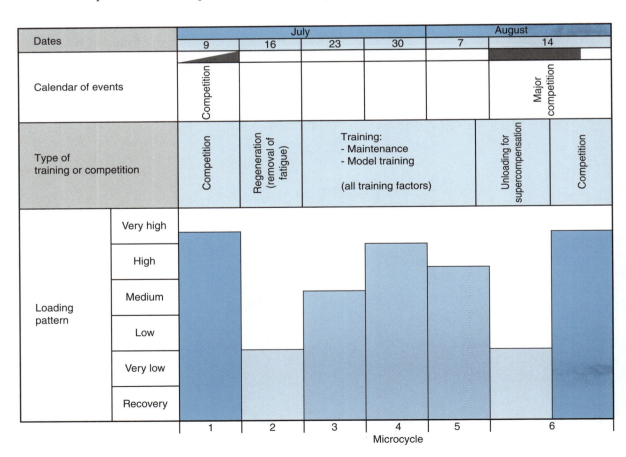

FIGURE 7.31 Macrocycle structure for two important competitions.

other competitions are planned in the microcycles between these two important dates. The results of the qualification contest are used as markers of progress toward the major contest and serve as guidelines for modifying before the major contest. If additional contests are planned between these two contests, the focus will be on performing well instead of training. Additionally, if the number of contests is increased during this macrocycle the athlete would experience a significant increase in fatigue, which might impede performance in the major contests at the end of the cycle.

In figure 7.31 the two competitions are separated by several microcycles. The first microcycle after the qualifying competition is a regeneration microcycle designed to dissipate fatigue and allow the athlete to recover from the stress of the first competition. The next three microcycles are used to fine-tune technical skills, tactical strategies, and physical capacity. These microcycles are designed to build the athlete's confidence in his abilities and develop the motivational levels necessary to produce a maximal performance at the major event on August 14. The 8 to 14 days prior to the August 14 competition are used for peaking (refer to figure 9.3 in chapter 9). During this time the training load is decreased to elevate the level of readiness and, as a result to decrease fatigue. If the peaking phase is structured correctly, performance will be significantly elevated.

Macrocycles for Unloading and Tapering for Competitions

The goal of unloading and tapering macrocycles is to remove fatigue to stimulate a supercompensation of performance. Optimal taper or unloading durations appear to be between 8 and 14 days and require a decrease in training load of about 40% to 60% (8). Four strategies for decreasing the load are available: linear, slow decay, fast decay, or step taper (12). The type and duration of taper are largely determined by the training load encountered in the weeks before the taper period. For example, if the training load is high, the taper or unloading period may require a longer duration and a greater reduction in training load. The basic tapering strategies appear to be effective in many sports including weightlifting, track and field, and swimming. Additional information on tapering strategies can be found in chapter 9.

Macrocycles for the Transition Phase

The transition phase is an important part of the annual training plan. A basic macrocycle structure for a transition phase is presented in figure 7.32. More details about the structure of the transition phase are provided in chapter 8.

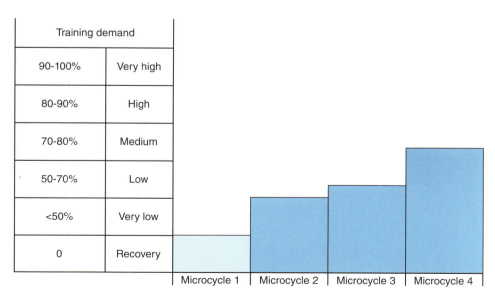

FIGURE 7.32 Loading pattern for a transition macrocycle.

Summary of Major Concepts

The microcycle is the most important and functional part of the annual training plan. The macrocycle is useful for dividing the annual training plan into smaller segments. Ultimately, the macrocycle directs the focus of the microcycle to fulfill the goals of the annual training plan.

A microcycle must provide variation in the training load (volume and intensity) to facilitate recovery. The technique used to create this variation in training load is based on the scientific principles related to the ability of the body to recover from training stress. The application of these microcycle models is based on many physiological factors that relate to the body's ability to tolerate, recover from, and adapt to training stress. If the training loads are varied appropriately, the athlete will be able to recover from and tolerate the training demand, which ultimately improves performance. Nevertheless, the microcycle program must not be interpreted rigidly; rather, adjustments can be made upon subjective feedback and objective data based on the athlete's individual response to the training loads. The acceptable levels of residual fatigue vary in accordance with the objectives of the training session and the phase of the annual plan.

It is important to vary the loading patterns between the microcycles. This allows the training load to be varied across the macrocycle so the athlete can deal with accumulated fatigue and avoid overtraining. The coach must appropriately sequence developmental, competition, recovery–regeneration, and peaking–unloading microcycles.

The microcycle and macrocycle are structured to direct training so that the athlete will achieve a physiological and psychological peak at the appropriate time. The training plan should be based on the concepts of bioenergetic specificity of training, muscle physiology, hormonal physiology, and the body's response to training stress. To better guide the training program, the coach should consider quantifying the training stress with the numerical intensity and volume system outlined in this chapter.

Periodization of the Annual Plan

8

Efficiency is one of the most desired qualities of any professional. To be efficient, coaches must be well organized and use periodization as a tool for planning an athlete's training. Even coaches who are extremely knowledgeable can compromise their effectiveness if they lack good planning skills. For this reason, this book focuses on periodization, which can be used by sports professionals to craft a wide variety of plans.

A well-organized coach has at his disposal several types of plans, including short-term plans (e.g., daily session plans), microcycles and macrocycles, and annual plans. At the beginning of a new year of training, the coach should create a blueprint, or annual plan. Although this plan has to be as detailed as possible, equally important for the coach is to also apply it in a very flexible manner. This actually means that based on the results in testing, training progress and eventual competitions, the original plan might be slightly or profoundly altered. The coach should reflect on the progress or stagnation of the evolution of performance of the athlete, and as a result, make changes in the plan. Be prepared to be flexible; planning and programming should not be rigid.

Annual Training Plan and Its Characteristics

The annual plan and its training phases are essential tools used to maximize an athlete's physiological adaptation, which is a prerequisite for improved performance. Without the progression of training demand from phase to phase, high performance cannot be achieved. During the last month of training (the transition phase), the plan will vary from the rest of the training year to reduce physiological and psychological stress, remove fatigue, induce regeneration, and prepare the athlete for the next year of training.

The goal of training is to induce physiological adaptations and maximize performance at specific points in time, usually during the main competitions of the year. To accomplish this goal, the athlete's physiological potential must increase at the appropriate time, thereby ensuring a greater potential for a high level of performance. The athlete's level of readiness for competitions requires a complex interaction of skills, biomotor abilities, psychological traits, well-planned nutrition, and the management of fatigue. The best approach for accomplishing these goals is to use periodized training that is logically constructed and appropriately sequenced.

The annual plan is the foundation for stimulating physiological and psychological adaptations while managing fatigue. In the context of this plan, the greatest challenge is peaking the athlete at the appropriate times throughout the training year. When working with inexperienced athletes, the coach will direct the training plan with little input from the athletes. Conversely, with elite athletes the coach should encourage input from the athletes when establishing the annual training plan's objectives and structure. By involving elite athletes in the planning process, the coach can create a positive environment in which the athlete can use the planning process as a motivational tool.

The annual training plan should contain at least three training phases: preparatory, competitive, and transition. The number of times these three phases are performed will depend on the type of plan used (e.g., monocycle, bi-cycle, tri-cycle, **multipeak**). The objectives and characteristics of these phases remain consistent regardless of how many times they are repeated throughout the annual training plan. To optimize the athlete's development throughout the annual training plan and elevate training potential and readiness for competitions, each training phase must be correctly sequenced, completely integrated, and properly structured.

Preparatory Phase

The preparatory phase is probably the most important phase of the annual training plan. This phase establishes the physical, technical, and psychological base from which the competitive phase is developed. The adaptations developed as a result of the increased volume of training in this phase will allow the athlete to better tolerate the increase in training intensity that occurs in the competitive phase. However, if the preparatory phase is inadequate, the athlete's ability to tolerate training and maximize performance during the competitive phase will be compromised. The preparatory phase has the following objectives:

- To acquire and improve general physical training capacity
- To improve the biomotor abilities required by the sport
- To cultivate psychological traits
- To develop, improve, or perfect technique
- To familiarize athletes with the basic strategic maneuvers mastered in the following phase
- To teach athletes the theory and methodology of training specific to the sport
- To develop an individualized and sport-specific nutrition plan

The preparatory phase lasts 3 to 6 months depending on the climate, sport, and type of annual plan used (e.g., monocycle, bi-cycle, tri-cycle, multipeak). For individual sports, especially the aerobic endurance sports (e.g., marathon, triathlon, Nordic skiing), the preparatory phase is approximately twice as long as the competitive phase; for team sports the preparatory phase may be somewhat shorter, but not less than 2 to 3 months, especially for younger athletes. For international-class players, however, this phase can only be 3 to 5 weeks long, for organizational reasons, such as their competition schedule. The preparatory phase is specific to each sport and distinctive for each subphase (table 8.1). For any sport, the preparatory phase should be divided into two subphases: general and specific preparation. For international-class athletes that use a multipeak plan (e.g., team or racquet sports), the general subphase is very short.

General Preparation Subphase

The general preparation subphase is used to elevate the athlete's working capacity, increase general physical preparation, improve technical elements, and enhance basic tactical abilities. The primary emphasis of this subphase is to establish a high level of physical conditioning, which will improve the athlete's physiological and psychological capacity to tolerate the demands of both training and competition. Regardless of the sport, a sound physical base is an essential component for the athlete. Typically, the base is established through the use of general and sport-specific exercises, rather than a reliance on sport-specific skill development. For instance, a gymnastics coach may dedicate the first two or three microcycles to the development of general and specific strength needed to master a certain technical element in the following cycles. This concept is valid for other sports in which certain physical attributes can limit technical progress. Many times the inability to develop technical skill is the result of an inadequately developed physical base. Therefore, it may be warranted to determine whether the athlete possesses adequate physical support for the technical performance of an element or skill.

TABLE 8.1 — Training Objectives for Each Subphase of the Preparatory Phase

Sport	Dominant training factor	Subphase: General preparation	Subphase: Specific preparation
Gymnastics	Physical Technical	General and maximum strength Technical elements	Specific strength and power Elements, half and skeleton of full routine
Rowing	Physical	Aerobic endurance Anatomical adaptation Maximum strength Muscular endurance	Anaerobic endurance Aerobic endurance Muscular endurance
Swimming (100 m)	Physical	Aerobic endurance Anatomical adaptation Maximum strength	Anaerobic endurance Aerobic endurance Maximum strength Maximum power
Swimming (800 m)	Physical	Aerobic endurance Anatomical adaptation Maximum strength	Aerobic endurance Anaerobic endurance Muscular endurance
Team sports	Technical Tactical Physical	Technical elements Individual and simple team tactics High-intensity exercise endurance General and maximum strength	Apply technical elements in game situations Team tactics Anaerobic endurance Power development

Throughout this subphase the plan includes a high training volume, consisting of exercises that require both general and specific effort. The goal is to improve working capacity and psychological drive (determination, perseverance, and willpower) necessary for the sport. For example, the development of aerobic endurance is the main objective for sports in which endurance is the dominant ability or a major contributor to performance (e.g., running, swimming, rowing, Nordic skiing, cycling). For these sports 70% to 80% of the total training time may be devoted to the development of aerobic endurance, which can be seen in the miles or kilometers covered in training. In sports for which strength, power, and speed are important attributes, this subphase will focus on the development of anatomical adaptations and maximum strength. Increasing the weight lifted or the volume load of training is an objective way to increase working capacity and induce adaptations necessary for the sporting activity.

The process is somewhat different for team sport athletes: While developing the physical base, these athletes must also spend substantial time developing technical and tactical skills. Although technical and tactical improvements are important aspects of the training process, the plan must not neglect the development of high-intensity exercise, endurance, strength, and speed because these components of the physical base lay the groundwork for future performance accomplishments.

In most sports, the type of training used in the preparatory phase, especially the general subphase, plays a major role in determining the athlete's performance capacity during the competitive phase. Insufficient emphasis on training volume during this subphase may account for poor performances, lack of consistency, and a decrease in performance capacity during the later portion of the competitive phase. Consequently, 25% to 33% of the training for the preparatory phase should be allocated to this subphase, with the rest of the preparation phase consisting of sport-specific preparatory activities. The duration of the general

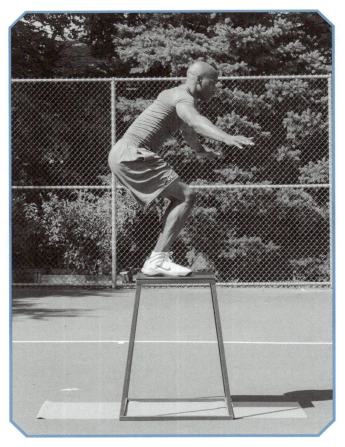

Establishing a high level of physical conditioning is important before beginning specific training tasks.

preparation phase will be longer for novice athletes and should be progressively reduced for advanced athletes. A characteristic of the general preparation phase for team sports is the priority given to physical training in the organization of the microcycles. During this phase, coaches often plan physical training in the morning, when players are recovered from the training of the previous day, and leave the afternoon for technical and tactical training.

Increasing training volume during the general preparation subphase is the primary emphasis; although training intensity is important, it is a secondary factor in the preparatory phase. Intensive training can be undertaken but should not exceed 40% of the total amount of training in this subphase, particularly for beginners and juniors. It is important to remember the objective of increasing working capacity during this subphase. With the increases in training, volume fatigue will increase markedly, and thus, preparedness will decrease greatly, reducing performance capacity. Therefore, it is inadvisable to compete during this subphase because the athlete will have a high level of fatigue, which will reduce performance capacity and increase the risk for injury (12). When the athlete is highly fatigued as a result of training, technical skills will be relatively unstable and the athlete's ability to perform specific tactical maneuvers will decrease. Competition during this subphase also can negatively affect the athlete's psychological status, and it decreases the amount of time that can be dedicated to developing the physiological base needed to expand the athlete's capabilities.

Specific Preparation Subphase

The specific preparation subphase, or the second part of the preparatory phase, represents a transition from an emphasis on physical development to an emphasis on competition-related activities. Like the general preparation subphase, the specific preparation subphase has the objective of increasing the athlete's working capacity. However, in this subphase training emphasizes sport-specific activities. Although the volume of work is high during this subphase, the primary emphasis (70% to 80% of total work) is on specific exercises related to the skills or technical elements of the sport. Toward the end of this phase the volume begins to progressively decrease, allowing for a gradual increase in the training intensity.

For sports in which intensity is important (e.g., sprinting, jumping, and team sports), the training volume may be lowered by as much as 40% in the later portions of this subphase. A different approach would be taken for sports that rely on technical mastery and coordinated movements (e.g., figure skating, diving, gymnastics). In these sports it is essential that the athlete continue to perfect and develop the technical proficiency necessary for success during the competitive phase. Similarly, in team sports, racket sports, and martial arts, the specific preparation subphase should focus on the development and improvement of sport-specific technical and tactical elements. This is accomplished with specific exercises that target the prime movers, movement patterns, and technical skills required by the sport. These exercises must be performed in such a way as to create a link between the physical attributes developed in the general preparation subphase and the technical and tactical skills necessary for successful competition. Although the major emphasis is on technical and tactical skill development, a secondary emphasis should be on maintaining general physical development. This secondary focus should contain only a few exercises for general development (a maximum of 20%) that contribute to the athlete's multilateral development.

As the athlete's training shifts toward specialized training, there should be progressive improvement in performance-based testing and athletic performance. In the later stages of this subphase, competitions can be used as evaluative tools that provide feedback about the athlete's preparation for competition, specifically her technical and tactical development. Information garnered from these competitions can be used to modify training plans to address specific deficiencies.

Competitive Phase

Among the main tasks of the competitive phase is the perfection of all training factors, which enables the athlete to compete successfully in the main competitions or championships targeted by the annual training plan. Several general objectives are addressed during the competitive phase, regardless of the sport:

- Continued improvement or maintenance of sport-specific biomotor abilities
- Enhancing psychological traits
- Perfecting and consolidating technique
- Elevating performance to the highest level
- Dissipating fatigue and elevating readiness
- Perfecting technical and tactical maneuvers
- Gaining competitive experience
- Maintaining sport-specific fitness
- Designing an individualized nutrition plan

As the athlete progresses to the competitive phase, it is important that the level of physical development established during the preparatory phase be maintained. Maintenance of the physical attributes developed in previous phases is important because they support the other training factors that are developed during the competitive phase. This can be accomplished by dedicating 90% of the total physical preparation activities to sport-specific activities, such as skill-based conditioning exercises and tactical drills in racquet and team sports. The remaining 10% of the planned physical preparation activities can come from nonspecific or indirect activities, such as active rest or game-based activities that are not directly related to the sport being trained.

The objectives established for the competitive phase are met by the use of sport-specific training activities that can include technical and tactical exercises. Included in this process may be the use of simulated, exhibition, and actual competitive events. It is essential that the training activities are sport specific to stimulate performance improvement, stabilization, and consistency. As the athlete progresses through the competitive phase, training becomes more intensive while training volume is decreased. For sports dominated by speed, power, and maximum strength (e.g., sprinting, jumping, throwing, weightlifting), training intensity can increase dramatically while the volume of training is progressively decreased. In endurance sports (e.g., distance running, swimming, cross-country skiing, canoeing, rowing), training volume can be maintained or only slightly lower than that seen in the preparatory phase. An exception to this practice occurs during the competitive microcycle, when intensity decreases according to the number of races and the level of competition.

As the athlete progresses through the competitive phase, the alterations to the training plan should elevate readiness to achieve high performance. The structure of the training plan will play a large role in stimulating these effects; if the plan is structured correctly, the athlete will optimize performance at the appropriate time. If performance begins to decline or becomes stagnant, it is likely that the amount of work was decreased too much, reducing physical capacity, or that the work was maintained at too high a level and fatigue is masking the potential performance gains. The modulation between work and performance appears to be an art based on science, and the integration of athlete monitoring and coaching experience will guide the decisions made during this phase of training.

The length of the competitive phase depends on the sport and the type of annual training plan. Long competitive phases (8 to 10 months) are typically seen in team sports as a result of the set league schedules and international championships. Conversely, athletes in individual sports have more freedom in determining their competitive schedule, allowing for more control over the length of the competitive phase and the structure of training leading into the major competition of the year. Regardless of the sport, one of the most important factors in determining the duration and structure of the competitive phase is the phase's start date. When structuring the competitive phase and its start date consider the following parameters:

- The number of competitions required to reach the highest performance (on average it takes between 7 and 10 competitions to achieve the highest performance results
- The amount of time or interval between competitions
- The duration of eventual qualifying meets
- The time required for special preparation before the main competition of the year
- The time needed for recovery and regeneration

When structuring the competitive phase of the annual training plan, it may be warranted to divide the phase into two subphases: the precompetitive subphase and the main competitive subphase.

Precompetitive Subphase

The precompetitive phase generally contains unofficial competitions or, in the case of team sports, exhibition games. Although this subphase is an integral part of the competitive phase, the objective is not to achieve the highest level of competition. This subphase should serve

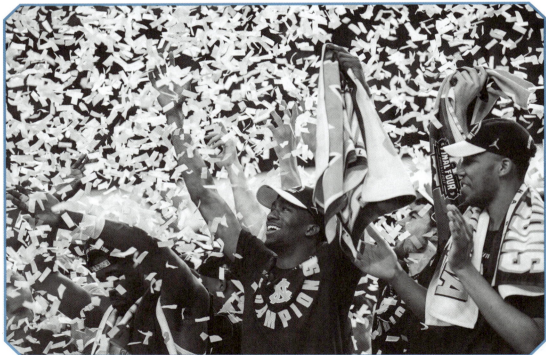

Annual training plans should be structured to account for the possibility of reaching a major championship competition.

as a training tool in which the athlete participates in exhibitions or unofficial competitions as a means of preparing for later events. One of the main reasons for the use of exhibition or unofficial contests is to allow for objective feedback about the athlete's training level and readiness for future contests. These competitions will allow for the evaluation of all technical, tactical, and physical skills under competitive conditions. Exhibitions and unofficial competitions should not significantly alter the training program, especially for elite athletes, because these contests provide a testing ground for the main competitive subphase, when the official contests begin.

Main Competitive Subphase

The main competitive subphase is dedicated strictly to maximizing an athlete's capacity and readiness, thus allowing for superior performances at the main contests. The number of training sessions contained in this subphase should reflect whether the athlete is participating in a loading or regeneration (unloading) microcycle. A loading microcycle may have 10 to 14 sessions per week, whereas an unloading microcycle will contain many fewer sessions, thus facilitating a decrease in fatigue and an elevation in preparedness prior to the competition. The training content of this subphase should be centered on sport-specific methods and the maintenance of specific physical development.

Although the training volume may still be high for endurance sports, the coach can reduce the training volume to 50% to 75% of the level of the preparatory phase for sports that require technical mastery, speed, strength, or power. While volume is decreasing, the intensity of training gradually increases, with the highest levels occurring 2 or 3 weeks prior to the main competition.

The stress curve will be elevated during the competitive phase as a result of the increased intensity of training and the stress of participation in competitions. The stress curve should have an undulating shape, reflecting the fluctuations between stressful activities (e.g., competitions, intense training sessions, social factors) and short periods of regeneration. The harder a competition or training session, the higher the stress curve and the longer the compensation phase needed to reduce the amount of accumulated stress or fatigue.

If possible, the coach should arrange competitions progressively in order of importance, concluding with the main competitions. Another organizational strategy is to introduce main competitions interspersed with lesser competitions that allow the athlete to continue to train without visible changes in the training plan (e.g., lowering volume or intensity) and without longer unloading periods to trigger peak performance.

By including six to eight microcycles prior to the main competition, the coach can focus the training program and daily cycle on the specific requirements of the competition. This will maximize the athlete's physical, technical, tactical, and psychological preparations for the main competition. Preparing the athlete for the specific competitive environment and demands will prevent any surprises and enhance the athlete's performance. In this portion of the competitive phase, 8 to 14 days of unloading will be used to peak the athlete (see chapter 9).

Unloading or Tapering Subphase The unloading or tapering subphase offers the best way to elevate the athlete's readiness and stimulate a supercompensation of performance that will increase the athlete's performance potential during the competition. Peaking is accomplished via manipulating both volume and intensity to reduce the accumulated fatigue stimulated from previous training and competition; this will allow the athlete to rest and regenerate before the major competition.

The unloading or tapering subphase, especially for individual sports, should last 8 to 14 days and can include various methods of reducing volume and training intensity (see chapter 9). The strategy for unloading during this subphase depends largely on the type of training undertaken and the individual sport. Classically, for endurance sports, it is advisable to reduce intensity and maintain volume because endurance athletes are better adapted to tolerate high-volume training than high-intensity training (figure 8.1). During the first microcycle

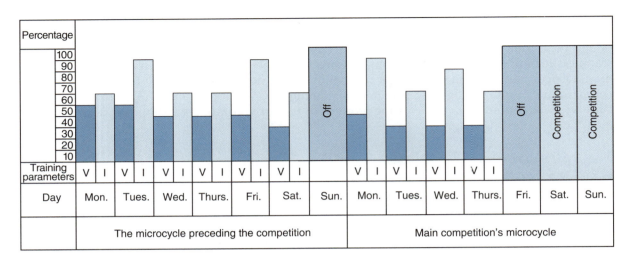

FIGURE 8.1 Unloading phase for an endurance sport.

Reprinted, by permission, from T.O. Bompa and C. Buzzichelli, 2015, *Periodization training for sports,* 3rd ed. (Champaign, IL: Human Kinetics), 327.

of unloading, the process will involve reducing the number of daily training sessions and modulating training intensity to begin the recovery process. The coach should eliminate all extraneous activities that can contribute to the athlete's fatigue and encourage the athlete to use free time to rest and recover for the impending competition. In this portion of the unloading period, it may be warranted to reduce the volume and frequency (two sessions per week) of strength training. Further reductions in the volume and intensity of training may be planned during the second microcycle of the unloading period. This can be accomplished by limiting strength training to one or two sessions, or by removing strength training completely depending on the sport. The volume and intensity of other training factors also should be reduced.

The same unloading approach is used for sports dominated by speed, power, or technical proficiency. In the first microcycle, the training volume is reduced by 40% to 50%, depending on the level of training undertaken prior to the taper. This period should include several short but high-intensity sessions to maintain the adaptations induced by previous training phases (figure 8.2). A two-peak microcycle structure may be used during the first microcycle of this subphase, but long rest intervals need to be included between repetitions to help

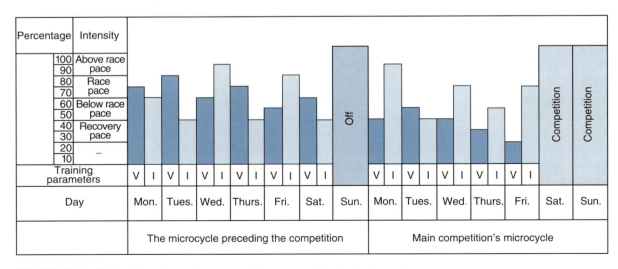

FIGURE 8.2 Unloading phase for a speed- or power-dominated sport.

Reprinted, by permission, from T.O. Bompa and C. Buzzichelli, 2015, *Periodization training for sports,* 3rd ed. (Champaign, IL: Human Kinetics), 327.

dissipate fatigue and stress. During the high-intensity training session, all exercises should be dynamic and of short duration and should contain medium- to high-intensity loading. The other sessions in the microcycle should alternate submaximal intensities between low and very low intensities. With these types of sports, the volume and frequency of strength training should be reduced while maintaining moderate to high intensities with slightly longer rest intervals. Complete removal of strength training may not be warranted because power and speed are highly dependent on strength levels.

During the second microcycle of this subphase, in which the main competition occurs, the coach continues to reduce training volume and the intensity of training. Only one peak occurs during the early portion of this microcycle. Across this microcycle the objective is to maximally reduce fatigue and stress while increasing preparedness and maintaining the physiological adaptations that have been established.

A slightly different approach may be used when working with team sports where both training volume and intensity are equally important. During the first microcycle of the unloading phase, the coach should reduce the work volume to produce the unloading effect (figure 8.3). This can be accomplished by progressively reducing intensity across the microcycle while having two intense training sessions of 50% to 60% of maximum. During the second microcycle of this subphase, the coach should continue to reduce the volume and intensity of training, reducing volume to a greater extent than intensity. This subphase can include a two-peak microcycle, where the first peak is performed at a higher intensity than the second (15% to 20% less than the first peak). Two days prior to the competition, the athlete should undergo short training sessions of low to very low intensities. For more details on tapering or peaking athletes for competition, refer to chapter 9.

Special Preparation Period The special preparation period can be organized separately or in concert with the unloading phase and contains activities designed to enhance performance in the most important competition of the year. The special preparation period can last between 3 and 7 days, depending on the characteristics of the competition. During this phase certain training aspects, especially tactical elements, are altered according to the latest information on opponents or the competitive schedule. The vast majority of the training in this phase follows the model concept, with the purpose of enhancing preparation for the upcoming competition. One aspect that has important implications for the final result is the special psychological preparations that target relaxation, confidence building, and motivation. However, these techniques should be used cautiously because overemphasis on psychological elements can impair performance. Each athlete is different and will require specific preparation activities to meet his individual needs.

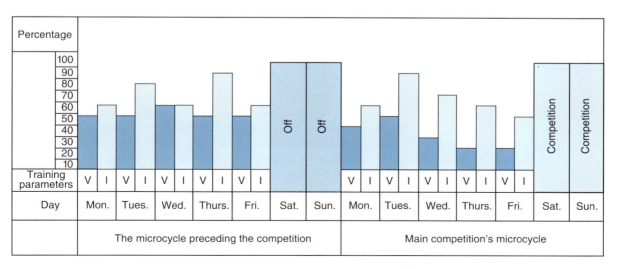

FIGURE 8.3 Unloading phase for a team sport.

Reprinted, by permission, from T.O. Bompa and C. Buzzichelli, 2015, *Periodization training for sports*, 3rd ed. (Champaign, IL: Human Kinetics), 329.

Transition Phase

After long periods of training, hard work, and stressful competitions in which both physiological and psychological fatigue can accumulate, a transition period should be used to link annual training plans or preparation for another major competition, as in the case of the bi-cycle, tri-cycle, and multicycle annual training plan. The transition phase serves an important role in preparing the athlete for the next training cycle. The athlete should start the new preparatory phase only when fully recovered from the previous competitive season. If the athlete initiates a new preparatory phase without full recovery, it is likely that performances will be impaired in future competitive cycles and the risk of injury will increase.

The transition phase, often inappropriately called the off-season, links two annual training plans. This phase facilitates psychological rest, relaxation, and biological regeneration while maintaining an acceptable level of general physical preparation (40% to 50% of the competitive phase). Training should be low key: All loading factors should be reduced; the main training components should be centered on general training, with minimal, if any, technical or tactical development. The transition phase generally should last 2 to 4 weeks but could be extended to 6 weeks, especially for younger athletes. Under normal circumstances the transition phase should not last longer than 6 weeks.

There are two common approaches to the transition phase. The first (incorrect) approach encourages complete rest with no physical activity; in this case, the term *off-season* fits perfectly. This abrupt interruption of training and the complete inactivity can lead to significant detraining even if only undertaken for a short period of time (<4 weeks). This detraining effect can cause a substantial loss in the physiological adaptations established in the previous months of training.

Some authors have suggested that an abrupt cessation of training by highly trained athletes creates a phenomenon known as **detraining syndrome**, relaxation syndrome (20, 21), exercise abstinence, or exercise dependency syndrome (18). This type of detraining appears to occur in athletes who either intentionally cease training or are forced to stop training in response to an injury. Detraining syndrome can be characterized by many symptoms including insomnia, anxiety, depression, alterations to cardiovascular function, and a loss of appetite (see the sidebar, Potential Symptoms of Detraining Syndrome, for additional symptoms). These symptoms usually are not pathological and can be reversed if training is resumed within a short time. If the cessation of training is prolonged, these symptoms can become more pronounced, indicating that the athlete's body is unable to adapt to this sudden inactivity. The time frame in which these symptoms manifest themselves is highly specific to the individual athlete; generally, it can occur within 2 to 3 weeks of inactivity and varies in severity.

Simply decreasing the level of training can also stimulate a detraining effect that will decrease physiological (table 8.2) and performance capacity. The magnitude of the detraining effects will be related to the duration of the detraining period. Short-term detraining, which occurs in less than 4 weeks, can result in some significant decreases in endurance and strength performance (15).

In endurance athletes, short-term detraining has been reported to result in a 4% to 25% decrease in time to exhaustion and a substantial reduction in endurance performance (20). It has been postulated that the reductions in endurance performance are largely dictated by the decline in cardiorespiratory fitness noted in response to short-term detraining (14). Maximal aerobic capacity can be reduced by 4% in as little as 4 days of detraining (28); decreased by 7% within 3 weeks of the cessation of training (4); and reduced by 14% in as little as 4 weeks of detraining (20). If the detraining period is extended to 8 weeks, aerobic capacity can continue to decrease up to 20% of pre-detraining values (21). These reductions in aerobic capacity are most likely related to specific alterations to the cardiorespiratory system, including decreases in blood volume, stroke volume, and maximal cardiac output (table 8.2). These detraining-induced physiological alterations appear to occur progressively and proportionally to the training status of the athlete; this suggests that highly trained endurance athletes will experience a greater magnitude of decline in both physiological and performance capacity.

TABLE 8.2 — Short-Term and Long-Term Detraining Effects

Physiological factors altered by detraining	Detraining characteristics	Short-term (<4 weeks)	Long-term (>4 weeks)
Cardiorespiratory	Maximal oxygen uptake	↓	↓
	Blood volume	↑	↑
	Submaximal heart rate	↑	↑
	Recovery heart rate	↑	↑
	Stroke volume during exercise	↓	↓
	Maximal cardiac output	↓	↓
	Ventricular mass and dimension	↓	↓
	Mean blood pressure	↑	↑
	Maximal ventilatory volume	↓	↓
	Submaximal ventilatory volume	↑	↑
	Oxygen pulse	↓	↓
	Ventilatory equivalent	↑	↑
	Endurance performance	↓	↓
Skeletal muscle	Capillary density	↓	↓
	Arterial-venous oxygen difference	—	↓
	Fiber type distribution	—	Altered
	Fiber cross-sectional area	↓	↓
	Type II:I area ratio	—	↓
	Muscle mass	—	↓
	EMG activity	↓	↓
	Strength-power performance	↓	↓
	Oxidative enzyme capacity	↓	↓
	Glycogen synthase activity	↓	—
	Mitochondrial ATP production	↓	—
Metabolic characteristics	Maximal respiratory exchange ratio	↑	↑
	Submaximal respiratory exchange ratio	↑	↑
	Insulin-mediated glucose uptake	↓	↓
	Muscle GLUT4 protein content	↓	↓
	Muscle lipoprotein lipase activity	↓	↓
	Postprandial lipemia	↑	—
	High-density lipoprotein cholesterol	↓	↓
	Low-density lipoprotein cholesterol	↓	↓
	Submaximal blood lactate	↑	↑
	Lactate threshold	↓	↓
	Bicarbonate level	↓	↓
	Muscle glycogen level	↓	↓
	Adrenaline-stimulated lipolysis	↓	↓

↓ = decrease, ↑ = increase, — = no data available; EMG = electromyographic; ATP = adenosine triphosphate; GLUT4 = glucose transporter-4.

Adapted from Mujika and Padilla 2000 (20, 21).

Potential Symptoms of Detraining Syndrome

- Increased occurrence of dizziness and fainting
- Nonsystematic precordial disturbances
- Increased sensation or occurrence of cardiac arrhythmias
- Occurrence of extrasystolia and palpitations
- Increased incidence of headaches
- Loss of appetite
- Increased incidence of insomnia
- Occurrence of anxiety and depression
- Profuse sweating
- Gastric disturbances

Adapted from Mujika and Padilla 2000 (21).

Short-term and long-term detraining can also produce marked alterations in strength and power performance. For example, 4 weeks of detraining in which strength training is completely removed from the training plan results in a 6% to 10% reduction in maximum muscular strength and a 14% to 17% decrease in maximum power generation capacity (15). These reductions in strength-power performance may be related to preferential atrophy of type II muscle fibers (13, 24) and a reduction in neural drive (1, 10). The reduction in the ability to express muscular strength and power characteristics depends on the magnitude of the reduction of muscle cross-sectional area and electromyographic activity.

The extent of strength and power performance and physiological detraining-induced maladaptation depends on several factors including the duration of detraining and the training status of the athlete. Although the largest decrease in the expression of muscular strength occurs during the first 4 weeks (10% decrease), extending the detraining period to 8 weeks will result in a continued performance reduction (11% to 12% decrease) (10, 20, 21). These reductions in performance appear to occur at a greater rate and magnitude in highly trained individuals compared with recreational athletes and untrained people; the latter appear able to maintain both strength and power performance in response to 2 to 3 weeks of detraining (13, 16, 22).

If training completely stops during the transition phase, it is likely, depending on the length of the phase, that the athlete will lose a substantial amount of the physiological adaptations gained from the previous training period. When this occurs, the athlete will spend a large portion of the next preparatory phase attempting to reestablish the physiological adaptations that were gained in the previous training period, which limits the athlete's ability to continue to improve. Conversely, if the athlete uses an active rest period during the transition phase, she will retain a larger portion of her physiological adaptations and continue to develop both physiological and performance capacities during the next general preparation phase.

In the second approach to the transition phase, active rest is used to minimize the loss of physiological function that occurs when passive methods are used. Active rest refers to participating in a compatible sport or using a period of low-volume and low-intensity training within the athlete's sport (25). By using this approach, the athlete will be able to minimize the loss of physiological adaptation and maintain some level of general fitness.

The transition phase begins immediately after the completion of the main competition and can last between 2 and 4 weeks. During the first week after the competition, active or passive rest can be used. Passive rest may be necessary if the athlete has injuries. If active rest is used during this microcycle, the volume and intensity of training are substantially reduced and may target movement patterns or activities that are not used in training. During the second to fourth microcycle of the transition phase (in a 4-week transition), the volume and intensity of training can remain low or increase slightly. The activity used for active rest must match the bioenergetic characteristics of the sport being trained for. For example, a cyclist may use cross-country skiing or running as a transition activity, whereas a volleyball player may use basketball. The transition phase is a period during which the athlete can recover physically and psychologically while minimizing the loss of fitness.

The transition phase has an additional purpose: During this phase, the coach and athlete should analyze the training program, performance results, and testing outcomes. This is an essential task because it will allow the coach and athlete to make specific changes to the athlete's next annual training plan.

Classifying Annual Plans

Figures 8.4 through 8.8 illustrate different models of annual training plans. Examination of figure 8.4 reveals several characteristics:

- It is a monocycle and therefore is appropriate for seasonal sports with one major competitive phase.
- The model is based on the specifics of training for speed and power sports such as sprinting, jumping, and throwing events in track and field.
- The volume and intensity curves may not be appropriate for sports that are dominated by endurance.

Annual training plans differ according to the requirements of the sport, and the classification of these plans largely depends on the number of competitive phases. Seasonal sports such as skiing, canoeing, cycling, triathlon, soccer, and sports with one major competition during the year usually require one competitive phase. These annual training plans can be

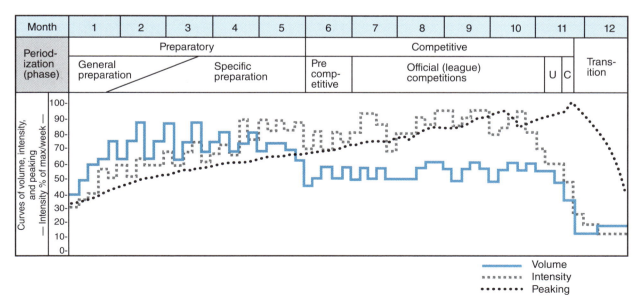

FIGURE 8.4 Monocycle for a speed and power sport. Please note that loading variations follow the concept of step loading.

U = unloading phase; C = competition.

classified as *monocycles*, because they contain only one competitive phase and one major peak (figures 8.4 and 8.5). These plans are divided into three major phases: preparatory, competitive, and transition phases. The monocycle plans shown in figures 8.4 and 8.5 include a preparatory phase in both general and specific phases of preparation. In figure 8.4, note the relationship between general and specific preparation: As one decreases, the other increases substantially. In some instances, such as in soccer, the general preparation phase can be very short or can be eliminated altogether, especially for national and international-class players.

The competitive phase in figures 8.4 and 8.5 is divided into several smaller subphases. The precompetitive subphase, which usually includes exhibition competitions only, comes before the main competition subphase in which all official competitions are scheduled. Before the most important competition of the year, two shorter subphases should be planned. The first is an unloading phase or taper, which is generally marked by lower volumes and intensities of training. This phase allows for the removal of fatigue and an elevation in physical and psychological potential, which creates a performance supercompensation effect. After this subphase a special preparation phase follows, during which technical and tactical changes can be made. This subphase can occur in conjunction with the unloading phase or can be a separate subphase.

The preparatory and competitive phases of the annual training plans are marked by some specific characteristics. During the preparatory phase and early competitive phase, training volume is emphasized with lower intensities according to the specifics of the sport. During the preparatory phase, the quantity of work is very high and the intensity of work is correspondingly lower. As the competitive phase approaches (figure 8.4), the training volume decreases to allow the athletes to use most of their energy for high-intensity training for speed- and power-dominant sports.

The monocycle model illustrated in figure 8.5 is an example of an annual training plan for endurance sports, where the bioenergetic contribution is 50%:50% (anaerobic:aerobic), or an even higher proportion for aerobic endurance. The dynamics of the volume of training demonstrate that aerobic metabolism is clearly dominant. Therefore, the training volume curve must be high throughout the competitive phase.

When working with sports that have two separate seasons (e.g., track and field, which has an indoor and outdoor season), a completely different approach is used to develop the

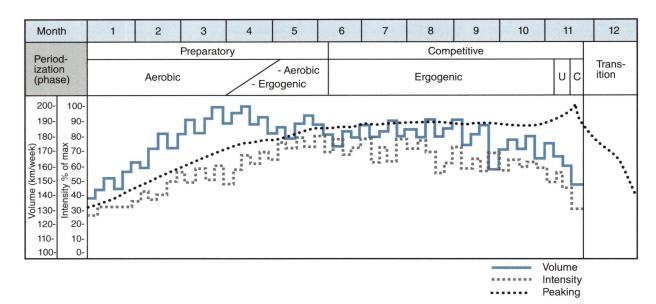

FIGURE 8.5 Monocycle for a sport in which endurance is the main requirement.

U = unloading phase; C = competition.

annual training plan. Because there are two distinct competitive phases, an annual training plan that contains two peaks, or a bi-cycle, is used. Figure 8.6 gives an example of an annual training plan with a bi-cycle structure that incorporates the following phases:

- *Preparatory phase 1:* The first preparatory phase, which should be the longest, lasts approximately 3 months and is broken into general and specific subphases.
- *Competitive phase 1:* The first competitive phase lasts about 2 1/2 months and brings the athlete to a peak performance.
- *Transition phase 1:* The first transition phase lasts approximately 1 to 2 weeks and is marked by a period of unloading to recover the athlete. This phase leads into the second preparatory phase.
- *Preparatory phase 2:* The second preparatory phase is shorter, but slightly more specific, than the first preparatory phase, lasting approximately 2 months. This phase has a much shorter general preparation subphase, with most of the training being performed in the specific preparation subphase.
- *Competitive phase 2:* The second competitive phase is slightly longer, about 3 1/2 months, and brings the athlete to a peak performance.
- *Transition phase 2:* The second transition phase is approximately 1 to 1 1/2 months long and is used to unload and recover the athlete. This phase links to the next annual training plan.

A bi-cycle plan contains two short monocycles that are linked by a very short unloading and transition phase. The approach is similar for each cycle except that the training volume in preparatory phase 1 is much greater than that in preparatory phase 2. Additionally, the level of readiness will be lower during competitive phase 1. For example, in track and field, the outdoor championships are considered to be more important that the indoor competitions, and so the second competitive phase of the annual plan should target this major competition. Thus, it is warranted to bring the athlete's readiness to its highest level of the year in the second competitive phase.

Although the bi-cycle annual training plan is useful for some sports, other sports such as boxing, wrestling, martial arts, and gymnastics may have three major competitions during

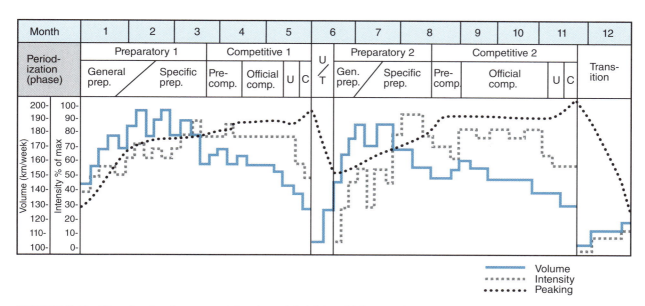

FIGURE 8.6 Bi-cycle plan for a sport (track and field) in which speed and power dominate.

Prep.= preparation; comp. = competitive; U = unloading; T = transition; C = competition.

the annual plan (e.g., national championships, a qualifying meet, and the international competition itself). Assuming each competition is 3 or 4 months apart, the athlete would have three competitive phases, which would create a tri-cycle annual training plan structure. As illustrated in figure 8.7, a tri-cycle plan incorporates the following sequence of training:

- *Preparatory phase 1:* Preparatory phase 1 is the longest preparatory phase of the annual training plan, lasting around 2 months. It contains both general and specific preparation subphases.
- *Competitive phase 1:* Competitive phase 1 is the shortest of the three competitive phases in the annual training plan, lasting around 1 1/2 months.
- *Transition Phase 1:* The first transition phase is very short and links the first competitive phase with the second preparatory phase. As with all transition phases, there is a period of unloading to allow the athlete to recover.
- *Preparatory phase 2:* Preparatory phase 2 is shorter than the first preparatory phase, lasting around 1 1/2 months. This preparatory phase only contains a specific preparation phase.
- *Competitive phase 2: Competitive* phase 2 is longer than the first competitive phase, lasting approximately 1 3/4 months.
- *Transition phase 2:* The second transition phase contains a short period of unloading designed to allow the athlete to recover from the fatigue accumulated during competitions. This transition is also short because it links competitive phase 2 to preparatory phase 3.
- *Preparatory phase 3*: This preparatory phase is a short preparatory phase lasting only about 1 1/2 months. As with the second preparatory phase, only the specific preparation subphase is used.
- *Competitive phase 3:* This competitive phase is the longest of the three competitive phases contained in the tri-cycle annual training plan (approximately 2 months). As such, this phase should peak the athlete for the most major competition of the year.

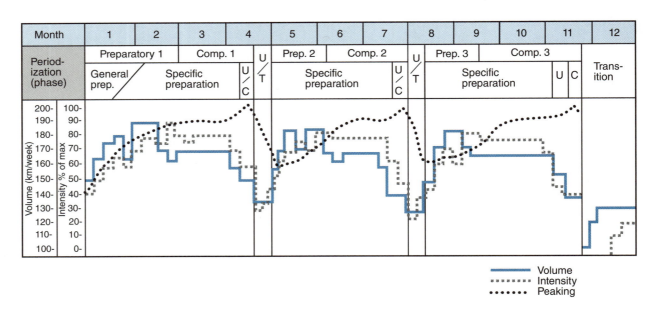

FIGURE 8.7 Annual training plan with tri-cycle structure.

Prep.= preparatory/preparation; comp. = competitive; U = unloading phase; C = competition; T = transition.

- *Transition phase 3:* This transition phase is the longest transition phase contained in the annual training plan, lasting approximately 1 month. It serves an important role in inducing recovery and preparing the athlete for the next annual training plan.

In a tri-cycle plan, the most important competition of the three should occur during the last cycle of the year. The first of the three preparatory phases should be the longest, during which the athlete builds the technical, tactical, and physical foundation from which the next two cycles are built. Because this type of plan is typically used with advanced athletes only, the first preparatory phase contains the general preparation subphase.

In an annual plan with a tri-cycle structure, the volume curve is the highest in the first preparatory phase. This highlights the importance of training volume in this phase. The intensity curve depicted in the tri-cycle structure (figure 8.7) follows a pattern similar to that seen in a monocycle. Both the volume and intensity curves decrease slightly for each of the three unloading phases that precede the main competitions. Within the annual training plan, the highest level of training should be planned for the third competitive phase to allow for the highest performances to occur at the main competition of the year.

Although the bi-cycle and tri-cycle structures are useful for many sports, other sports such as tennis, martial arts, boxing, and gymnastics may have four or more competitions that require multipeak performance (figure 8.8). In these situations, the preparatory phase, which is crucial for the development of technical and tactical skills as well as specific biomotor abilities, is shortened significantly. Advanced athletes who have developed a strong foundation of training during the early years of their athletic development may find it easier to cope with such a heavy competitive schedule, but young athletes may have a hard time coping with such a stressful schedule. This may be a reason why so many young players burn out before winning a major tournament.

Month	1	2	3	4	5	6	7	8	9	10	11	12
Type of training	1	2	3	4	1	2	3	4	1	2	3	4	1	2	3	4

FIGURE 8.8 A hypothetical multipeak annual training plan for tennis.
1 = preparatory phase; 2 = intensification, or competition; 3 = transition/recovery.

Developing a multipeak annual plan (figure 8.8) is a challenging task. This is especially true for sports like professional tennis where the preparatory phase is very short and often planned prior to major tournaments. In figure 8.8, the 1s represents a very short preparatory phase that also focuses, in the early week, on regeneration. The rest of these short preparatory cycles should also have the scope of improving specific biomotor abilities. Since the dominant ability in tennis is power, the coach should do the utmost to train it prior to the next tournament. Although figure 8.8 represents a scenario often seen in tennis, coaches should be very selective regarding the number of tournaments a player attends. This type of plan is often used by young players whose background is quite superficial, and their capacity to tolerate physical and psychological stress might not be high enough for this type of annual plan. This is why younger and inexperienced players are exposed to injuries and losses that may make some players withdraw from tournaments.

Selective Periodization

Far too often the annual training plans developed for elite athletes are used for young athletes who lack the training experience and physiological maturity to tolerate intensive competitive schedules. This is one reason why periodization of training should be individualized. The coach should consider the athlete's readiness for intensive competitive schedules, using the following guidelines:

- A monocycle is strongly suggested as the basic annual training model for novice and junior athletes. Such a plan has a long preparatory phase during which the athlete can develop foundational technical, tactical, and physical elements without the major stress of competitions. The monocycle is the typical annual plan for seasonal sports and sports for which endurance is the dominant biomotor ability (e.g., Nordic skiing, rowing, cycling, and long-distance running).
- The bi-cycle annual training plan is typically used for advanced or elite athletes who can qualify for national championships. Even in this scenario, the preparatory phase should be as long as possible to allow for the development of fundamental skills and physiological potential.
- The multipeak annual training plan is recommended for advanced or international-level athletes. Presumably, these athletes have a solid foundation that allows them to handle an annual plan that contains three or more peaks.

The duration of the training phases depends largely on the competitive schedule. Table 8.3 provides guidelines for distributing the training weeks contained in each training phase.

TABLE 8.3 Guidelines for the Distribution of Weeks for Each Training Phase Contained in the Classic Types of Annual Training Plans

Annual plan structure	Total weeks per cycle	Number of weeks per phase		
		Preparatory	Competitive	Transition
Monocycle	52	≥32	10-15	5
Bi-cycle	26	13	5-10	3
Tri-cycle	17-18	≥8	3-5	2-3
Multipeak	52	15-18	22-30	7-8

Stress and Periodization

The ability to manage the stress that accumulates as a result of training and competition is an important factor that underlies successful athletic performances. Training-induced stress can be considered a summation of both physiological and psychological stressors and can be elicited by both internal and adverse external influences. Therefore, it may be warranted to focus on the training effects induced by the training plan rather than the work being completed. The training plan must consider the development of fatigue, which is a by-product of training, and how to monitor or evaluate its effect on performance.

Periodization is an important tool in the management of fatigue that accumulates in response to physiological, psychological, and sociological stressors resulting from training and competition. In creating the annual plan, the coach needs to consider the effects of both training and competition on the development of fatigue and the level of stress experienced by the athlete. If structured carefully, the annual plan will manage this fatigue and reduce levels of fatigue during major competitions, when stress can be very high. Figure 8.9 shows how stress may vary across an annual training plan. Note that stress does not have the same magnitude throughout the annual plan, which is a distinct advantage of periodized training.

The stress curve in figure 8.9 parallels the intensity curve in that the higher the intensity, the higher the level of stress. The shape of the stress curve also indicates that stress is lowest during the transition phase and increases throughout the preparatory phase. In the competitive phase of training, levels of stress will fluctuate in response to competitive stress and short periods

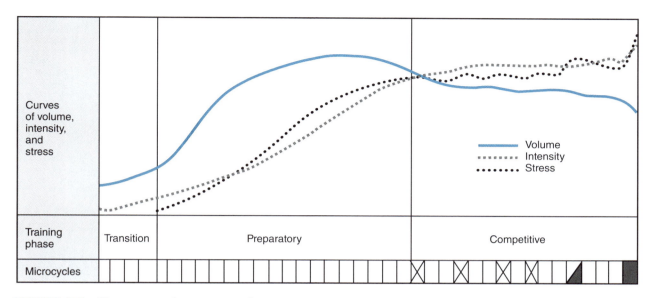

FIGURE 8.9 Stress curve for a monocycle.

of regeneration. During the preparatory phase, the magnitude of the stress curve is a result of the relationship between training volume and intensity. Although the volume or quantity of training is high, the intensity is low because it is difficult to emphasize a high amount of work and an elevated intensity simultaneously (with the exception of weightlifting).

Training intensity is a prime contributor to stress. Therefore, the coach should consider decreasing the athlete's level of stress during the preparatory phase by emphasizing volume more than intensity. However, it is likely that the high volumes of training typically seen in the preparatory phase also produce a significant amount of metabolic stress (19) and large hormonal disturbances (17), which can result in high levels of fatigue.

The stress curve throughout the competitive phase undulates in accordance with competitive, developmental, and regeneration microcycles. The number and frequency of competitions during the competitive phase clearly can have a negative impact on the athlete's level of stress. Frequent competitions can increase the athlete's level of stress, and the coach must allow a few days of regeneration following these competitions. To further deal with the stress of the competitive phase, a short period (2 or 3 days) of unloading prior to the competition may be warranted.

In addition to alternating high- and low-stress activities, the athlete can use relaxation techniques to cope with stress. Equally important is having a specific nutritional plan produced by a specialist; certain foods may have a positive effect on coping with fatigue and psychological stress. The ability to tolerate stress is highly individual, and athletes who have difficulty dealing with stress may need to use motivational and relaxation techniques. The athlete's ability to tolerate stress depends largely on the training plan. The coach must structure the training plan to include phases of regeneration that use relaxation and visualization techniques to help the athlete tolerate training and competitive stress.

The athlete's psychological state depends largely on his physiological status. If the athlete is experiencing high levels of fatigue, this accumulated stress appears to negatively affect psychological status (6). The better physiologically prepared the athlete, the greater the likelihood that he has a positive psychological status. A periodized training program that is structured correctly will ensure superior physiological preparedness, psychological readiness, stress management, and mental training.

While an athlete may be able to manage stress during a monocycle, this is likely not the case for tri-cycles and it is especially not the case for multipeak annual plans. The same can

	Sunday	Monday	Tuesday	Wednesday	Thursday	Friday	Saturday	Sunday
S/T	Peak	R/R	Train/U	Peak	R/R	Train	Train/U	Peak
a.m.	Pre-game arousal activities	Off (Physiotherapy)		Pre-game arousal activities				Pre-game arousal activities
p.m.	Game	Individual physical and psychological assessment of stress; physio techniques	Pre-game tactical training and power training	Game	Same as Monday p.m.	High-intensity training Drills for speed and agility Technical-tactical drills with high intensity	Technical and pre-game tactical training	Game

FIGURE 8.10 A suggested microcycle for a team sport with games planned on Sundays and Wednesdays.

S/T = scope of training; R/R = recovery/regeneration/stress management; train/U = training and unload to reach supercompensation for the game.

be said about most team sports, which often have an annual plan that lasts 10 months. In the case of team sports, careful considerations should be given to each microcycle, as the players may experience a cumulative effect of stress that can compromise the goals planned for the week. Figure 8.10 suggests a plan for a two-game microcycle and the activities programmed for the players so that they can better cope with and tolerate physical and psychological stress.

Chart of the Annual Training Plan

Now that the basic concept of periodization and the main objectives of each training phase and subphase have been presented, an annual training plan can be constructed. Charting an annual training plan requires an understanding of the relationships between the training components and the stress that these factors impart upon the athlete. During this process decisions must be made that consider the timing of major competitions, the ratio of training factors contained in each phase, and the sequencing of the training phases. Successful training planners are able to use their knowledge about training and its physiological responses to develop training plans that will induce specific outcomes.

Annual training plans for all athletes are constructed with the same basic steps; however, each plan, and thus the chart, must be individualized to the physiological specifics of the sport and the athlete's needs. Several examples of annual training plan charts are provided in this text. Please note that the following charts represent a progression from simple to more intricate. It is important to follow the progression presented here, to fully prepare to create such charts.

Chart of a Monocycle Annual Training Plan

The monocycle, the first example of a training chart, represents a very simple form of an annual plan for a hypothetical junior basketball team (figure 8.11). At the top part of figure 8.11, the planner can note the dates of the plan, the coach, and the team; in the second line, the planner can checkmark the weekends in each month when there are games scheduled. Since basketball is played in many countries from the fall through the spring months (October to mid-April, in figure 8.11), the first month in the plan is June and the last part of the plan ends in mid-April. The remaining weeks in April and the month of May are reserved for a transition phase. The month of June is the first month of an informal and flexibly applied preparatory phase. Remember that summer is also a vacation away from school. However, for dedicated players, summer can also be used as a preparatory phase, where the players can work (2 to 3 times per week) on overall flexibility

Chart of the Annual Plan

Type:
Coach:

Dates	Months	June	July	August	September	October	November	December	January	February	March	April	May
	Weeks												
Competitions	Domestic					■■■■■	■■■■				■■■		
	International												
	Location												
Periodization	Training phase	Preparatory						Competitive					Transition
	Strength	AA		M x S	P			Maintain					
	Endurance	Aerobic		Ergogenesis									
	Speed	General speed		Specific speed									
	Nutrition												
	Testing dates			▪					▪				
	Medical control dates			▪								▪	

FIGURE 8.11 Annual training plan for a junior basketball team. As needed, adjust the suggested plan to the specific conditions including the plan's duration and its flexible application (e.g., length of the transition phase).

AA = anatomical adaptation type of strength training; aerob. = aerobic-type endurance training; M x S = maximum strength; P = power; nutrition = please introduce in the above chart the elements (such as a high carbohydrate intake) of the nutrition plan as suggested by a nutrition specialist.

185

and strength training (anatomical adaptation [AA] type with emphasis on strengthening the ligaments and tendons).

The next second in figure 8.11, marked "Competitions," is used to specify the schedule of the games the coach has selected for the year (here, from October to mid-April as represented by the shaded squares). In the space reserved for the location of the competition, add the actual name of the place where each game is played.

Once the dates and locations of the competitions are recorded on the training chart, the coach has to decide the key elements of periodization. The annual training plan is divided into training phases, working from right to left. In figure 8.11 the line for periodization contains the three classic phases: preparatory (June to the end of September), competitive (early October to mid-April), and transition (late April to the end of May). Next, decide the duration and type of training for each training phase. Since the players in this example are high schoolers, the periodization of strength has a longer anatomical adaptation phase, followed by two short maximum strength and power phases. The same types of training will be maintained throughout the competitive phase. Endurance training (mostly aerobic) and general speed drills start at the same dates as anatomical adaptation, followed by game-specific endurance (ergogenesis) and speed training which are necessary to ready the players for the games to come.

A very important concern for junior athletes is nutrition. Consult a nutritionist to create a nutrition plan for the players, or a specialist who is familiar with the nutritional needs during a teenager's years of growth and physical development. Next, complete the lines for testing dates and medical control dates. Every coach should test the abilities of her players during the first week of the plan. Two more testing dates should be utilized at the end of December or early January and during the first week of the transition. Medical control, at the beginning and end of the annual plan, is necessary to evaluate the health status of each player.

Chart of a Bi-Cycle Annual Training Plan

Figure 8.12 represents an example of a bi-cycle training plan for high school swimmers. Traditionally, swimming has two major competitions and therefore two peaks per year (short course during winter and long course during the summer). The main criteria for deciding the two peaks of the year and, as such, the intrinsic training phases, depends on the dates of the main competitions of the year. Please note the two distinctive competitive phases in figure 8.12, each of them culminating with a national championship (end of February and end of August). All other competitions are scheduled every second week, an advantage that follows a training requirement: compete, recover, train, supercompensate for the next race, and compete again. This method of programming training and competitions allows the coach to avoid overtraining.

Periodization of training phases and of the dominant abilities follows the same methodology, as discussed in chapter 5. Please note that each cycle of competitions is followed by a transition phase. Note also the criteria for dividing each cycle into macrocycles, such as the schedule of competitions and the duration of training phases for strength, speed, and endurance training. The bottom of the chart offers a place to decide the dates for medical control and testing, which are traditionally placed at the beginning of a program and at the end of most training phases for the periodization of dominant biomotor abilities.

Chart of a Tri-Cycle Annual Training Plan

Once there is comprehension of a monocycle and bi-cycle, the coach can work on understanding a hypothetical tri-cycle, which is often used for martial arts, artistic sports, and some seasonal sports. A tri-cycle can be used even in Alpine and Nordic skiing, where competitions such as the national championships, major international championships, World Cup, or Olympic Games can be the top three peaks of the year. Figure 8.13 represents a hypothetical tri-cycle for martial arts, where the three major peaks are scheduled for April 26, August 2, and December 13. Note that the peak on November 8 is a peak of intensity only, not a peak of shape for the year.

Chart of the Annual Plan

Type:
Coach:

Dates		Months	October				November				December				January				February				March				April				May				June				July				August				September			
		Weeks																																																				
Competitions		Domestic						■					■				■			■																			■			■	■	■			■						
		International																																																				
		Location																	Nat. champ.																									Nat. champ.									
Periodization		Training phase	Preparatory 1															Competitive 1							T			Preparatory 2											Competitive 2												T	
		Strength	AA		MxS				M-E										Maintain							AA			MxS				M-E							Maintain												
		Endurance	AE						AE-AN							Specific											AE				AN							Event-specific										AE			
		Speed														Event-specific																								Event-specific													
		Psychological																																																				
		Nutrition																																																				
		Macrocycles	1			2			3				4				5				6				7			8			9				10				11			12				13				14		
		Microcycles	1	2	3	4	5	6	7	8	9	10	11	12	13	14	15	16	17	18	19	20	21	22	23	24	25	26	27	28	29	30	31	32	33	34	35	36	37	38	39	40	41	42	43	44	45	46	47	48	49	50	51	52
		Testing dates	■						■					■																	■				■																			
		Medical control dates																																																			■	■

FIGURE 8.12 Bi-cycle training plan for high school swimmers.

AA = anatomical adaptation; AE = aerobic; AN= anaerobic; MxS = maximum strength; T= transition; M-E = muscle endurance (capacity to perform many repetitions against a low to medium load).

Note: Some lines in figure 8.12 are empty. This means that the coach, psychologist, and nutritionist must specify the terminology to be used in those spaces.

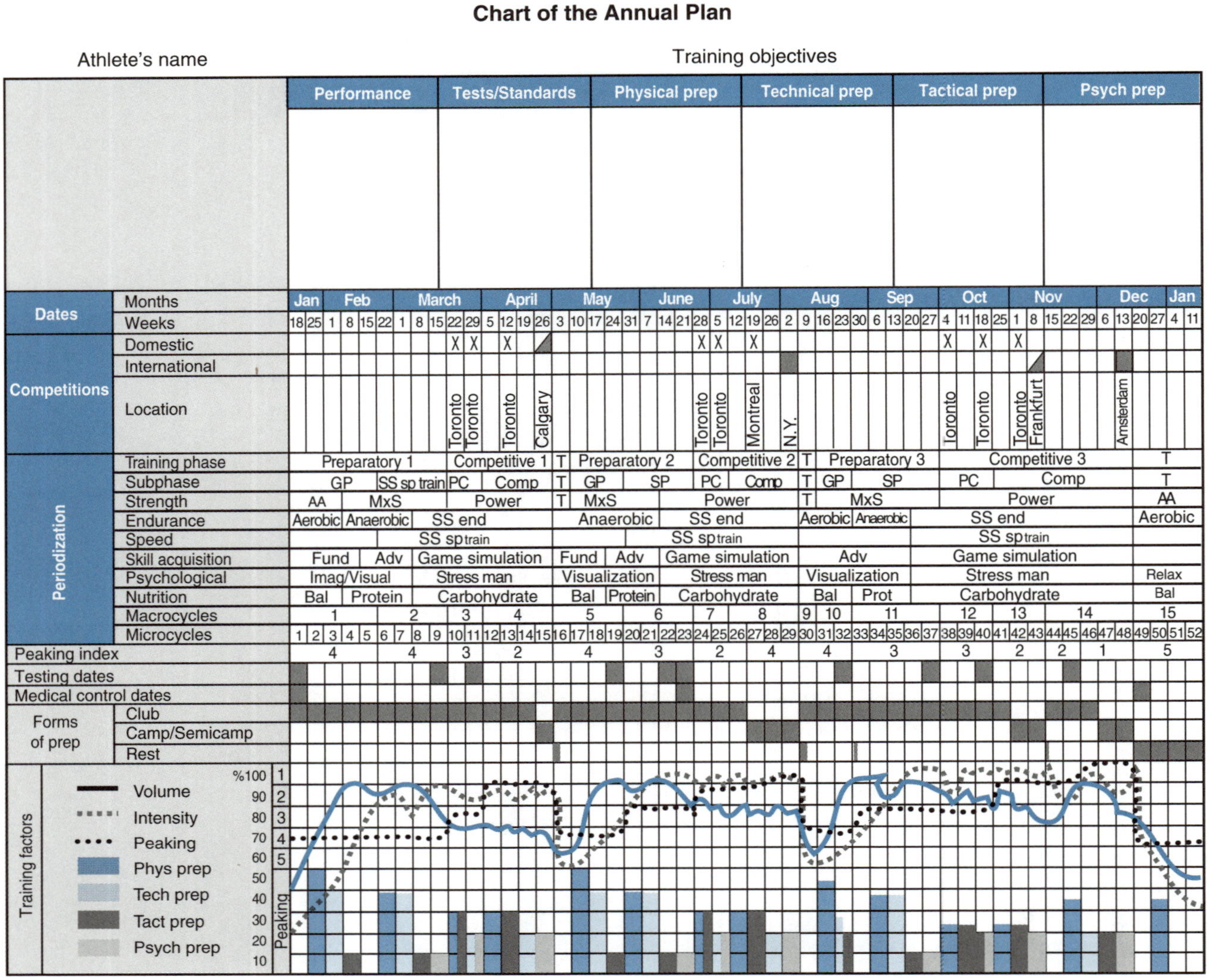

Chart of the Annual Plan

FIGURE 8.13 Tri-cycle annual training plan for martial arts.

Prep. = preparations; comp. = competitive; T = transition; GP = general preparation phase; SS sp. train = sport-specific speed training; PC = precompetition phase; SP = specific preparation phase; AA = anatomical adaptation; MxS = maximum strength; SS end. = sport-specific endurance; fund. = fundamental; adv. = advanced; imag./visual = imagery and visualization; stress. man. = stress management; relax = relaxation; bal. = balanced.

Secondary competitions have to also be planned prior to each peak. Ideally, these competitions should be organized based on the difficulty of opponents, with the lowest difficulty planned at the beginning of the competitive phase and the most challenging opponent faced toward the end. To best monitor fatigue, most competitions are planned two weeks apart, with a short recovery phase immediately after each competition and 2 to 3 days of lower intensity to facilitate supercompensation.

Figure 8.13 can also be used to plan additional information, such as skill acquisition, psychological techniques, and nutrition. Employ the expertise of a sport psychologist and nutritionist to help define and achieve specific goals for the athlete. Underneath periodization, there is a line where peaking index can be specified for each training phase. See the next section for more information on the peaking index.

At the bottom of figure 8.13 are three curves: one for volume, one for intensity, and one for peaking. Methodologically speaking, during the early part of the preparatory phase the volume of training has to be emphasized so that a strong physiological foundation is built.

This strong base will result in proper adaptation of the body and mind, so that the athletes will be able to tolerate work and manage fatigue during each cycle. At the same time, the intensity curve is lower since an athlete cannot tolerate high volume or high intensity at the beginning of the annual plan.

Athletes usually begin a new annual training program with workload percentages between 30% and 50% of maximal work capacity, depending on their performance levels. The curve that represents the volume of training is progressively elevated through the preparatory phase, reaching its summit at the end of the general preparation phase. Conversely, during the specific preparation phase, the curve that represents the amount of volume decreases progressively, below the curve that depicts intensity. This curve trails the training volume curve through the preparatory phase, and then the gaps opens up by the middle of the competitive phase. Both curves undulate more during macrocycles with many competitions.

The intensity is generally higher during the early part of a microcycle that precedes a competition; it decreases as the competition approaches, to allow the athlete to rest and regenerate before the competition. When volume of training is high, intensity of training is generally lower. If both volume and intensity are high, the potential for overtraining increases markedly (7).

During the early part of the macrocycle before the main competition, volume increases, reflecting an emphasis on high-quality work. Toward the end of this macrocycle the volume decreases, usually in the last two microcycles prior to the next macrocycle. Training intensity is at first slightly lower than training volume but then elevates progressively as the competition approaches. During unloading, however, both curves may drop slightly depending on the type of taper being used. Traditionally, intensity is not elevated much for endurance sports, allowing both volume and intensity to be stressed equally. However, international-class athletes with a stronger foundation and endurance base can tolerate a higher intensity even during the competitive phase (with a slightly reduced volume). This approach to training for endurance athletes is necessary if higher performance is expected. Sports characterized by dynamic activities that express high power outputs will require that intensity be elevated to levels higher than the training volume curve. As for the short subphase of competitions, volume is down and intensity is up, signifying that most competitions are intense.

The **peaking curve**, or readiness curve as it is sometimes called, is a direct result of the interplay between volume and intensity, which will affect the athlete's level of fitness or fatigue. The peaking curve generally trails both volume and intensity curves through the preparatory phase in response to the fatigue that is developed in this phase. The peaking curve then elevates during the precompetition and competitive subphases in response to the reduction of fatigue that occurs as volume is decreased. The peaking curve represents the athlete's potential for high-level performance as well as his level of fatigue.

In the sample chart for an annual plan (figure 8.13), the magnitude (not the percentage of each curve) signifies the emphasis placed on volume and intensity. Expressing these curves in percentages rather than in relation to each other is more complicated; therefore, only experienced coaches training elite athletes should use that method of expression. Similarly, the stress curve is not included in the figure because its shape is affected by (and therefore resembles) the intensity curve; competition dates also affect the stress curve.

Peaking Index

The new parameter introduced in figure 8.13, the peaking or readiness index (2, 3, 29), represents the athlete's level of readiness to compete and reflects the athlete's physiological, technical, tactical, and psychological status (table 8.4). To modulate the athlete's level of readiness, the training factors must be manipulated to dissipate fatigue, thus elevating the athlete's potential to perform well. In this process competitions must be prioritized. It would be impossible to peak for every competition because fitness would begin to decline, attributable to spending too much time at low volumes or intensities of training. Thus varying levels of emphasis should be placed on specific competitions. Except for high-priority

TABLE 8.4 Description of the Peaking Index

Peaking index	Level of readiness (%)
1	100
2	90
3	70-80
4	60
5	≤50

competitions, it is not essential for the athlete (especially elite athletes and teams) to peak for every competition. In sports in which the competitive phase is long and there are many competitions, it is not feasible to achieve a true peak for each competition, game, or match.

The peaking index will be modulated by alterations in training load (volume and intensity) and will reflect the athlete's level of fatigue, which directly affects preparedness. High levels of fatigue will decrease preparedness, whereas low levels of fatigue will increase preparedness. However, if fitness declines too much in response to prolonged periods of low volume and intensities of training, preparedness will decline.

The athlete should achieve her highest level of readiness (peak) for the main competition at the end of the competitive phase. Therefore, it may be warranted to approach many of the competitions in the competitive phase of the annual training plan without peaking, effectively training through the competition and using minimal unloading strategies prior to these competitions. If a coach used peaking strategies that include unloading for every competition in the competitive phase, it would reduce the athlete's physiological capacity and readiness to perform across the season. However, this does not mean the athlete will not focus on each game. Rather the athlete and coach must determine the optimal approach to take or the degree of unloading to use prior to the competition.

Coaches of team sports should use the greatest amount of unloading when targeting the most important competitions or the three strongest opponents in the competitive schedule. In figure 8.13 this is indicated by peaking index level 1 and represents a situation where the athlete's level of readiness must be at its highest. To achieve this level of readiness, the athlete would have to use specific peaking strategies (see chapter 9). Peaking index level 2 represents a level of readiness that is approximately 90% of that experienced in level 1. This index would be used when playing the top two-thirds of the league, excluding the top three to five teams. To achieve this level of readiness, the athlete would use less reduction in training volume and intensity compared with level 1. When playing against nonthreatening teams in a league game or during precompetitive games, athletes would use peaking index level 3 (70% to 80% of maximal readiness). The training plan should emphasize technical and tactical objectives rather than winning during precompetitive games. It may be necessary to achieve this level of readiness in the special preparation subphase of a bi-cycle or tri-cycle plan. Peaking index level 4, indicated as 60% of maximal readiness, represents a level of readiness typically seen in the preparatory phase, when the athlete is undertaking high training loads and is not prepared to compete. Peaking index level 5, which represents 50% or less of maximal readiness, is typically seen during the transition phase at the end of the annual plan, when the training workload is at its lowest level during the annual plan, as are levels of fitness and fatigue.

The peaking index line in figure 8.13 represents the appropriate index for each macrocycle and serves as a guide by which the index curve is drawn. The peaking index will fluctuate or undulate in parallel to the fatigue or stress levels generated by training, and will increase in correspondence with the unloading microcycles. As the training becomes more specific and intense, from general preparation to specific preparation and throughout the competitive phase, the peaking index will improve.

The peaking index can be adapted to reflect a sport-specific level of readiness. Table 8.5 shows how the peaking index can be adapted to reflect a sport-specific level of readiness for individual sports, using the best performance of the athlete as a reference.

The peaking index will be modulated by alterations in training load (volume and intensity) and will reflect the athlete's level of fatigue, which directly affects readiness. High levels of fatigue will decrease an athlete's capabilities, whereas low levels of fatigue will increase readiness. However, if degree of preparedness declines too much in response to prolonged periods of low volume and intensities of training, athlete's performance capabilities will visibly decline.

TABLE 8.5 — Adaptation of the Peaking Index to Individual Sport Performance

Peaking index	Level of readiness (%)	Sprinter (100 m PB: 10 s)	Level of readiness (%)	Powerlifter (deadlift PB: 250 kg)
1	100	10.00-10.05 s	100	250-247.5 kg
2	99-99.5	10.06-10.10 s	97-98	242.5-245 kg
3	98-98.5	10.11-10.20 s	95-96	237.5-240 kg
4	97-97.5	10.21-10.30 s	93-95	232.5-235 kg
5	≤97	≥10.31 s	≤94	≤230 kg

PB = personal best.

Chart for a Multipeak Annual Training Plan

Creating a multipeak chart for an annual plan is a very challenging task, even for experienced coaches. The example illustrated by figure 8.14 is a clear demonstration of the planning reality in professional tennis, where there are year-round opportunities to play at various tournaments. The prize money advertised by organizers can often be an unrealistic temptation for many players. This is why many players fall into the mistake of registering for

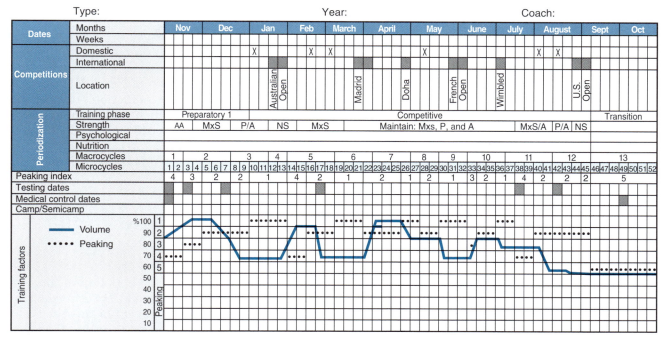

FIGURE 8.14 Multipeak annual plan for tennis.

X = secondary important tournament; AA = anatomical adaptation; MxS = maximum strength; P/A = power/agility; maintain = maintain maximum strength, power, and agility; NS = no strength during the U.S. and Australian Opens. The same proposal is suggested for the duration of other important tournaments.

Note: In the case of tennis, speed is actually agility and endurance is actually specific training that coaches should express in duration of time; therefore, this chart does not include lines for speed and endurance.

too many tournaments, when they are unprepared for the stress associated with traveling, playing, and being eliminated in the early part of the tournament, then traveling again to another tournament. Often these illusions can result in unpleasant, frustrating injuries. Thus, the proposed multipeak annual plan for tennis recommends the coach and player be very discerning when selecting the number of tournaments.

The top line of figure 8.14 is used to specify the months of the plan. Remember that after the last tournament, the U.S. Open in this example, the player can take a deserving vacation of 7 weeks for recovery and regeneration (labeled as T, or Transition, in figure 8.14). Use the second line to specify the weekend date (Sundays) in each square. The date of Sunday, which is the end of the week, always specified in a chart of an annual plan. The selected tournaments are noted in the line for domestic competitions, signified with an X for secondary importance tournaments. The fourth and fifth lines can be used to specify major tournaments, culminating with the U.S. Open.

The segment of the chart dedicated to periodization is used to specify training phases: the preparatory phase from early November to early January, the competitive phase from early January to first week in September, and the transition phase for the rest of September and all of October. The competitive phase notes the following tournament selections: Australian Open, Madrid, Doha, French Open, Wimbledon, and the U.S. Open. An essential line is dedicated to periodization of strength, where two types of strength are proposed: anatomical adaptation and maximum strength, which are so essential in tennis. Without dedicating time to maximum strength, the player will have a hard time improving power and agility, both of which are directly dependent on the improvement of maximum strength. Note that from Madrid to after the Wimbledon tournament, there is a long maintenance phase with time for maintaining maximum strength and power. Remember, what is not trained will detrain; if maximum strength deteriorates, power and agility will be directly affected, and speed and power on the court will be affected too. Periodization also includes two essential plans: psychological and nutrition. Coaches should use specialists in the area of sport psychology and nutrition to determine the specific needs for tennis.

The line for periodization of macrocycles involves specifying the duration of each phase, as dictated by the periodization of strength and the dates of the tournaments. Use the line for microcycles only as a reference date for the level of training state and level of peaking of the athlete. To better understand peaking index, please refer to its explanation earlier in this chapter. Testing and medical control dates are also highlighted in their specific line. Finally, the curves of volume and intensity are specified at the bottom of the chart. The elevation of each curve reflects the level necessary to stress training volume, intensity, and peaking, and should follow the load dynamic of the macrocycles. Try this type of planning and learn from it to improve planning for the following year.

Criteria for Compiling an Annual Plan

Compiling an annual training plan is an essential part of the training process because this plan provides the guidelines by which training is directed. The ideal time to establish the annual training plan is at the end of the transition phase before the initiation of the next training year. After the athlete completes the main competition of the year, her improvement and physiological and psychological responses to the training plan can be analyzed and evaluated. Her rate of improvement or progress, competition performance, and tests also can be analyzed at this time. The information garnered from this analysis will influence the objectives established for the next training year as well as the structure of the training plan. The coach will use these observations coupled with the upcoming competitive schedule to establish the next year's training plan.

Each year's competitive schedule, including national and international events, is set by the national or international federation. Each regional organization bases its competition

Elements of an Annual Training Plan

1. Performance model analysis (ergogenesis, biomechanics and strength, speed, and endurance characteristics for the athlete's level of competition)
2. Retrospective analysis
3. Performance prediction
4. Objectives in the areas of performance, physical preparation, technical and tactical preparation, nutrition, and theoretical and psychological preparation
5. Competition calendar
6. Tests and standards
7. Periodization model (including the chart of the annual plan and the structure of the macrocycles)
8. Preparation model
9. Athlete or team organization and administration model (including budget and equipment needs)

calendar on this schedule. These dates should be available by the transition phase of the previous year's annual training plan; otherwise, the next year's annual training plan cannot be established. In many instances individual sport federations do not issue competitive calendars until one or two months within the preparation phase. In that case the coach will design the annual plan by basing the competitive phase on that of the previous year. The plan will be later adjusted when the competitive calendars are out. Once the annual training plan is established, individual or small-group training plans can be developed. The annual training plan established by the coach should be clear and concise and must present the appropriate technical information.

The quality of an annual plan directly reflects the coach's methodological knowledge, his experience, and the latest innovations in training theory. The coach must stay abreast of these factors by reading scientific literature, attending conferences, networking with other coaches, and closely observing the training process of his athletes. The coach will modify and adapt the annual training plan in parallel with his increased knowledge and experience. The more organized the coach, the easier this process will be.

In some instances, the coach may be asked by the national sports association or funding organization to present a model of the next annual training plan. Such a model should be well organized and well thought out and must account for the main parameters of training. The following sections outline a model of an annual plan that contains all of the needed elements. An outline of the components contained in the presentation of a training program can be found in Elements of an Annual Training Plan.

Performance Model Analysis

In the performance model analysis, the first element that should be presented is a needs analysis in which the scientific and methodological aspects of the sport are presented in the context of the training needs. To do so, a coach should take into account the biomechanical and physiological characteristics of the sport and analyze the contribution of each biomotor ability to performance (figure 8.15).

Strength

Performance Model Analysis	
Ergogenesis	
Dominant energy system:	
Anaerobic alactic %:	
Anaerobic lactic %:	
Aerobic %:	
Strength	
Specific strength*:	
Prime movers:	
Muscular actions of the prime movers:	
ROM:	
Speed	
Linear	Nonlinear
Acceleration	
Maximum speed	
Speed endurance	
RSA	
Rest between reps	
Passive	Active
Complete	Incomplete
Endurance	
Continuous	
Intermittent	
Specific	

FIGURE 8.15 Chart of performance model analysis.

*Between maximum strength (MxS), power (P), power endurance (PE), muscle endurance short (MES), muscle endurance medium (MEM), and muscle endurance long (MEL). This is the strength that must be developed before the competitive season and then maintained.

ROM = range of motion; RSA = repeated sprint ability.

1. Select the type of strength. Determine which of the following qualities of strength are specific to the event: power; power endurance; or short, medium, or long muscle endurance. The increase of the chosen quality or qualities will be the ultimate goal of the entire periodization of strength. Remember that for the endurance types of strength (of a more metabolic nature), the morpho-functional adaptations to training require longer exposure to the stimuli than is the case for the neural adaptations. This factor directly affects the length of the conversion phase, and therefore the time remaining for other phases, as the program designing process works backward from the endpoint.

2. Determine the appropriate duration of the anatomical adaptation period based on the athlete's characteristics (including his or her athletic development stage and strength training experience) and the time available for an introductory phase.

3. Decide whether or not to implement a period devoted to hypertrophy in light of the characteristics of the athlete and of the sporting event.

4. Select the exercises to use in training. Strength and conditioning coaches should select training exercises according to the specifics of the sport, the athlete's needs, and the phase of training. Each athletic skill is performed by prime movers, which can differ from sport to sport, depending on the specific skill requirements. Therefore, coaches must first identify the prime movers, then select the strength exercises that best involve those muscles. At the same time, they must consider the athlete's needs, which depend on her background and individual strengths and weaknesses. Because the weakest link in a chain always breaks first, compensation exercises (also referred to as accessory exercises) should be selected to strengthen the weakest muscles. The selection of exercises is also phase specific. Normally, during the anatomical adaptation phase, most muscle groups are employed to build a better and more multilateral foundation. As the competitive phase approaches, training becomes more specific, and exercises are selected specifically to involve the prime movers. Thus, coaches must analyze the sport movements in order to determine exercises and loading parameters. The following factors should be considered:

   - Planes on which the movements take place (sagittal, frontal, transverse)
   - Force expressed at various joint angles within the sport-specific range of motion (i.e., the zone that must be most affected by the development of the specific strength)
   - Muscle groups producing the movements (i.e., the prime movers, which also must be most affected by the development of the specific strength)
   - Muscle actions (concentric, eccentric, isometric)

5. Choose the methods to use in each macrocycle and the progression of training means. Details about training methods and progression are provided in chapter 10.

Speed

1. Evaluate the number, intensity, and duration of sprints or quick actions.
2. Consider the differences between, and the contributions of, each of the following qualities of speed: alactic speed (acceleration, maximum speed); lactic speed short (repeated sprint ability, or RSA); and lactic speed long (speed endurance). Note: Lactic speed long (speed endurance) is an expression of lactic power in which speed is maintained for more than 8 s. In contrast, lactic speed short (repeated sprint ability or RSA) is an expression of alactic capacity in which sprints under 6 s are repeated with partial recovery until they become an expression of lactic power short, which also heavily engages aerobic power during short rest intervals to restore phosphates through aerobic phosphorylation.
3. Evaluate the type (active or passive) and duration of recovery between sprints or fast actions.
4. Evaluate whether speed is expressed linearly or nonlinearly.
5. Choose the methods to use in each macrocycle and the progression of training means.

Endurance

1. Use scientific literature to determine the contributions of each energy system to the sport activity (at the competitive level of the team or athlete):
   - Anaerobic alactic (ATP-CP)
   - Anaerobic lactic (LA)
   - Aerobic (O_2)
2. Evaluate whether an activity is continuous or intermittent.
3. Determine the working intensity zones for endurance and the progression to be used throughout the training program.
4. Choose the methods to use in each macrocycle and the progression of training means.

The coach can make use of online resources (e.g., www.pubmed.gov) to find relevant scientific literature about the metabolic, biomechanical, and neuromuscular characteristics of the sport. Online videos, of the competition level of the athletes being coached, can be used for biomechanical analysis purpose.

Retrospective Analysis

In this section the coach presents personal or team information (e.g., sport, gender, age, height, weight, body composition). To properly craft the performance predictions and objectives for the upcoming season, the coach must thoroughly analyze performance and behavior in the previous season. Performance achievements refer to competitive performance as well as performance on tests and standards. This information can be presented in a table (table 8.6).

TABLE 8.6 Hypothetical Analysis of Test Results for a Female Javelin Thrower

	Performance	Planned	Achieved
Objectives	1. Distance thrown	51.50 m	52.57 m
	2. 30 m dash	4.80 s	4.7 s
	3. Standing long jump	2.4 m	2.4 m
	4. Overhead, two hands, medicine ball throws (6.6 lb, or 3 kg)	18 m	21.4 m

Note: The factors presented are only examples; other factors (e.g., markers of muscular strength, changes in body composition, body mass) would be presented.

After analyzing the past year's competitive performances, objectives, and tests or standards, the coach can determine the athlete's state of preparation by analyzing each training factor. For physical preparation, the coach can analyze whether the indices of general and specific biomotor abilities development corresponded with the specific needs of the sport and whether they adequately supported the technical, tactical, and psychological preparation. Such information can be collected from competitions and test results, linking any improvement or decline in technical or tactical performance with the athlete's rate of progress or regress as reflected in test scores. Often, improvement will prevail during the preparation phase, but regression occurs during the competitive phase as a result of inconsistent and inadequate physical preparation. Thus, the coach would continue specific physical preparation throughout the competitive phase and test the athlete's progress consistently in each macrocycle, to collect objective data regarding the dynamics of physical preparation.

When examining technical preparation, the coach should evaluate the technical proficiency of the athlete and to what extent technical training and ability affected the athlete's performance. The coach should assess the effectiveness of past technical elements to determine whether to use them in the future. The time dedicated to improving technical elements directly reflects the athlete's level of technical proficiency and the fineness of the skill acquisition. Because muscular strength affects technical proficiency (5), the coach should determine whether the athlete has sufficient strength to undertake the technical elements required by the sport.

An analysis of tactical preparation should reveal whether tactical maneuvers were properly chosen and suited to the characteristics of the team, and whether they led to the solution of game problems. To conclude the retrospective analysis, the coach should indicate which, if any, of the past year's strategic tools should be eliminated, maintained as part of the team's strategies, or perfected so that the team's efficiency will improve in the next training year.

The coach also has to investigate the athlete's psychological preparation and behavior and quality of nutrition plan, and how these factors affected the final performance. In assessing the athlete's behavior, the coach would consider what happened during and outside of training (e.g., consider social factors); often it is the case that some elements outside of training significantly affect training and competitive performance.

Finally, the coach needs to collaborate with training specialists (e.g., strength and conditioning coaches, exercise physiologists, sport scientists, nutritionists, physiotherapists) to determine how the strategies used in the previous year affected the athlete's performance capacity. The conclusions of the retrospective analysis are then used to predict future progress and performance and to establish specific training and competitive objectives for the new annual training plan.

Performance Prediction

One of the coach's important duties is determining the skills and abilities that need to be developed and the performances that need to be achieved between the date of planning and the main contests. Performance prediction is a reference from which the objectives and standards for the annual training plan are generated. Achieving these objectives and standards increases the athlete's likelihood of attaining the highest possible competitive performance. For instance, a gymnastics coach scores routines and technical elements to see whether they are difficult enough to warrant a 15.01 average score (total points of 120.1 in the all-around), which is needed for a gymnast to place in the top six at the women's national championships. Following such an analysis, the coach decides what technical elements need to be incorporated from the previous year's routines and the skills that may need to be added to achieve the predicted score during the next training year. This prediction must consider the gymnast's ability and skill level in order to be realistic.

Performance prediction for team sports is more difficult than for individual sports because there are many more factors that can affect performance. Among the few aspects that the coach can predict are the technical elements, tactical maneuvers, and level of ability that the players must acquire to improve performance during the next year's annual training plan.

For sports in which performance is objectively and precisely measured (e.g., track and field, weightlifting, track cycling), performance prediction is easier. With these sports the coach examines the best results achieved in the previous training year and uses the athlete's rate of improvement to predict the level that the athlete can attain in the next training year. For example, the performances of men rowing in a major regatta can be predicted with this process (table 8.7). Using these predictions and considering the athletes' abilities and potential for improvement, the coach can set the standards for his or her crews and the placing expectations for a specific regatta (table 8.8). Using performance prediction, the coach sets realistic objectives for each training factor and prepares the chart of the annual training plan.

TABLE 8.7 Performance Prediction for Three Events for the Places of Male Rowers in the Olympic Games (Events Listed in Speed Order)

Event	Performance (min) by place			
	I	II-III	IV-VI	VI-IX
Eight	5:38	5:41	5:45	5:50
Coxless four	6:05	6:09	6:13	6:17
Single skull	6:53	6:56	6:58	7:04

TABLE 8.8 Minimum Performance Prediction and Placing Expectation in a Major Regatta

Event	Performance (min)	Predicted place
Eight	5:45	VI-VIII
Quad	5:58	VI-VIII
Coxless four	6:12	III-V
Coxed four	6:20	VII-IX
Double skull	6:30	III-V
Coxless pair	6:50	V-VI
Single skull	7:10	VII-IX
Coxed pair	7:15	VI-IX

Objectives

In both the annual training plan and the planning projection, the objectives must be presented in a methodological sequence with precise and concise language. The objectives are established based on past performances, test standards achieved, the rate of improvement for skills and performance, and the dates of the main competitions. In setting objectives, the coach must consider the dominant training factor and the factors that are poorly developed and thus limit the athlete's competitive and training potential. Then the coach determines the order of training priorities according to the limiting factors (e.g., physical, technical, nutrition plan, or psychological preparation).

The methodological sequence and presentation of each training factor are as follows:

1. Performance objective
2. Physical preparation (e.g., strength, speed, endurance, flexibility, or coordination)
3. Technical preparation (offensive and defensive skills)
4. Tactical preparation (offensive and defensive individual and team tactics)
5. Psychological preparation
6. Nutrition plan
7. Theoretical preparation

This does not mean that the coach should stress each factor in this sequence. Rather she should give priority to those factors for which the athlete is proportionately underdeveloped and those that are primary to all athletes participating in the sport.

While setting objectives, the coach should consider and state the probability (percentage chance) of achieving those objectives, especially the performance objective. Although this process relies on objective facts, it may be warranted to consider subjective assessments (e.g., the athlete's reserve, improvement potential, and psychological traits). Objectives for a hypothetical volleyball player are presented in table 8.9.

TABLE 8.9 Objectives for a Volleyball Player

Performance factors		
Item	**Objective**	**Probability of achievement**
Performance	Take first place in the junior national championships.	80%
	Place in the top six in the senior national championships.	50%-60%

Training factors		
Item	**Factor**	**Objective**
Physical preparation	Strength	Improve leg strength to increase jumping ability.
	Speed	Improve short speed to facilitate quicker footwork for blocking and defense.
	Endurance	Improve power endurance required in long games and tournaments.
	Flexibility	Improve both shoulder and ankle flexibility.
Technical preparation	Serving	Improve serving consistency.
	Spiking	Improve spiking accuracy.
	Blocking	Improve blocking ability.
Tactical preparation	Offense	Improve spiking in a 6-0 system.
	Defense	Improve timing and quickness of blocking.
Psychological preparation		Develop the ability to play calmly and with confidence following a mistake.
Nutrition		
Theoretical preparation		Know all penalties that the referee may call.

Competition Calendar

Establishing the competition calendar is an important aspect of the annual training plan. The competitive schedule is established by the coach in accordance with the events scheduled by the national, conference, or international governing body. In this process, competitions are selected that best suit the athlete's needs, level of development, performance capacity, skills, and psychological traits. Although athletes should contribute to the planning process, especially elite athletes, the coach has the decisive role in establishing the competitive schedule.

The major championship or main competitive objective of the training year is the central factor used to establish the periodized training plan and the competitive calendar. Other official and unofficial competitions should be of secondary importance. However, these competitions serve an important role in allowing the coach to assess the athlete's development and preparation level for the main competitions targeted by the annual plan. These competitions are spread over the competitive phase and are most prominent during the precompetitive subphase. Competitions should not be scheduled early in the preparatory phase because the focus during this phase is on physical preparation and skill development rather than performance. Ideally, major competitions and secondary competitions are alternated in the plan. Although team sports have many league or official games, competitions are sometimes scarce in individual sports. To maintain the unity of the annual training plan throughout the competitive phase, the coach should consider organizing preparatory competitions that can be integrated into the training plan.

When arranging the competitions in the annual plan, the coach must consider the principle of progressive increase in training load, in which preparatory competitions of secondary importance must lead into major competitions that are more challenging. Although this method is ideal, it is not always possible, especially in team sports in which sport governing bodies set the competition calendar. The number of competitions in the competition calendar can have a profound effect on the ability of the athlete to achieve the performance objectives. A heavy, demanding competition schedule, as often occurs in team sports, may result in a premature elevation in performance readiness that in turn leads to a less than optimal performance at the end of the competitive phase when the major contest is planned. Conversely, participating in too few competitions can decrease readiness for competitions and prevent the athlete from achieving the planned performance objective. Therefore, planning can become a delicate balancing act between too many and too few competitions in the calendar. Two important criteria can be used to establish the optimal number of competitions: the nature of the sport and the athlete's performance level or developmental status. For sports in which the effort is intense and for athletes with low performance capabilities, 15 to 25 competitions per year may suffice. With elite athletes, especially those involved in team sports (e.g., premier league soccer), more contests (>30) may be planned.

Once the competition schedule is established it should not be changed, because the entire annual training plan is based on this schedule. Coaches who work with high school or university athletes should not plan any competitions, especially important ones, during examination periods. Similarly, athletes should not participate in any official or demanding competitions during the last two microcycles before the main contest (tapering phase). During these two microcycles, the coach and athlete should focus on training and make relatively few changes based on results of the previous secondary competitions. Each contest, whether primary or secondary, will tax the athlete physically and mentally. Recovery and regeneration must be built into the training plan, especially after secondary contests that lead into the main competitions targeted by the annual training plan.

Tests and Standards

The evaluation of specific tests and standards related to a sport is a crucial part of developing a periodized training plan. These evaluations need to be organized, systematic, and consistently performed across the annual training plan to garner detailed information about the athlete's progress. Monitoring training by using tests and standards provides the coach an objective means with which to quantify the athlete's evolution, potential for stagnation, or risk of performance deterioration. By monitoring training, the coach can evaluate the dose–response relationship, and thus optimize the training load to help the athlete achieve optimal performance at the appropriate time.

An athlete monitoring program can include specific physical tests that are periodically performed by the athlete to evaluate markers of the athlete's progress. More specific testing can be used to identify the athlete's strengths and weaknesses. Test results are then evaluated in relation to established performance standards. To ensure the effectiveness of a testing battery, the tests used must be valid (measure what they are supposed to measure), reliable (repeatable), and related to factors that affect the actual competitive performance. To truly understand the athlete's status, the coach must select diverse tests that evaluate more than just competitive performance results (23). For example, swimming performance is affected by speed, stroke mechanics, and start and turning ability. In addition, physiological factors such as anaerobic power and capacity, muscle power and flexibility, and general and specific endurance affect swimming performance. Actual swim performance should also be evaluated, but time should not be the only focus. The coach should examine technical proficiency at each training session, as it can then offer insight into the athlete's progress by relating technical skill level with competitive performance (23). Therefore, to monitor a swimmer's preparation, the coach should periodically use tests that address these factors. A large amount of research has been conducted that correlates specific tests with performance in specific sporting activities, and this research can be used to establish performance-based testing procedures.

The testing battery should be based on metabolic specificity (bioenergetics), sport specificity (biomechanical or movement pattern), and the athlete's training status (11). Athletes should be familiarized with the testing procedures but should not directly train to master the test because this distorts the evaluative ability of the test itself. Obviously, the test may contain an activity that is germane to the training process and is frequently encountered during the training plan. For example, a common exercise used to train lower-body strength is the back squat, and this same exercise is often used to evaluate lower-body strength. So

Main Objectives of the Tests Contained in an Athlete Monitoring Program

- To monitor the athlete's rate of improvement in specific biomotor abilities or skills
- To determine skill status and ability level, which can then be used to guide training
- To determine the athlete's training content
- To determine the athlete's strengths, weaknesses, and limitations
- To test improvement in tactical skills or maneuvers
- To evaluate body mechanics and movement skill (analytically, at the very beginning of the preparation, then at each training session afterward)
- To determine appropriate standards in all training factors
- To evaluate and develop psychological attributes or traits
- To evaluate the athlete's potential for overtraining
- To evaluate the impact of the nutrition plan on performance and body composition
- To monitor the dose–response relationship in the training plan

in this instance an athlete would train the back squat to develop leg strength and use a one-repetition maximum test with the back squat to evaluate maximum strength.

The testing battery should be concise (four to eight performance tests) and the tests should be highly related to the sport in question. For example, Stone and colleagues (27) reported that maximum strength as assessed by the snatch and isometric midthigh pull is strongly related to throwing ability in university shot put and weight bag throwers. Therefore, it makes sense to evaluate maximum strength throughout the annual training plan of university throwers. Haff and colleagues (9) used a biweekly testing battery that included assessments of body mass, body fat, lean body mass, hormonal responses to training, and force–time curve characteristics (peak force, rate of force development with isometric and dynamic movements) in elite women weightlifters. The testing battery was simple to perform, and changes in the force–time curve characteristics were related to the training plan. Interestingly, the maximization of peak force and peak rate of force development were shown to be related to weightlifting performance (8). Thus, this simple battery of tests was able to differentiate the level of preparedness of these athletes.

The tests used across the annual training plan and the dates of testing should be decided when the coach constructs the annual training plan. The first tests should occur during the first microcycle of the preparatory phase. By conducting the test at this time, the coach can determine the athlete's level of preparation and make any modifications to the annual training plan. Each macrocycle targets specific objectives, and testing can be conducted to determine whether these objectives are accomplished. Therefore, some form of testing should be conducted during 1 or 2 days at the end of each preparatory phase and precompetitive subphase macrocycle. This testing is used to evaluate the athlete's preparatory status during these phases. If the test results reveal consistent improvement, the original training structure should be maintained. Conversely, if the results indicate stagnation or decrease in the specific test measures, then the coach may need to modify the next training cycle. The coach must be careful when evaluating testing data because the phase of training may cause expected decreases in specific performance characteristics. For example, during the general preparation phase where training volume, work load, and fatigue are the highest, one might expect declines in markers of maximum power-generating capacity. On the other hand, during the competitive phase one would expect elevations in power-generating capacity. During the competitive phase of the annual training plan, testing sessions should be planned only if the time between two competitions is 4 to 5 weeks. During this phase the competitions themselves provide ideal opportunities to evaluate the athlete's training status. Regardless of which phase of the annual training plan the testing sessions occur in, the coach must keep detailed records about the athlete's test results. The more organized the data, the easier it is to perform a longitudinal analysis of the athlete's rate of improvement and adaptation to the training plan.

In the written plan, the coach should indicate the test for each training factor using different colors or symbols. The coach should establish standards for each test, especially for physical and technical factors, while compiling the annual plan. Standards from the previous training year can serve as reference points for achieving each standard. This progression should reflect the athlete's rate of improvement and level of adaptation to the program. For novice athletes who are just beginning a structured training program, the results of the first testing session can be used as the reference point for further planning.

The coach must be careful when establishing standards because they provide incentives for preparation and progress. Standards must present a challenge but also must be realistic enough that the athlete can achieve them. For athletes who are aiming for high levels of performance, the standards must resemble those of other top athletes. There are two types of standards; evolutionary standards and maintenance standards. Evolutionary standards are slightly superior to the athlete's potential and stimulate increases in performance; maintenance standards aim to preserve an optimal level of preparation. The time frame of training that progresses the athlete toward these standards should include a maximum of two macrocycles between each testing period. If the athlete has not achieved the standard within two macrocycles, the coach must determine why. For simplicity, the results of the tests and standards can be presented in a table (table 8.10).

TABLE 8.10 Tests and Standard for a Preparatory Phase of Training in University Throwers

Tests	Measures		August 23	September 20	October 18
Biometrics	Body mass	(kg)	101.0	101.5	103.0
	Lean body mass	(kg)	78.3	78.8	80.2
	Body composition	(%)	21.9	21.5	21.5
Isometric midthigh pull	Peak force	(N)	2,881	2,894	3,002
	Peak rate of force development	(N/s)	15,047	18,873	18,000
Resistance training	Snatch	(kg)	61.8	65.5	67.7
Throwing	Shot put	(m)	11.99	12.25	12.63
	Weight bag throw	(m)	11.55	12.43	12.97

Adapted from Stone et al. 2003 (26).

N/s= Newtons per second; N= Newtons

Periodization Model

The periodization of the annual plan provides the model to follow in training. The competition schedule should be used as a foundation from which the most suitable annual plan is constructed (monocycle, bi-cycle, tri-cycle, or multipeak structure). After selecting the annual plan structure in accordance with the competition calendar, the coach determines the duration of each phase and subphase of training (figure 8.16). After placing each training phase, the coach sequences the macrocycles in accordance with the periodization of biomotor abilities. Each macrocycle states the direction of the training process. The coach can further specify the training process by inserting the progression of biomotor ability development or specifying the periodization of certain training means.

Preparation Model

The preparation model is a synopsis of the entire annual training plan. It delineates the main qualities and quantitative parameters used in training and the percentage increment per parameter between the current and previous annual plans. The coach must link the preparation model with the whole structure of the annual plan and its objectives. An experienced coach might predict the duration and number of workouts required to develop the necessary skills and abilities to accomplish the objectives. A preparation model can be structured as shown in table 8.11.

The model presented in table 8.11 assumes that to reach a higher performance level, the athlete must increase his aerobic and muscular endurance. This is accomplished by elevating training volume, prolonging the preparatory phase, and increasing the number of training

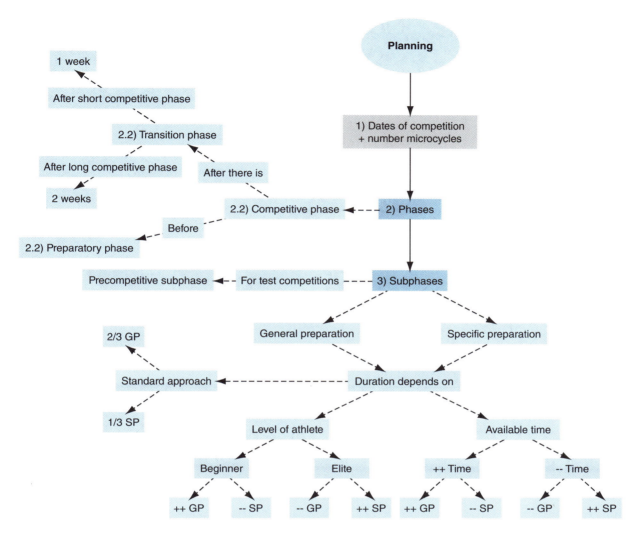

FIGURE 8.16 Flow chart of the compiling of the annual plan.

GP = general preparation; SP = specific preparation.

Courtesy of Dott. Giovanni Altomari, ISCI-SSC.

sessions to correspond with an increase in the total number of hours spent training. Also, modifying the ratio between different methods and types of training will enhance muscular endurance and aerobic endurance.

To improve both aerobic and muscular endurance through strength training and special water exercises, the training content can be altered with the guidelines presented in table 8.12. The breakdown per training phase may occur as in table 8.13. In addition to including these sections of an annual plan, the coach should consider the team or club's organizational and administration structure, including the budget and equipment needs.

TABLE 8.11 Preparatory Model for a 400 m Swimmer

Training factor	Symbol/units	Volume (%)	Change over previous year (%)
Type of annual training plan	Monocycle		
Periodization			
Duration of annual plan (days)	322	100	>8
Preparatory phase (days)	182	56.5	<5
Competitive phase (days)	119	37	<3
Transition phase (days)	21	6.5	
Macrocycles (n)	9		
Microcycles (n)	46		
At the club	41		
At national camp	3		
Abroad	2		
Competitions (n)	7		
International	2		
National	4		
Regional	1		
Training lessons (n)	554		>6
Hours of training	1,122		<8.4
Tests (n)	16		
Medical controls (n)	3		
Specific training (days)	266	82.6	>3
Swimming (km)	2,436		>6
Nonspecific training (days)	14		>2
Running (km)	640	4.4	>2
Strength training (kgm)	460,000		>14
Games (h)	28		>1
Rest (days)	42	13	<8

TABLE 8.12 Model of Training Content for the Annual Plan and Alterations of Each Element Compared With the Previous Year

Content	Content of annual plan (%)	Change from previous year (%)
Anaerobic endurance and speed	2	<6
Muscular endurance	16	>2
Racing tempo endurance	32	0
Aerobic endurance over medium distance	24	>2
Aerobic endurance over long distance	20	>2

TABLE 8.13 Alterations of Training Content and Its Percentage per Training Phase Between the Previous and Current Annual Plan

Content	Preparatory phase (%)	Change (%)	Competitive phase (%)	Change (%)
Anaerobic endurance and speed	5	<4	8	<2
Muscular endurance	10	>2	16	>3
Racing tempo endurance	20	<2	36	<2
Aerobic endurance over medium distance	30	>3	20	>2
Aerobic endurance over long distance	35	>5	20	>4

Summary of Major Concepts

The annual training plan is the cornerstones of a well-structured training program. Irrespective of the coach's knowledge of sport science, if his planning and organizational skills are poor, his training effectiveness will be low. The fundamental concept for good annual planning is periodization, especially structuring the phases of biomotor abilities development. The periodization of strength, speed, and endurance represents the manipulation of different training phases with specific goals, organized in a specific sequence, with the ultimate scope of creating high levels of sport-specific adaptations. When this happens, the athlete is physiologically equipped to perform at her best.

A good understanding of periodization will help the coach produce better annual training plans, using the chart to direct the training process. The competition schedule should guide the structure of the training phases. The periodization of nutrition and psychological training should be integrated into the annual training plan as well. The coach can tailor the annual plan chart to meet the needs of the athletes.

Peaking for Competition

9

Athletes, coaches, and sport scientists work continually to facilitate the development of physiological adaptations that underlie optimal performance. Athletes undergo rigorous training plans that require them to train at high loads, interspersed with unloading phases, to optimize performance at major competitions. Peaking an athlete's performance usually is accomplished by reducing the training load for a predetermined time prior to major competitions. This period of reduced training is termed a **taper**. To optimize performance at the appropriate time and achieve peak condition, coaches and athletes must understand how to integrate tapers and competitions into the annual training plan.

Training Conditions for Peaking

Achieving superior athletic performance is the direct outcome of an athlete's morphofunctional adaptations to various types of stimuli, represented by the training process. The training process is organized and planned over various phases, during which an athlete reaches certain training states. Peaking for a competition is complex, and the athlete cannot realize it on short notice; rather, the athlete attains it in a sequential, cumulative manner and must make progress through other training states before the state of peaking occurs.

Figure 9.1 displays the evolution of peaking during a monocycle annual plan. A detailed explanation of each term will bring better understanding of the concept of training states. **Degree of training** represents the foundation on which the coach may base other training states. As a result of organized and systematic training, the athlete's biomotor abilities development reaches a high level, as does his acquisition of skills and tactical maneuvers. These improvements are reflected through above average results as well as high standards in all tests toward the end of the preparatory phase. An athlete who has reached a high degree of training is, therefore, someone who has achieved a high level of physical and psychological adaptation to the coach's training programs and has perfected all of the pertinent biomotor abilities required by the sport or event. Thus, degree of training and preparedness are synonymous. When the level of adaptation is low, other training states are adversely affected (e.g., psychological and readiness for competitions); this decreases the magnitude of athletic shape and, implicitly, the reachable level of peak of performance.

Preparedness may be general or specific. General preparedness signifies a high adaptation to different forms of training; specific preparedness signifies the athlete has adapted to the specific training requirements of a sport. It is on such a solid base or degree of training during the competitive phase that the athlete attains the state of athletic shape. Papoti and colleagues wrote, "A high level of preparedness is determined by fairly stable factors, whose training effect realization require a long

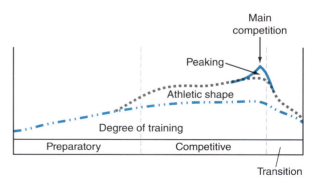

FIGURE 9.1 Accumulation and elevation of training states throughout training phases in a monocycle.

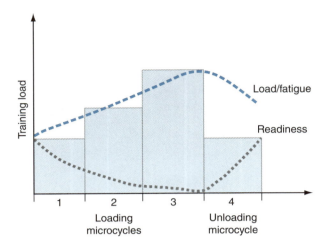

FIGURE 9.2 The fluctuation of the readiness curve is opposed to that of the training load: as the load increases throughout a macrocycle, the level of readiness decreases; as the training load is decreased during unloading microcycles, the level of readiness increases. The highest level of performance is achieved when preparedness and readiness curves meet.

period of time, and thus is not subject to sudden changes: the development of biomotor abilities, the capacity of functional systems, the level of technical-tactical skills, and so on" (53b).

During the competitive phase, athletes are often heard to say that they are in good or bad shape. The state of **athletic shape** (or readiness[1]) is an extension of the degree of training, during which the athletes may perform and attain results close to their maximum capacity, depending on the degree of dissipation of residual fatigue while maintaining her level of preparedness.[2] This paramount training state, which is achieved through specialized training programs (including the cycling unloading of training to reduce fatigue), precedes and incorporates the process of peaking for the main competition of the year. The state of athletic shape is the basis from which the athlete initiates peaking, or the moment during which a high level of preparedness and the highest level of readiness coincide (figure 9.2).

Peaking, as the highlight of athletic shape, results in the athlete's best performance of the year. It is a temporary training state in which physical and psychological efficiencies are maximized and the levels of technical and tactical preparation are optimal (high preparedness), while the absence of residual fatigue (readiness) allows the athlete to produce the highest possible performance.

Peaking

The ultimate goal of an athlete's training plan is to optimize performance in specific competitions throughout the training year. This goal is accomplished through careful sequencing of the annual training plan. The foundation for peaking an athlete's performance is established during the preparatory and competition phases of training, when the athlete builds her physical, tactical, and technical training base (64, 65). During the later portions of the competition phase of training, the process of peaking an athlete for specific competition is initiated (figure 9.3). Peaking, or tapering as it is sometimes called (64, 65), is a complex process that can be affected by many factors including the training volume, frequency, and intensity (19). If the taper is implemented correctly, peaking occurs in response to the physiological and psychological adaptations induced by the training plan (19, 41). The taper is one of the most critical phases of an athlete's readiness for competition (19). Tapers are widely used by athletes from various sports to gain a performance edge over their competitors (10, 21, 24, 26, 34, 35, 38, 50, 63).

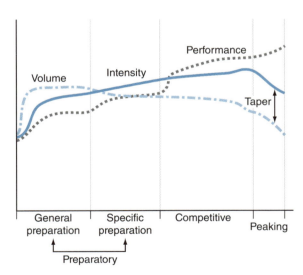

FIGURE 9.3 Dynamics of volume, intensity, and performance level throughout an annual plan.

---

[1] The state of "readiness to perform" is achieved on the base of a high level of preparedness and [...] its formation is quite rapid [...]. Differently from the state of preparedness, readiness is affected by considerable fluctuations," according to Papoti and colleagues (53b).

[2] Athletic shape is formed by stable and unstable components. The unstable components are those that affect the degree of readiness to perform of the athlete. The interaction between the stable and unstable components of the athletic shape determines the dynamics of competition performance," according to Matveyev (32b).

Defining a Taper

Many definitions have been used to describe how an athlete's training plan is modified in the final days before a competition (4, 39, 41, 44, 59, 62). When attempting to peak an athlete for competition, the coach reduces the workload prior to the competition (41). The reduction in workload that is used during this time is considered a taper (4, 41, 61). Traditionally, a taper is simply defined as a reduction in training workload prior to a competition (58). Mujika and Padilla (40) defined a taper as "a progressive non-linear reduction of the training load during a variable period of time, in an attempt to reduce the physiological and psychological stress of daily training and optimize sports performance" (p. 80). This definition expands on the traditional definition by including some implications for the design of the taper (41).

Primary Aim of a Taper

The goal of a taper is to optimize the athlete's performance at a specific time (4, 19, 41, 59). This is usually accomplished by systematically reducing the training load to decrease the cumulative fatigue (both physiological and psychological) that is generated in response to training while maintaining sport-specific fitness (41). The taper allows the athlete to reduce the internal load (residual fatigue), thus elevating performance (41, 61). This contention is supported in the scientific literature, which shows that accumulated fatigue is reduced during a taper period while readiness slightly increases (35), thereby improving performance. As fatigue is dissipated in response to the taper, the athlete may realize significant positive psychological alterations, such as a reduction in perception of effort, improved mood, a reduction in sense of fatigue, and an increased sense of vigor (20, 41, 56). These findings indicate that at the initiation of a taper, the physiological adaptations to the training program have already occurred (41) and are probably masked by accumulated fatigue (60), whereas the psychological adaptations will occur in response to the taper. Thus, the taper is a mechanism for decreasing both physiological and psychological fatigue, allowing for performance gains.

Premise of Tapering

The **fitness–fatigue relationship** is a central concept underlying the appropriate implementation of a taper (5, 60). An athlete's readiness to perform is variable because it is directly affected by changes in the levels of fitness and fatigue generated in response to training (6, 64, 65). Readiness is optimized by using training plans that maximize the fitness response while minimizing the development of fatigue (54). When training workload is high, readiness is low as a result of a high level of accumulated fatigue.

The premise behind a taper is to dissipate accumulated fatigue (achieving a higher level of readiness) while retaining fitness (preparedness). Because the level of acquired fitness is relatively stable over several minutes, hours, and days, it is considered to be a slow-changing component of athletic preparedness. Conversely, fatigue is considered to be a fast-changing component because it is highly variable and is affected by physiological and psychological stressors (64, 65). Thus, when the training load is decreased during a taper, the accumulated fatigue is dissipated somewhat rapidly, whereas physical potential is maintained for a given duration depending on the type of taper used and the total workload preceding the taper (4, 5).

Although the premise behind a taper is somewhat simple, the implementation of a taper is complex. If the duration of the taper is too long, the level of readiness achieved by the training program can dissipate, resulting in a state of detraining (40) and a reduction in performance level (figure 9.4). This reduction in training load can be considered a compromise between the extent of the training reduction and the duration of this reduction (61), which combine to determine level of readiness to perform. If, for example, the training workload

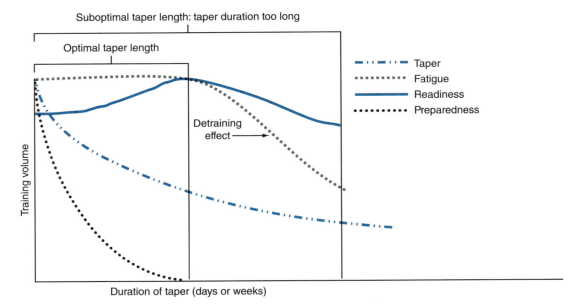

FIGURE 9.4 Interrelationship of fatigue, preparedness, readiness, and taper length. During the taper fatigue decreases rapidly, while preparedness is maintained for a little longer depending on the composition of the taper and the preceding workload. However, if the taper extends for too long, preparedness will dissipate until detraining occurs.

prior to the taper was very high, a greater reduction or duration of a taper would be necessary to maximize the decrease in fatigue required to elevate readiness (30, 61). Thus, the taper is more than simply reducing the training load; it involves integrating many factors to elevate the athlete's readiness and optimize performance.

Factors Affecting a Taper

There are many strategies for including a taper in an annual training plan (4). The key component of each of these strategies is to alter the training plan to reduce training load (i.e., training volume, intensity, and even frequency). The effectiveness of these reductions in training load will depend on the duration of the taper (59) and its relationship to the training load that preceded the taper (61). If the taper lasts too long, both fatigue and physical potential (preparedness) will be decreased, which would lead to detraining (40). In this situation, performance would not increase, and the taper would be deemed ineffective. Therefore, the coach must understand the interactions of training intensity, volume of training, training frequency, and the duration of the taper.

Training Intensity

The scientific literature indicates that when reducing volume and frequency during a taper, it might be warranted to maintain or slightly elevate the training intensity (4, 24, 30, 34, 41, 50, 59). It appears that the training intensity during the taper is closely related to the ability to maintain training-induced performance adaptations during periods of reduced training load (17, 58). It has also been suggested that the training intensity is a key factor in maintaining training-induced physiological adaptations during the taper (4, 44). When examining endurance training studies, researchers have noted that lower training intensities ($\leq 70\%$ $\dot{V}O_2max$) during the taper period tend to result in a decrease or maintenance of endurance performance (25, 33). Conversely, when higher intensities ($\geq 90\%$ $\dot{V}O_2max$) are included in the taper, performance tends to increase (58). Similarly, when examining strength and power training, investigators have determined that maintaining intensity during the taper, while decreasing training volume, enhances strength (11, 27) and power performance (6b, 31b). Thus, it seems warranted to maintain the training intensity during the taper period and adjust the workload by manipulating training volume or frequency or the duration of the taper (41, 59) (see Recommended Tapering Strategies).

Training Volume

Reducing training volume during a taper to reduce the training load is the method that is probably the most discussed in the scientific literature (4, 19, 34, 41, 59, 61). The volume of training can be decreased during a taper by reducing the duration of each training session, reducing training frequency, or both (4, 41). Decreasing the duration of each training session is preferable to reducing the training frequency, because the former appears to exert a greater effect on the effectiveness of a taper (4).

The pretaper training volume will dictate how much training volume must be decreased during the taper period to maximize performance outcomes. Tapers that range between a 50% and 90% reduction in training volume have been reported in the scientific literature on swimming (28, 36, 37, 42, 62), running (22, 23, 25, 33, 38, 39, 58), cycling (32, 47, 48, 57), triathlon (2, 49, 63), and strength training (11, 27). In well-trained endurance athletes (e.g., cycling and running), a standardized 50% to 70% reduction in training volume has been reported to maintain or increase training-induced adaptations (22, 23, 25, 32, 33, 57). Progressive tapers that result in a 75% reduction in training volume appear to optimize taper-induced outcomes, compared with a 50% reduction in training volume (38). It appears that low-volume tapers result in better physiological and performance outcomes, compared with moderate-volume tapers (58).

The scientific literature indicates that a 41% to 60% reduction in training volume during the taper results in optimal performance improvements (4). However, the percentage reduction in training volume is related to the pretaper training workload and the planned duration of the taper. If the training load prior to the taper is heavy, then a greater reduction in training volume, of the magnitude of 60% to 90% of pretaper loads, may be warranted to dissipate fatigue (41, 61) (see Recommended Tapering Strategies). If training volume is substantially reduced, a shorter duration of taper may be warranted to offset the loss of training-induced adaptations that would result in a decrease in physical potential performance (30). See table 9.1 for a summary of the factors that influence training volume during the taper.

Recommended Tapering Strategies

- Use tapering strategies to dissipate fatigue, maintain physical capabilities, elevate readiness, and improve performance.
- Create individualized taper strategies that last between 1 and 2 weeks.
- Maintain moderate to high training intensities during the taper to avoid detraining.
- Decrease training volume by 41% to 60% of pretaper volumes. If extensive training precedes the taper, it may be warranted to decrease training volume by 60% to 90% of pretaper volumes.
- Maintain training frequency at 80% or more of pretaper frequencies.
- Use progressive, nonlinear taper models.
- Expect performance gains of approximately 3% in response to the taper.

Adapted from Mujika and Padilla 2003 (41), Mujika 1998 (34), and Bosquet et al. 2002 (4).

TABLE 9.1 — Factors Affecting Training Volume in the Taper

	Characteristic	Effect on taper volume
Load of pretaper Macrocycle	High	Greater reduction
	Low	Smaller reduction
Taper duration	Short	Greater reduction
	Long	Smaller reduction
Type of load reduction	Linear	Higher mean volume; lower final volume
	Step	Lower mean volume; higher final volume

Training Frequency

Reducing training frequency is another popular method for reducing the training load during a taper (14, 18, 41, 59). Several studies report that reductions of the magnitude of 50% of pretaper training frequencies can increase performance (18, 28). Decreases in training frequency for 2 weeks have been shown to result in maintenance of training-induced physiological and performance outcomes in athletic groups (22, 23, 25, 32, 33, 41, 44, 50, 57). This literature indicates that modulating training frequencies might be a successful method for altering training volume.

Although physiological adaptations can be maintained with 30% to 50% of pretaper training frequencies in moderately trained individuals, it has been suggested that highly trained athletes may need a greater frequency of training during the taper period to maintain technical proficiency (41). These findings indicate that training frequency should be maintained at 80% or more of pretaper training values to optimize performance outcomes and

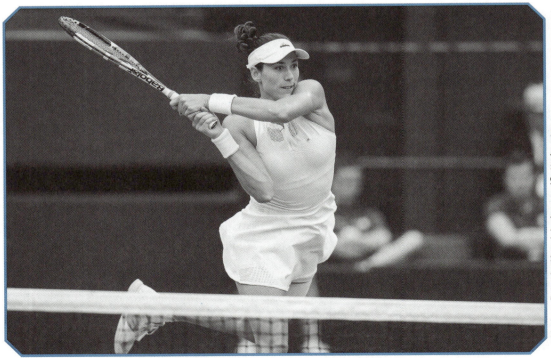

Tapering training can help an athlete peak for a key competition.

maintain technical proficiency (4, 41) (see Recommended Tapering Strategies). For alactic power sports (60m dash, jumps and throws in track & field, diving) a lower training frequency during the taper, achieved by placing more off days within the microcycles, could favour the myosin heavy chain rebound to the fast IIX phenotype, thus improving performance. It is a common practice in high-level team sports to plan 2 or 3 days off from training either during the first week of the taper or between the first and second weeks.

This approach is taken because team sport athletes usually enter the taper period before tournaments or cup finals in an overreaching state due to the long competitive season. For this reason, for professional and national teams, sports medicine practitioners are strongly advised to check the athlete's testosterone-to-cortisol ratio and level of free testosterone (possibly checking them throughout the season for comparative purposes). The results give strength and conditioning coaches more information to use in establishing training load during the taper for each player.

Duration of Taper

The duration of a taper is probably one of the most difficult things to determine (41), because many factors affect the taper. For example, the pretaper training workload can significantly affect the length of the taper necessary to dissipate training-induced fatigue and elevate readiness (61). The amount of volume reduction or the pattern of reduction during the taper affects the duration needed to elevate readiness while maintaining high adaptation level (preparedness). If a larger reduction in training volume is used, then a shorter duration of taper would be warranted (30, 61). Other factors (e.g., body weight, gender, weekly training hours, and load-reduction strategy) influence the way the taper is planned (table 9.2).

Physiological, psychological, and performance improvements have been reported in the scientific literature for 1- to 4-week tapers (4), preferably 1-2 weeks for well-trained athletes. Several authors suggest that 8 to 14 days are necessary to dissipate fatigue and avoid the negative effects of detraining that might occur with a longer taper (4, 30). However, it appears that the duration of a taper is highly individualized (4, 41) as a result of differences in physiological and psychological adaptations to reductions in training load (4, 35, 43). Therefore, it is recommended that the taper duration be individualized for each athlete (see Recommended Tapering Strategies).

TABLE 9.2 Factors Affecting Duration of the Taper

Characteristics		Effects on the duration of the taper
Body weight	High	More lasting
	Low	Less lasting
Gender	Male	More lasting with less time dedicated to strength maintenance
	Female	Less lasting with more time dedicated to strength maintenance
Load of pretaper macrocycle	High	More lasting
	Low	Less lasting
Load reduction strategy during taper	Linear	More lasting
	Step	Less lasting
Weekly training hours	High	More lasting (>15 hours)
	Low	Less lasting (<10 hours)

Types of Tapers

Various taper formats have been proposed in the literature (4, 41). Tapers can be broadly defined as either **progressive** or **nonprogressive**. A progressive taper is marked by a systematic and progressive reduction in training load, whereas a nonprogressive taper uses standardized reductions in training load (41). Different loading characteristics can exist within each category of taper.

In a progressive taper, the training load is reduced in either a linear or an exponential fashion. Progressive tapers can be classified into three types: a linear taper, a slow exponential taper, and a fast exponential taper (figure 9.5) (41). The linear taper normally contains a higher mean training load than the loads seen in either a slow or fast exponential taper. A slow exponential taper tends to have a slower reduction in training load and higher training loads than those seen in a fast exponential taper (41). Fast exponential tapers appear to result in greater performance gains than linear or slow exponential tapers (2, 41, 63). For example, a comparison between fast and slow exponential tapers revealed that the fast exponential taper resulted in a 3.9% to 4.1% greater increase in markers of performance (41).

The nonprogressive taper, also called a step taper (2, 34, 41, 63), is accomplished with standardized reductions in training. This taper is often marked by sudden decreases in training load (61), which can increase the likelihood of a loss of physical potential during the taper (2). **Step tapers** have been shown by many studies to improve both physiological and performance adaptations to training (13, 17, 22, 23, 25, 32, 41, 51). However, the literature indicates that step tapers are less effective than either slow or fast progressive tapers (2, 4, 63). For example, Mujika and Padilla (41) reported that step tapers result in a 1.2% to 1.5% increase in markers of performance, whereas exponential tapers result in a 4.0% to 5.0% increase in performance. Authors usually recommend that an exponential taper be used when attempting to peak an athlete's performance for a competition (4, 41, 61).

The selection of the type of progressive taper will depend on many factors including the training load prior to the taper (61) and the duration of the taper (19). However, it appears that the fast exponential tapers should be selected in most instances (41) (see the Recommended Tapering Strategies).

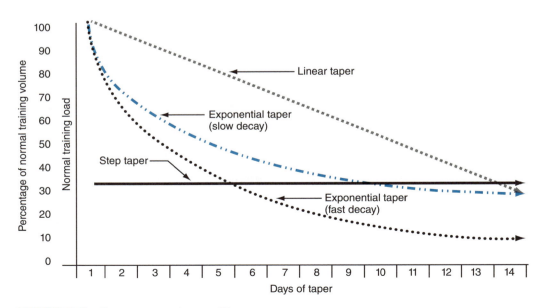

FIGURE 9.5 Four common types of tapers.

Adapted from Mujika and Padilla 2003 (41).

Expected Performance Improvements

The primary goal of any taper is to elevate performance at the appropriate time (4, 34, 41). Small improvements in performance may result in distinct differences in placing at the Olympics. For example, Mujika and colleagues (43) reported that the difference between the gold medal and fourth place in swimming at the 2000 Sydney Olympics was only 1.62%, and the difference between third and eighth place was only 2.02%. At the 2004 Athens Olympics, the difference between first and third place in weightlifting was 1.96% (women = 2.21%; men = 1.73%). These data show that very small elevations in performance can have a great impact on performance outcomes and may mean the difference between winning and losing.

When examining the scientific literature, it has been reported that a properly implemented taper can result in significant improvements in performance (0.5% to 11.0%) and muscular strength and power (8% to 25%) in runners, triathletes, cyclists and swimmers (16, 24, 32, 38, 41, 48, 53, 58, 63). When specifically examining competition measures, it appears that a 0.5% to 6.0% (~3.0%) increase in performance can be expected in response to a preevent taper (41). Mujika and colleagues (43) reported that during a 3-week taper prior to the 2004 Sydney Olympics, swimming performance was elevated by 2.2%. Interestingly, the magnitude of this taper-induced increase in swimming performance was similar to the differences between first and fourth place (1.62%) and third and eighth place (2.02%) (4, 43).

Regarding muscular strength, it appears that a taper can result in a 2% to 8% increase in performance. Izquierdo and colleagues (27) reported that a taper protocol results in a 2.0% increase in back squat and bench press performance. A larger increase in strength performance in response to a taper protocol was reported by Coutts and colleagues (7), who found that a three-repetition maximum back squat strength increased by 7.2% and three-repetition maximum bench press increased by 5.2%. Gibala and colleagues (11) reported a 3% to 8% increase in maximal isometric and dynamic force-generating capacity.

A properly implemented taper can result in significant increases in performance. The magnitude of the performance gains will be related to many factors, especially the type of taper selected (41). The appropriate taper may result in an elevation of performance (about 3.0%) that differentiates between first and third place at the Olympic Games, because the magnitude of taper-induced gains in performance is similar to that of the difference between first and third place in many sports.

Competition Phase of the Annual Plan

The competition phase of the annual training plan is a complex training entity, with the objective of reaching the state of readiness for the major competitions of the year. This is facilitated by using tapering and peaking methods as well as effective planning of competitions. Although the competitive period usually contains many competitions, a true peak of performance can only be maintained for about 7 to 14 days (52b); this suggests that the competition phase must be planned carefully to optimize the athlete's performance.

Classifications of Competitions

Competitions can be classified into two broad categories: (1) major or official competitions and (2) preparatory or exhibition competitions.

Major competitions are the athlete's most important competitions (e.g., national championships, world championships, Olympic Games). These contests require the athlete to be at peak performance and often provide the guidelines for organizing the athlete's annual training plan, especially for individual sports. Preparations for a major competition usually include a taper to dissipate accumulated fatigue and enhance the athlete's readiness.

Preparatory or exhibition competitions are used to test the athlete and attain feedback regarding specific aspects of training. These competitions are integral to the preparation of the athlete and are an important part of the training plan. Often athletes will place these

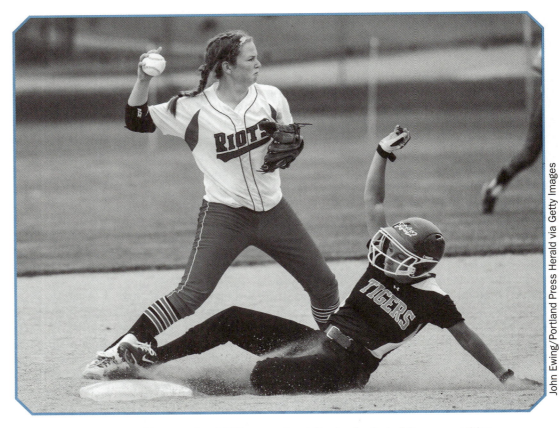

Minor competitions and exhibition events at the beginning of the competition calendar are good ways to gauge how a training plan is working.

types of competitions at the end of the unloading microcycle without using any specific tapering strategies. Many coaches use these competitions to test some aspect of the athlete's development, such as technical, tactical, or a given biomotor ability. Victory is not always the focus of these types of competitions; rather, they are undertaken as very high-intensity training sessions. However, victory in these competitions may yield valuable information about the athlete's level of readiness which may then lead to alterations to the training plan.

Planning for Competition

The most important step in developing the annual training plan is to establish the competitive schedule for the athlete or team and to determine which competitions require peak form. The competition schedule is established by the sport's governing body and culminates with the national, continental, or world championships. When determining the competitive schedule, the coach needs to select specific competitions that can be considered preparatory or exhibition contests and are scheduled to target specific training objectives. These contests are used as hard training days that target specific skill sets, so they can serve as important tools for preparing the athlete for major competitions.

Many coaches make two large mistakes when planning the competitive schedule for their athletes. The first mistake is to have the athlete participate in every available competition; this interrupts the athlete's training and her ability to develop the physiological, technical, and tactical skills required for major competitions. The second major mistake is attempting to peak the athlete for every competition. If the athlete attempts to peak too frequently, she likely will need a large number of restoration-based training sessions and will not undergo enough actual training to enhance physiological, tactical, or technical characteristics. It is recommended that the athlete attempt to peak by using specific tapering strategies for only a very few competitions (two or three) and that the remainder of the competitive schedule consist of competitions of secondary emphasis preceded by a short unloading of 2 to 3 days (figure 9.6). Both of these common coaching errors can be avoided if the coach plans an appropriate competitive phase of training.

There are several ways to plan the competitive phase of training (52). If the athlete is preparing for one specific competition, the coach should use a simple competition training period; if two or more competitions are being prepared for, a complex competition training period is used (52). The number of macrocycles in the competitive period is dictated by the complexity of the competition phase of training (simple versus complex) and the athlete's needs (52).

Two methods for planning the competitive phase of the annual training plan are traditionally used: the grouping and the cyclic approach. The grouping approach is a method of planning 2 or 3 weeks in a row, during which the athlete takes part in tournaments or competitions or participates in several events or races per weekend. As illustrated in figure 9.8, this approach is usually followed by several microcycles (3 or 4 weeks) that are dedicated to training and allow the athlete to prepare for another 2 or 3 weeks of grouped competitions.

In the example illustrated in figure 9.7, the athlete or team participates in a group of competitions spread over a 2-week period during the early part of the competitive schedule. During these 2 weeks, races or games may be held during each weekend. The first microcycle following these competitions is of low intensity, with the first 2 or 3 days of the cycle targeting a low training load designed to stimulate regeneration. After the first 2 or 3 days of the cycle are completed, the training load is increased, typically resulting in one peak of training load at the end of the microcycle. The next two and a half microcycles are dedicated to demanding training, followed by a short 2- or 3-day unloading period that leads into the next 3 weeks of competitions. The next major competition occurs on August 21 and is designated as the qualifying competition for the championships that are held on September 25. Because the August 21 contest is a major competition that serves as a qualifier for the championships, an 8- to 14-day exponential taper is used to elevate performance. After the athlete completes the qualifying competition, she enters a regeneration microcycle, followed by 2 to 2.5 weeks

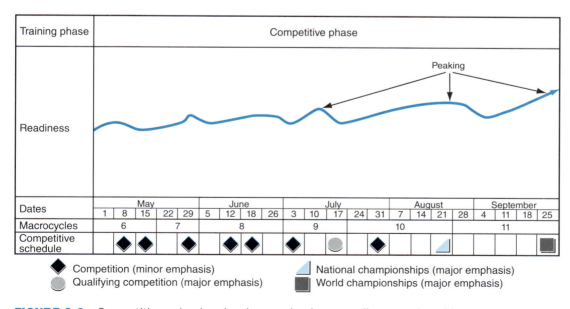

FIGURE 9.6 Competitive calendar showing emphasis on readiness and peaking.

of hard training before undertaking another taper. If the schedule is structured correctly, performance will be optimized at the championships.

The grouping method usually is best suited for individual sports where only a few major competitions are undertaken throughout the annual training plan. With team sports, the grouping method may only be useful when teams approach national championships, international competitions, or official international tournaments. Leagues of most team sports use a cyclic approach to determine the competitive schedule.

In the cyclic approach, competitions are spaced at regular, repeating intervals (figure 9.9). In figure 9.9, the vast majority of the competitions occur each weekend during macrocycles 8 and 9. This pattern of competition is often seen in American football, where competitions usually occur each weekend throughout the fall. The last two macrocycles (10 and 11) contain

Training phase	Competitive phase																			
	May					June				July					August				September			
Dates	1	8	15	22	29	5	12	19	26	3	10	17	24	31	7	14	21	28	4	11	18	25
Macrocycles	6			7			8				9				10				11			
Competitive schedule				◆	◆					◆	◆	◆				◢						■

◆ Competition (minor emphasis)

◢ Qualifying competition (major emphasis)

■ Championships (major emphasis)

FIGURE 9.7 Competitive schedule based on the grouping approach.

Competition Is Not a Substitute for Training

Many coaches maintain that participation in competitions elevates an athlete's preparation level. Although this is true to a certain extent, a coach should not expect to achieve an elevated level of physical potential and correct peaking through competition only, as coaches often attempt in some professional sports. Participation in competitions, especially during the precompetitive phase when exhibition contests are planned, does assist athletes with reaching a high state of readiness for the main competition of the year. During such competitions, they have the opportunity to test all training factors in the most specific way. To consider the competition as the only mean of improvement, however, deteriorates quality of training by curbing the main cycle of activity, which is training, unloading, competition, and regeneration (figure 9.8). Furthermore, some coaches, by omitting either the unloading before competitions or the regeneration afterward, are increasing the injury potential of their athletes, while never allowing them to compete in a state of readiness.

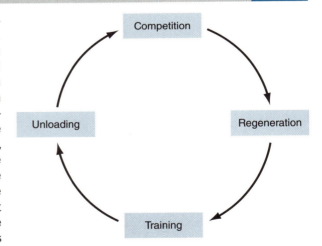

FIGURE 9.8 Cyclic pattern of the activities that induce good performance for competitions, while avoiding injuries.

the two major competitions of this competition phase. In American university football, the competition in macrocycle 10 would be the conference championships, whereas the contest in macrocycle 11 would be a national championship or bowl game. Because each microcycle throughout macrocycle 8 and 9 ends with a game, a one-peak microcycle structure may be warranted. This peak or increased training load would occur on Tuesday or Wednesday. An unloading period would be used (1 or 2 days before each game) to dissipate fatigue and prepare the athlete for competition. Coaches who work with individual sports should consider using the cyclic approach in the lead-up to the major competitions (figure 9.10). In this approach the coach may take the athlete to competitions that occur every 2 weeks to

FIGURE 9.9 Competition schedule for a team sport based on a cyclic approach.

FIGURE 9.10 Cyclic approach for a cross-country skier.

gain information about the athlete in competitive situations. This will allow the coach to modify the training plan based on the feedback garnered from the periodic competitions.

In the cyclic approach, the first half of the week after a competition would contain a lower training load to enhance recovery, whereas the second half of the week would contain higher training loads (figure 9.11). The microcycle preceding the next competition would be structured so that the higher training loads are encountered earlier in the week (i.e., Tuesday or Wednesday) and unloading would occur in the second half of the week to facilitate recovery for the weekend competition. However, this is only an example of how a microcycle could be formatted; many different formats are available based on the type of taper and the competitive season. Although these two major approaches are often used to design the competitive phase of training, it is likely that the cyclic and grouped approaches can be combined when planning for competitions.

Competition Frequency

Determining the frequency of competitions is a complex undertaking. Factors such as the athlete's characteristics, training age, and sport contribute to the frequency and number of

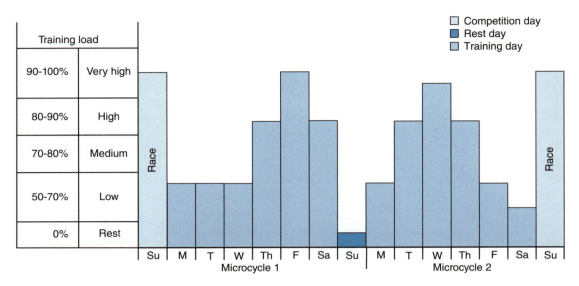

FIGURE 9.11 Microcycle structure for training between competitions during the cyclic approach.

competitions undertaken each year. The coach also must consider the length of the competition phase, given that a longer phase would allow a greater number of competitions.

A primary determinant of the number of competitions undertaken by athletes is their age and training experience (9). The less experienced the child or youth athlete, the less frequently he should compete (9). If the athlete's training is centered on multilateral development, the young athlete will increase the number of competitive starts progressively as his skills develop and as his training plan increases the emphasis on specialization (45, 55). Kauhanen (29) suggested that as the young athlete becomes more trained, the number of major competitions should increase each year (table 9.3). During these years, secondary or minor competitions are still undertaken to help develop the athlete's skills in competition. With young athletes the primary emphasis is the development of the skills that will be used in competition as they become more trained.

TABLE 9.3 Suggested Types and Number of Competitions for Young Athletes

Age (yr)	Type of competitions	Organized competitions/yr
4-7	No formal competition; just for fun	—
8-11	Informal competitions to stress skill form rather than winning; participate in other sports just for fun	Team sports: 5-10
12-13	Organized competitions in which the goal is to achieve certain physical, technical, or tactical goals rather than winning	Team sports: 10-15 Individual sports: 5-8
14-16	Participate in competitions without pushing to reach the best performance possible	Team sports: 15-20 Individual sports: 8-10
17-19	Participate in junior competitions to qualify for state and national championships; get ready to reach peak performance at the senior competitions	Team sports: 20-35 Individual sports: short duration, 20-30; long duration, 6-8

Reprinted, by permission, from T.O. Bompa and M. Carrera, 2015, *Conditioning young athletes* (Champaign, IL: Human Kinetics), 220.

A second factor determining the frequency of competitions is the characteristics of the sport. In team sports the length of the season can have a great impact on the number of competitions held. For example, a top team in the football Premier League may compete in roughly 60 competitions over approximately 270 days, which roughly equates to competing every 3 1/2 to 4 1/2 days (8).

Individual sports athletes usually have greater flexibility in the selection of competitions because these athletes usually compete less frequently than athletes in team sports. Dick (8) suggested that the buildup and principle competition period in track and field should consist of about 7 to 10 competitions. Any additional competitions would be used for lower-level training (8). Table 9.4 offers some very rough guidelines concerning the number of competitions for novice and advanced athletes. Regardless of the athlete or sport, the coach must consider the interrelationships of training, recovery, and peaking.

When constructing the training plan for the competitive phase, the coach must consider the sequence and frequency of competitions and how they relate to the time allowed for recovery after competition (46). The more frequently the athlete competes, the less time she will have to train for the next competition (8, 15). Therefore, overly frequent competitions can impede the athlete's development because each competition undertaken can result in fatigue, which must be dealt with by reducing training loads.

The coach should plan for two to four major competitions during the competitive phase of the training year. These competitions will most likely include qualifying meets for the year's main competition. The training plan should also include secondary competitions that are used as hard training sessions and to test the athlete's ability. The coach and athlete should think of the competitive schedule as a buildup to the major competition (table 9.5). However, the schedule must allow time between the preparatory (exhibition) competitions and the major competitions. The optimal sequencing between training, competition, and recovery during this phase will depend on the time interval between each competition.

Regarding the time interval between competitions, Bompa (3) and Harre (15) recommended the following:

- Undertake competitions only when the athlete is capable of achieving set objectives for each training factor: physical, technical, tactical, and psychological.

TABLE 9.4 Suggested Number of Competitions per Year in Athletics (Track and Field)

Event	Novice athletes Winter	Novice athletes Summer	Elite athletes Winter	Elite athletes Summer
Sprinters, hurdlers, jumpers, and throwers				
Specialized event	3-4	12-16	3-5	16-20
Other events and sports	2-3	4-6	1-3	3-5
Middle distance				
800-1,500 m	—	4-8	2-3	10-16
Short distances	2-3	8-10	2-4	8-10
Distance running and walking				
Marathon	—	1	—	2-3
31 mi (50 km) walk	—	6-8	—	8-10
Combined events				
Decathlon	—	1-2	—	2-3
Heptathlon	—	1-2	—	2-4
Individual events	2-4	10-12	3-5	12-16

TABLE 9.5 — Objectives for the Competitive Subphase

Competitive subphase	Objectives	Means of implementation
Precompetitive	1. Improve performance. 2. Gain experience. 3. Determine strengths and weaknesses. 4. Test technique and tactics.	1. Enter competitions of lower difficulty. 2. Increase frequency of competitions (team sports). 3. Use short unloading (3 to 7 days).
Competitive (league or official competitions)	1. Elevate readiness. 2. Prepare for qualifying competitions.	1. Adjust the macrocycle structure to the level of the opponent (team sport). 2. Use different unloading strategies according to the importance of the competition (individual sports). 3. Participate in competitions of increasing demands (individual sports).
Taper (major competitions)	1. Maximize readiness. 2. Compete at highest level in major competitions.	1. Use specialized preparation methods such as a taper to prepare for major competitions.

- Carefully select and schedule competitions so that they progressively increase in difficulty.
- Select challenging competitions because unchallenging competitions do not motivate the athlete.
- Challenge the athlete by placing him against opponents with superior capabilities.
- Avoid entering too many competitions. Participating in too many competitions, especially those that require substantial travel, will result in an improperly dosed competitive and training schedule, which will reduce physical and psychological potential.
- Sequence the competitive schedule in a progressive fashion, allowing for readiness to be maximized at the main competition of the season. This will allow the athlete every possibility to perform at her highest level at this contest.
- Allocate adequate time between competitions to allow the athlete time to train and correct any technical flaws noted in secondary or exhibition competitions.
- Instruct the athlete to perform at his highest level only in the main competitions of the training year. Think of the other competitions as sequential progressive steps that bring the athlete's physiological capacity, technical skill, tactical ability, and psychological state (and thus performance) to the very highest level.

As shown in table 9.6, the progressive decrease in volume and intensity of all training activities during the competitive phase, as well as the increased use of recovery techniques, helps the athlete replenish energy stores, achieve supercompensation, relax mentally, and build motivation to attain her best possible results in the competition targeted for peak performance. The strategy presented in table 9.6 must be applied for the duration of the tapering period, to ensure maximum neuromuscular benefits prior to major competitions. During this time, the focus shifts to recovery and regeneration through proper rest, nutrition, supplementation, and soft tissue therapies (e.g., deep massage, myofascial release). In terms of training, this is a time to reap the benefits of well-planned preparation and competitive periods.

TABLE 9.6 — Training and Recovery Strategies and Benefits During the Taper

Strategies		Benefits
Dynamics of volume	• Decrease total distance or duration by 40% to 60%. • Decrease number of reps. • Increase rest interval to full recovery. • Don't introduce new exercises.	• Achieve supercompensation of all physiological systems. • Increase readiness of the neuromuscular system. • Facilitate replenishment of energy stores.
Dynamics of intensity	• Reduce intensity by 5% to 10% for power sports and 20% to 30% for endurance sports, especially in the first week. • Raise intensity a few days before competition.	
Neuromuscular stimulation	• Use neuromuscular system potentiation methods.	• Induce pre-peaking neuromuscular state. • Increase recruitment of fast-twitch (FT) muscle fibers. • Increase discharge rate of FT fibers. • Maximize arousal of the neuromuscular system. • Increase reactivity of the neuromuscular system.
Recovery methods	• Use soft tissue management techniques (e.g., deep massage, myofascial release). • Control heart rate variability (HRV) values to ensure proper recovery dynamics. • Control sleep quality (e.g., use the Sleep as Android app). • Use psychological relaxation, motivation, and visualization techniques (e.g., hypnosis, which can induce a deep state of relaxation and faster nervous system recovery). • Ensure proper nutrition and sport- specific food supplementation.	• Improve soft tissue compliance and joint mobility. • Increase readiness of the neuromuscular system. • Relax mentally. • Increase confidence. • Increase arousal. • Replenish energy stores. • Sustain maximal power output throughout competition.

Identifying Peaking

To identify peaking, specifically in individual sports, one of the most objective criteria seems to be the dynamics of the athlete's performances (32c). Researchers used athletes from sprinting and mid-distance running as subjects (N = 2,300) for a longitudinal study about establishing zones of calculation for peaking. Considering the past year's personal best performance as a reference point (or 100%), zone 1, or the zone of high results, consisted of performances not more than 2.0% lower than the reference point. Medium results were those within 2% to 3.5% deviation of best performance. Low performances within 3.5% to 5% deviation were in zone 3. Finally, zone 4 consisted of poor results, or performances with a deviation of more than 5% from the previous year's best. The authors concluded that when an athlete can achieve performances within 2% (zone 1) of best, then she is in high athletic shape, close to a peak performance. From this point on, athletes easily facilitate peaking and achieve outstanding performances. Of course, these percentages can be adapted to reflect the significance to the event (tables 9.7 and 9.8).

TABLE 9.7 — Peaking Zones for an International-Level Marathoner*

Marathoner PB 2:10:00 (h/min/s)	Peaking zone
2:10:00-2:12:36	1 (up to 2%)
2:12:37-2:14:33	2 (2%-3.5%)
2:14:34-2:16:30	3 (3.5%-5%)
>2:16:30	4 (>5%)

*According to the classification of Matveyev, Kalinin, and Ozolin (32c).
PB = personal best.

TABLE 9.8 — Peaking Zones Adapted for an International-Level Sprinter

100m Sprinter PB 10.00 (s)	Peaking zone
10.00-10.10	1 (up to 1%)
10.11-10.20	2 (1-2%)
10.21-10.30	3 (2-3%)
>10.30	4 (>3%)

PB = personal best.

Maintaining a Peak

The time required to reach zone 1 is an important factor for peaking. Although this might differ according to each athlete's abilities, the average time an athlete needs to elevate the capacity from a precompetitive level to the aptitude of zone 1 is four to six microcycles. The athlete may not see dramatic increases during the first three or four microcycles because hard work that stresses intensity results in a high level of fatigue, which restricts the achievement of good performances. Following the last one or two microcycles, however, when the athlete has adapted to the training load and a slight decrease in the stress of training allows supercompensation to occur, higher performance is feasible. Although the duration of this transitory phase from lower performances to zone 1 varies according to many factors, it also varies according to the specifics of each sport and the coach's approach to training.

The duration of peaking, as well as zone 1, may be affected by the number of starts or competitions the athlete experiences. The longer the phase with weekly competitions, the lower the probability of duplicating high results. Many competitions do not necessarily lead to good and progressively higher performances. Often, there is a contrary effect, and results decrease toward the end of a competitive phase, when championship competitions are usually planned. A critical phase often begins after the eighth microcycle with competitions. This does not necessarily mean that performance is compromised toward the end of the competitive phase. On the contrary, it should draw the coach's attention to the need for better alternation of stressful exercises with regeneration activities. In addition, it should bring the coach's attention to the methods and means of selecting and planning competitions during precompetitive and competitive phases. This should be significant to some university coaches, especially for team sports, in which the competition schedule is loaded with many games, even during the preparatory phase. The individual training program each athlete follows, and the duration and type of training performed during the preparatory phase, have substantial influence on the duration of peaking. The longer and more solid the preparatory phase, the higher the probability of prolonging the athletic shape and peaking.

Assuming that the coach led and organized an adequate training program, the duration of zone 1 may be 1 to 2 months. During this time, the athlete may facilitate two or three peaks, in which he achieves high or even record performances. Researchers suggest that the duration of peaking may be up to 7 to 10 days because the nerve cells can maintain optimal working capacity for that long (52b). As previously stated, following each peaking for a top competition, a short phase of regeneration is strongly desirable, followed by training. Failure to do this will likely reduce the duration of zone 1. This approach is a reminder that there is a need to alternate stress with regeneration, an interplay of dramatic importance in training.

Summary of Major Concepts

Throughout the training phases, an athlete reaches higher levels of biomotor abilities development and technical and tactical skills, which form a training state called degree of training or preparedness. This training state is the stable component of the athletic shape, which is also affected by the exposure to high-intensity, specific training and competition, as well as the presence of residual fatigue. Residual fatigue greatly influences the athlete's readiness to perform, or her capability of manifesting preparedness through high performance, and ultimately her ability to reach a peak of performance.

The appropriate use of tapering strategies is essential for the athlete to achieve peak performance. The athlete cannot achieve a true peak for every competition he enters. Therefore, the coach must carefully craft the competitive schedule to include two to three major competitions per competitive phase. All other competitions should be considered preparatory competitions in which the athlete uses the competitive environment as a training tool to reach his best athletic shape. If, however, a team sport athlete participates in competitions that occur in a cyclic pattern, the coach should consider training strategies that allow the athlete to recover, train, and dissipate fatigue before each contest. As with individual sports, the culmination of the competitive team sports calendar should be a major contest, such as conference or national championship, at which the athlete reaches a physiological and performance peak.

The goal of a tapering strategy is to reduce training-induced fatigue and elevate readiness. When appropriately applied, the taper can improve performance approximately 3%, which can make a large difference in the competitive outcome. To implement the taper, the coach should decrease the training load in an exponential fashion and decrease training volume as well, by about 41% to 60% in most instances. If, however, the pretaper training load is very high, a greater reduction in training volume (60% to 90%) may be warranted. When training volume is reduced, training frequency should be maintained at 80% or more of the pretaper values. The taper should last approximately 8 to 14 days. If the pretaper training workload is excessive, a longer taper may be warranted; however, another strategy is to use a fast exponential taper that involves larger decreases in volume. During the taper period the training intensity should be maintained or slightly increased to allow the athlete to maintain the physiological adaptations achieved during the pretaper training.

PART III
TRAINING METHODS

Strength and Power Development

10

Strength and power-generating capacity are critical factors in determining success in a wide variety of sports, particularly in all team sports and sports that are dominated by speed. Contemporary scientific data reveal that strength and power are also important for sports with a large endurance component, such as long-distance running or cross-country skiing. Given the importance of muscular strength and power in so many sports, the coach and athlete must understand how the development of strength and power can affect performance. The coach and athlete need to understand the principles associated with resistance training to effectively use resistance training to enhance performance.

The Relationship Between the Main Biomotor Abilities

Athletic performance is dominated by combinations of strength, speed, and endurance. Most sport activities can be classified as having a predominant biomotor ability. Figure 10.1 illustrates a theoretical structure where strength or force, speed, or endurance is the dominant biomotor ability. For example, endurance is generally considered the dominant biomotor ability necessary for success in long-distance running. Every sporting activity has a dominant biomotor ability (figure 10.2). However, contemporary research suggests that sporting activities can be affected by several of the biomotor abilities (137, 140). This can be clearly seen by the fact that strength appears to influence both running speed (13, 24, 36) and endurance (114). For example, leg strength and power appear to be significantly related to sprint speed, with the strongest and most powerful athletes being able to run the fastest (13, 24, 36). Support for the influence of strength on endurance can be seen in the literature. Research shows that adding strength training to the training programs of long-distance runners

Physiological Bases for Speed and Agility

Nobody can be fast and agile before being strong. The start in sprinting and changes of direction in racquet and team sports are typical strength actions. The fastest sprinters apply a great deal of strength against the starting blocks at the instant of starting the race. Changes of direction, on the other hand, rely on strong eccentric force to decelerate and equally strong concentric force to accelerate. Do you want to be a fast and agile athlete? Increase your strength.

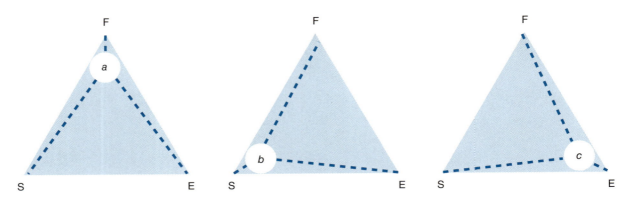

FIGURE 10.1 Relationships between the main biomotor abilities, in which (a) strength, (b) speed, and (c) endurance dominate.

F = strength or force; S = speed; E = endurance.
From Florescu, Dumitrescu, and Predescu 1969 (50).

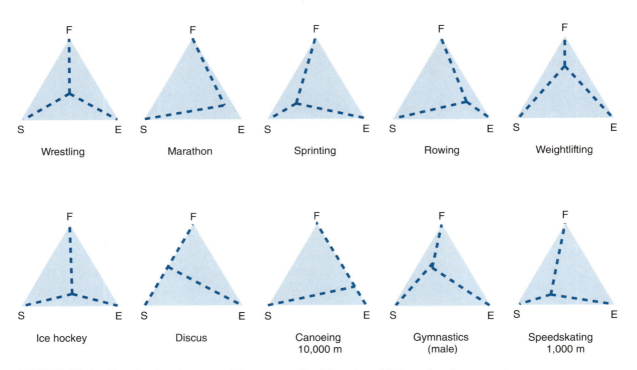

FIGURE 10.2 The dominant composition among the biomotor abilities of various sports.

F = strength or force; S = speed; E = endurance.

(106, 140), Nordic skiers (91, 139, 141), or cyclists (15) results in significantly greater improvements in performance, compared with focusing only on endurance training. Recent evidence suggests that stronger, more powerful athletes perform better on performance tests designed to evaluate agility (21, 143).

Based on this data, a hypothetical model can be constructed in which strength is connected with many of the factors that have been shown in the literature to improve performance in a variety of sporting activities (figure 10.3). Because strength affects the other biomotor abilities and almost all facets of athletic performance, strength should be considered to be

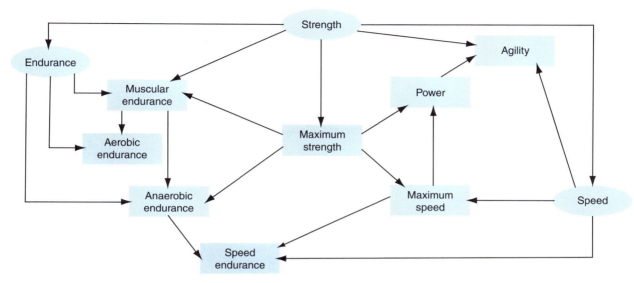

FIGURE 10.3 Interaction of biomotor abilities and various aspects of sport performance.

the crucial biomotor ability (20). Therefore, to maximize athletic performance, strength should always be trained in concert with the other biomotor abilities.

Strength

Strength can be defined as the maximal force or **torque** (rotational force) that a muscle or muscle group can generate. Strength is better defined as the ability of the neuromuscular system to produce force against an external resistance. For example, muscular strength has been related to sprint performance (13, 24, 36), American football performance (14, 55), soccer performance (32, 62, 90, 170), volleyball performance (47, 130), ice hockey performance (92), rugby league performance (58), and aerobic exercise performance (15, 91, 106, 140). These data seem to support the contention that muscular strength is a major contributor to most sport activities. Therefore, the appropriate application of resistance training can alter the neuromuscular system in a way that improves the athlete's capacity to produce force and improves sporting performance (69, 175, 176).

Force, Velocity, Rate of Force Development, and Power

When examining sport activities, the ability to generate force against an external resistance seems very important (127). Newton's second law of motion supports the importance of force-generating capacity (i.e., strength) (see the Equations sidebar), in that this law reveals that the product of mass and acceleration is equal to force (equation 1). If one rearranges this equation, it is easy to see that to increase the **acceleration** of an object, one must apply a greater force. Because increases in acceleration result in increases in **velocity**, it is also easy to conclude that a high force-generating capacity or strength level is needed to achieve high velocities of movements (180). Support for this idea can be seen in the literature, which demonstrates significant relationships between speed and muscular strength (13, 24, 36).

Equations

Equation 1 $F = M \times A + W$

F = Force
M = Mass of an object
A = Acceleration of an object
W = Weight of mass attributable to the effects of gravity

Equation 2 $RFD = \Delta F / \Delta T$

RFD = Rate of force development
ΔF = Change in force
ΔT = Change in time

Equation 3 $Power = F \times D/T$

Power = W/T
Power = $F \times V$
F = Force
W = Work
T = Time
V = Velocity

Further examination of the interaction between force and velocity suggests that an inverse relationship exists, whereas external resistance increases the movement velocity subsequently decreases (figure 10.4) (110, 208). The application of a periodized strength training program has the potential to alter the **force–velocity curve** (43, 104, 109, 110, 128, 135). The literature suggests that heavy strength training induces adaptations that are different than those seen with explosive strength training (74, 75, 110, 202). For example, the implementation of a strength training program that focuses on the use of heavy loading has a greater potential to alter the high-force portion of the force–velocity curve (figure 10.5), whereas

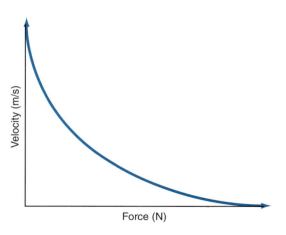

FIGURE 10.4 Force–velocity relationship.

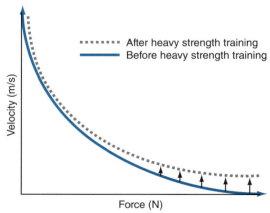

FIGURE 10.5 Theoretical alterations to the force–velocity curve by heavy strength training.

the implementation of explosive strength training exercises will alter the high-velocity portion of the curve (figure 10.6) (110).

The effect of explosive strength training on the high-velocity portion of the force–velocity curve is supported by evidence suggesting that explosive strength training has the potential to alter an athlete's explosive strength or **rate of force development** (RFD) (2, 66, 75, 76, 94). The RFD indicates how fast force is developed and is calculated by dividing the change in force by the change in time (193) (see equation 2). It appears that the ability to generate a high RFD is very important for sport activities that involve explosive movements (e.g., sprinting, jumping, throwing) and require force to be generated during a limited time frame (~70 to 250 ms). In general, this time is substantially less than the time necessary to reach maximum force (>250 ms) (9, 67, 159). However, maximum strength and the RFD are interrelated (9, 133) and both are associated with sporting performance, as both variables appear to relate to the ability to cause acceleration, which affects movement velocity (180).

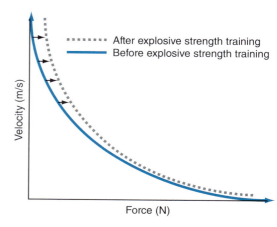

FIGURE 10.6 Theoretical alterations to the force–velocity curve by explosive strength training.

Both force and velocity are important in human movement, because the product of these two variables is power (110, 180) (see equation 3 on p. 232). Maximum force-generating capacity appears to be a major effector of power-generating capacity (157, 159). Schmidtbleicher (157, 159) suggested that as the load (which the athlete is overcoming) decreases, the effect that **maximum strength** has on power generation also decreases. He suggested that as this occurs, the RFD becomes more important (157, 159, 180).

It has been speculated that power-generating capacity, or the rate of performing work, is the single most important characteristic in sport (69, 110, 127, 157, 180). In fact, the power-generating capacity of various athletes appears to differentiate between levels of sporting performance (14, 55). Two types of power output are relevant in sporting performance: maximum power output and average power output. Maximum power output is most related to short-duration maximal performances such as jumping, sprinting, weightlifting, changing direction, and striking (11, 12, 69, 110, 127, 180, 188). Conversely, average power output is related to the performance of repetitive tasks such as endurance running (136), cycling (183), and Nordic skiing (139).

Factors Affecting Strength

Strength can be defined as the ability of the neuromuscular system to produce force against an external resistance (180). The maximum strength that an athlete can exhibit depends on seven key concepts: (1) the number of motor units involved (recruitment), (2) the motor unit firing rate (rate coding), (3) the amount of motor unit **synchronization**, (4) the use of the stretch shortening cycle, (5) the degree of neuromuscular inhibition, (6) the muscle fiber type, and (7) the degree of muscle hypertrophy (174, 180).

Motor Unit Recruitment

Motor unit recruitment relates to the number of motor units called into play (39, 86). When more motor units are activated, the amount of force generated by the muscle then increases (69). Recruitment usually occurs in an orderly pattern from smaller to larger motor units (86). Henneman and colleagues (86) in their seminal work established what is known as the **Henneman size principle,** which suggests that the size of the motor unit dictates its activation. This work established that larger motor units have a higher activation threshold and are activated after smaller motor units. It is also widely accepted that larger motor units are activated in response to higher external loads (48, 69). However, the motor unit recruitment pattern is affected not only by the force exerted (69) but also by the contraction speed (69), type of muscle contraction (44), and the metabolic state of the muscle (103, 134).

Motor Unit Rate Coding

Rate coding deals with the motor unit firing frequency (39). One unique aspect of rate coding is that the force generated by a muscle increases without recruiting additional motor units (69). Van Cutsem and colleagues (192) suggested that rate coding plays a significant role in determining the speed of voluntary contractions. Support for this contention can be seen in several investigations showing that higher motor unit firing rates are associated with higher rates of force development (2, 51, 192, 194). It appears that explosive high–power output exercises (e.g., plyometrics, power throws, jump squats) have the potential to alter the rate coding of motor units because these exercises tend to increase the motor unit firing rate (39, 69).

Motor Unit Synchronization

Motor units fire in response to low-intensity muscle actions with brief dynamic twitches that result in an **asynchronous** motor unit firing patterns (180). Asynchronous motor unit firing occurs as a result of one motor unit deactivating while another activates. Conversely, motor unit synchronization occurs as a result of the simultaneous activation of numerous motor units (59, 116) and historically has been suggested to result in an increased force output (135). Recent research suggests that motor unit synchronization may not directly enhance maximum force output or maximum strength (160, 204). The relationship between motor unit synchronization and force production capacity is partially supported by the literature, which demonstrates a higher incidence of motor unit synchronization in strength-trained athletes (162). However, it appears that motor unit synchronization may exert a stronger influence on the rate of force development (160). Support for this contention can be seen in recent research, which suggests that motor unit synchronization plays a role in force development during rapid muscle contractions (160). Motor unit synchronization may exert its greatest influence on performance of activities that require the simultaneous activation of multiple muscles at the same time, such as running, where during the propulsion (push off) phase, the gastrocnemius, soleus, glutei, hamstrings and quadriceps muscles all participate (160).

Stretch Shortening Cycle

A stretch shortening cycle (SSC) is defined as a combination of eccentric and concentric muscle actions (114, 115). A stretch shortening cycle could be considered a plyometric muscle action (180) because an eccentric muscle action (lengthening of the muscle) occurs prior to the concentric muscle action (shortening of the muscle) (115). The most well-known effect of the stretch shortening cycle is an enhancement in performance (concentric muscle action) during the final phase of the cycle (37, 114, 115). The performance enhancement resulting from a stretch shortening cycle most likely occurs because of storage of elastic energy during the eccentric phase (28, 115), activation of the stretch reflex (116), and optimization of muscle activation (3, 19). Several investigations have suggested that strength training improves maximum strength as a result of an improved ability to activate stretch shortening cycles (3, 37).

Neuromuscular Inhibition

Neural inhibition can occur as a result of neural feedback from various muscle and joint receptors that can reduce force production (59, 180). For example, it appears that the **Golgi tendon organ**, which operates as a protective mechanism, prevents the generation of harmful muscular forces during maximum or near-maximum efforts (59). If neural activation patterns of these protective mechanisms are altered, disinhibition may occur, and force-generating capacity may increase (107). Support for this argument can be seen in the work of Aagaard and colleagues (3), in which 14 weeks of strength training with heavy loads significantly reduced neuromuscular inhibitory responses. The resultant decrease in inhibition may partially explain some of the increases in force-generating capacity seen as a result of training (3).

Muscle Fiber Type

Cross-sectional studies suggest that strength and power athletes have high percentages of **type II muscle fibers** (fast-twitch; 53% to 60%) (56, 57, 77, 80, 148, 184). This is important because the muscle fiber type characteristics of an athlete play a significant role in the athlete's ability to exhibit maximum strength and power-generating capacity (56, 57, 148, 149, 185). For example, Fry and colleagues (56) reported that the type II fiber concentration of weightlifters is significantly correlated to the maximum weight lifted in the snatch ($r = 0.94$) and the clean and jerk ($r = 0.78$). The fiber type distribution of an athlete also appears to be significantly related to the athlete's vertical jump ability ($r = 0.79$). Conversely, athletes who participate in endurance sports generally have higher percentages of **type I muscle fibers** (slow-twitch) (17, 185), which have been shown to correspond to higher maximum oxygen consumption rates (17) and lower maximum force-generating capacities. Thus, the athlete who possesses higher concentrations of type II muscle fibers appears to have an advantage in sport

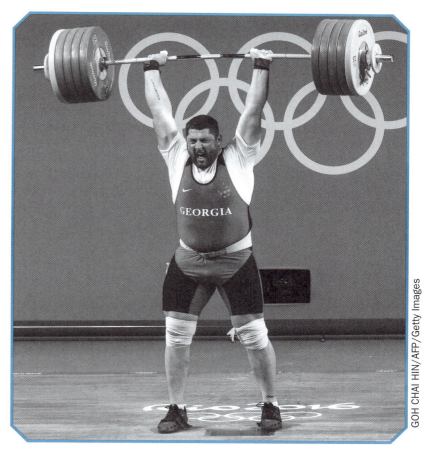

Strength is affected by many factors, including fiber type and the degree of muscle hypertrophy.

activities that require high levels of strength and power. Conversely, having a higher percentage of type I muscle fibers is advantageous to endurance exercise performance.

Muscle Hypertrophy

An increase in muscle cross-sectional area is thought to contribute to the increases in muscle hypertrophy seen in response to strength training (1, 51). Increases in the cross-sectional area of a muscle increases the number of contractile units and thus increases force-generating potential (10, 51, 198). Type II muscle fibers exhibit a greater plasticity, which is demonstrated by the faster rate of hypertrophy seen in response to training and the faster rate of atrophy seen with detraining (51, 78).

Physiological Adaptations to Strength Training

The physiological adaptations to a strength-training program can be categorized as being either neurological or morphological (51). Neurological adaptations include factors such as changes in motor unit recruitment patterns (69), motor unit synchronization (108, 132, 161-163), motor unit firing rate (39), and reflex activation (51). Morphological changes relate to changes in whole muscle size (34), muscle hypertrophy (34, 138), muscle fiber type transitions (200), and alterations to muscle architecture (164). The degree to which these two broad categories contribute to adaptations can be influenced by many factors such as training status (156), type of exercises used in the training program (29, 138), genetic makeup (23, 33, 100, 142, 189), age (101), and gender (101).

It has been suggested that the development of strength in the early phase of training is most affected by neurological factors, whereas in the longer term training adaptations are limited by the morphological factors (156, 196). The time when neurological factor adaptation predominates seems to be between 6 and 20 weeks from the initiation of a strength training program, depending on the type of exercise and the structure of the strength training program (29, 156, 196). This time frame can be altered depending on the complexity of the exercises used in the strength training program (29). Chilibeck and colleagues (29) suggested that complex exercises that involve more than one joint (e.g., squat, **power clean**, pulls) may require more time for neural adaptations to be manifested. Those investigators noted that the neurological adaptations in the upper arm occurred very rapidly, because hypertrophy was noted after 10 weeks of performing the biceps curl. Conversely, significant hypertrophy was not noted in the legs until after 20 weeks of leg press training. These data indicate that the exercises used in strength training may mitigate the degree to which neurological or hypertrophic factors predominate. The experience with intermediate and advanced strength athletes (powerlifters, weightlifters), increasing their strength and power levels year after year despite not gaining in body mass, indicates that neurological factors, especially intermuscular coordination, may have a predominant role in force production over the long term.

Neurological Adaptations

With the initiation of a strength training program, the primary adaptations that affect performance relate to motor learning and coordination (153). These adaptations appear to be very specific to the movement pattern and the sequence of muscle contraction (51), which suggests that the expression of strength requires a degree of skill.

Strength training has the potential to alter the motor unit recruitment patterns (69, 192), motor unit rate coding (2, 39, 69), and degree of motor unit synchronization (162). The type of training undertaken in a strength training program plays a role in determining neurological adaptations. For example, explosive strength training with high loads (e.g., jump squats) has been shown to lower the motor unit recruitment thresholds (69, 192) and increase the motor unit rate coding (2, 39, 192). A high loads strength training program has the potential to increase motor unit synchronization (160) and reduce neural inhibition (3). These neurological adaptations appear to alter force-generating capacity and the rate of force generation, which both can affect sports performance.

Morphological Adaptations

The occurrence of muscle hypertrophy in response to a strength training program results in changes to the muscle architecture (164). These architectural alterations can increase contractile material, which in turn can increase force production capacity (51). The most significant morphological change noted in most strength training studies is an increase in muscle hypertrophy (3, 51, 71, 79, 87, 164, 172). Most short-term strength training studies demonstrate significant hypertrophy of type II muscle fibers (1, 41, 95, 190, 198, 200), whereas long-term studies demonstrate hypertrophy of both type II and type I fibers (78, 123). Muscle hypertrophy is marked by significant increases in the cross-sectional area of the skeletal muscle fibers, which can result in an increase in contractile material (51) and an increase in the angle of pennation of the muscle (1). These two morphological adaptations significantly enhance muscular strength adaptations in response to a strength training program (1, 51).

A further consideration when looking at the morphological adaptations of the muscle is the training intervention (53). It appears that explosive strength training has the potential to significantly increase type II fiber size, significantly altering the ratio of type II to type I muscle fiber cross-sectional area, which favors maximum strength and power-generating capacity (53, 70, 180). Support for this contention is presented by Fry (53), who demonstrated that the ratio of type II to type I content is greater in weightlifters than in powerlifters and bodybuilders. These data suggest that the type of strength training used has the potential to dictate the types of morphological changes expressed by the skeletal muscle.

Another potential positive morphological adaptation to a strength training program is an alteration in the muscle fiber type (51, 200). The most consistent fiber type adaptation seen in response to a training program is a reduction in type IIx fiber distribution with a concomitant increase in type IIa distribution, especially if the training is anaerobic lactic (27, 79, 172, 200). The results of these studies may be predicated by the analytical techniques used. Newer analytical techniques suggest that muscles exhibit an even greater plasticity and thus may express greater alterations in response to training or detraining (60, 124, 191, 200).

Contemporary research has examined **myosin heavy chain** (MHC) content when identifying muscle composition (51, 53, 124, 200). MHC composition is closely associated with the classic fiber typing methods (53). However, current literature reveals that in addition to the major categories of MHC (type I, type IIa, and type IIx), there exists a pool of hybrid fibers (type I/IIa, type I/IIa/IIx, and type IIa/IIx). This pool of hybrids can be altered by strength training (200), endurance training (191), and bed rest (60). As this pool is modified, the percentage of type IIx, IIa, or I fibers can be altered, which partially explains the fiber type compositions of different classifications of strength athletes (table 10.1).

TABLE 10.1 Fiber Type Distributions of Various Strength-Trained Athletes

Population	Fiber type distribution (%)			
	I	IIa	IIx	Hybrids
Recreationally active young people (39, 172, 203)	41	33	6	20
Strength-trained men (9, 172, 203, 205)	34	58	<1	8
Strength-trained women (205)	35	53	<1	12
Bodybuilders (39)	27	47	9	17
Weightlifters (58)	35	64	1	NA

NA = not available.
Note: All percentages based on myosin heavy chain data.

Type of Strength

Various types of strength can be targeted within a strength training program. Understanding the relationship between strength and the performance characteristics of the sport will allow the coach to construct training programs that transfer strength development into performance gains. Some types of strength to consider are as follows:

- *General strength:* **General strength** refers to the strength of the whole muscular system. This strength is the foundation for the strength program and must be developed for ultimate performance to be achieved. Coaches can focus on general strength during the preparatory phase of training or during the first few years of training in novice athletes. If general strength is not adequately developed, the athlete's progress may be impeded.
- *Specific strength:* **Specific strength** relates to the motor patterns of muscle groups that are essential to a sport activity, as well as their ergogenesis. Athletes usually work on specific strength at the end of the preparation phase.
- *Power:* **Power** is the ability to develop force rapidly and at high velocities. This is essential in most sports, especially in athletics, team, and racquet sports. This type

of strength is best developed during the specific preparation phase and within the competition phase of training.

- *Maximum strength:* Maximum strength refers to the highest force the neuromuscular system can generate during a maximum voluntary contraction. Maximum strength is demonstrated by the highest load that an athlete can lift one time. Maximum strength has been related to factors such as muscle endurance, weightlifting performance, and speed.
- *Muscle endurance:* **Muscle endurance** is the ability of the neuromuscular system to produce force in a repetitive fashion over extended periods of time. The total number of repetitions that can be lifted with a specific load is a marker of muscle endurance.
- *Absolute strength:* **Absolute strength** refers to the amount of force that can be generated regardless of body weight. In some sports (shot put, American football, or the super-heavy weight class in weightlifting and wrestling), the athlete must achieve a very high level of muscular strength. An athlete's absolute maximal strength capacity can be measured with one repetition maximum testing (one-repetition maximum). Knowledge of the athlete's maximum capacity is necessary to calculate the training loads needed within a periodized training system.
- *Relative strength:* **Relative strength** is the ratio between an athlete's maximum strength and his body weight. The ratio for evaluating relative strength is calculated by the athlete's absolute strength divided by his body weight (178).

Methods of Strength Training

Strength training entails using various loads and methods to develop muscular strength and power. Depending on the goals of a strength training program, various methods of applying resistance can be used (see Methods of Strength Training Application). The preferred method of strength training combines the use of free weights with other methods of developing strength and power such as plyometrics, medicine ball work, and agility training. Using multijoint, large muscle mass exercises (e.g., cleans, arm pulls, squats) provides greater transfer to the athlete's sporting events compared with single-joint, small muscle mass exercises.

When designing a strength training program, the coach should consider the concept of progressive overload. In progressive overload, the loading structure is altered as the muscle adapts to the training stimulus (49). Progressive overload can be accomplished through the manipulation of many of the training variables, such as changing the loads used, altering the number of repetitions or sets in the training program, varying the frequency of training, altering the rest interval between sets or repetitions, and changing the exercises in the training program.

Manipulation of Training Variables

An effective strength training program systematically manipulates many training factors in a periodized fashion. Coaches can optimize the training plan by methodically managing the volume and the intensity of training. Early in the training plan, during the preparatory phase, volume will be higher, intensity will be lower, and sport-specific training will be minimized. As the athlete moves closer to the competitive phase, there is a general downward shift in training volume and an increase in training intensity and sport-specific training. Although the manipulation of volume and intensity of training is extremely important, it is also important to manipulate other variables associated with the training plan, such as the frequency of training, the order of exercises, the interset rest intervals, and the exercises selected.

Methods of Strength Training Application

- *Body weight:* Body weight resistance can be used to increase strength because of the actions of gravity on the body. Body weight exercises include a vast variety of exercises, all of which use the body as a resistive load. Some examples are push-ups, pull-ups, chin-ups, dips, and stair climbing.
- *Elastic bands:* When they are stretched, elastic bands can create resistive forces. A potential problem with this strength training device is that as forces exerted against the elastic band increase, the resistance becomes greater and the movement slower (83). With activities such as jumping, these devices apply less force at the initiation of the jump and greater force before the athlete has left the ground, which does not model the loading patterns typically found in sport. Similarly, since the resistance of the bands increases as the athlete stretches them, acceleration, so essential in sports, is impeded. Conversely, using a weighted vest or jumping with free weights applies the force consistently throughout the movement, which better translates to sports performance and is a more effective training practice (83). The only applications for elastic bands in sport training are in water sports, as they mimic the increase of resistance encountered as the arm of the swimmer or the oar of the rower get deeper in the water, or as a tool for accommodating resistance in strength exercises used for power training if the ballistic method is not utilized.
- *Weighted objects:* Weighted objects can include medicine balls, power balls, kettlebells, and bags of sand. Resistive force is created mostly by the force of gravity.
- *Weight stack machines:* With weight stack machines, resistance is provided by the action of gravity on the resistance. The direction of the force is controlled by the use of pulleys, cables, cams, and gears. It has been suggested that such machines do not match human strength curve patterns (83).
- *Fluid resistance machines:* Fluid resistance machines create resistive forces by moving the body or apparatus through a fluid, moving fluid past an object, moving fluid around an object, or moving fluid through an orifice (83). The fluid used in these devices can be either a liquid or a gas. One problem with fluid-based resistive devices is that they do not provide for eccentric muscle actions, nor for acceleration, which may limit the device's effectiveness (20, 83).
- *Free weights:* Free weights, such as dumbbells and barbells, are considered the gold standard of strength training. Free weights most closely match the human strength curve (83, 174) and use gravity to apply the resistive forces.
- *Isometric:* Isometric methods apply resistive forces in which the contractile forces equal the resistive forces. An example of an isometric muscle action is pushing with maximal forces against an immovable object.

In past years some training equipment producers have promoted many gadgets that are far from effective in sports training: from balance training (e.g., BOSU balls) to gadgets and machines that use elastic bands resistance. Under the guise of modern training, the new devices are strongly promoted on the market, misleading many novice coaches. This exaggeration goes so far as to suggest that even for a warm-up or some flexibility exercises (e.g., hurdles), the athlete needs to purchase a new device! Many gadgets are very ineffective and strain the budget of most sports clubs.

TABLE 10.2 Example of Volume Calculation

Exercise	Sets		Repetitions	Load (kg)	Volume load (kg)	Metric ton	Short ton
Power clean	3	×	5	125	1,875	1.875	2.067
Squat	3	×	5	160	2,400	2.400	2.646
Clean grip Romanian deadlift	3	×	5	140	2,100	2.100	2.315
				Total	6,375	6.375	7.028

To calculate the number of metric tons divide the volume load (in kg) by 1,000. To calculate the number of short tons, divide the volume load (in kg) by 907.2.

Volume

Volume of training can be quantified as the amount of work performed and can incorporate total training hours, number of kilograms lifted, **metric ton** or **short tons** lifted per training session, phase of training or per year, and the number of sets and repetitions completed. In the literature, volume is traditionally represented as a metric ton. A metric ton is equivalent to 2,204.6 lb (1,000 kg), whereas a short ton is equal to 2,000 lb (907.2 kg). The volume of a training session is calculated by multiplying the weight lifted by number of sets and the number of repetitions, which yields a volume load value (table 10.2).

The total workload in an annual training plan can approach 3,726 metric tons for elite weightlifters (7), with 2,789 metric tons in the preparatory phase and 937 metric tons in the competition phase. The number of metric tons encountered in a training session depends on the sport being trained for, the developmental status of the athlete, and the phase of training. As the athlete becomes more developed, he can tolerate higher training session or microcycle volume loads. It is common for weightlifters to train with 10 to 60 metric tons in a microcycle (7, 45). The microcycle volume can vary drastically depending on the sport and the phase of training (table 10.3).

Training Intensity

The **training intensity**, or load, relates to the amount of weight or resistance being used. The intensity of a training session can be calculated by dividing the volume load by the total number of repetitions completed.

The load used in strength training is best expressed as a percentage of one-repetition maximum (1RM) (111). Some strength and conditioning professionals recommend using repetitions to failure with repetition maximum zones (e.g., 1-3RM, 8-12RM, or 13-15RM) as a method for determining training intensity (27, 49). However, using training to failure in the development of maximum strength has been consistently questioned and is not the optimal method for loading during strength training (20, 102, 144, 173). This contention is supported by research from Izquierdo and colleagues (102), who suggested that training to failure brings about fewer improvements in muscular strength compared with not training to failure. Additional support for this argument was offered by Peterson and colleagues (144), who clearly showed in their meta-analysis that training to failure does not maximize strength gains. Thus, it appears that loading is best determined as a percentage of 1RM.

Examining different percentages of 1RM can help in the creation of a loading structure (table 10.4). In this structure, loading intensity zones (figure 10.7) can be quantified in relationship to their emphasis on muscle endurance, power generation, and maximum strength. Maximum strength is most likely emphasized with loads 70% of 1RM or greater, whereas muscle endurance is emphasized with loads between 20% and 50% of 1RM. Mus-

TABLE 10.3 Suggested Volume in Metric Tons of Strength Training per Year

Sport or event	Volume per microcycle			Volume per year	
	Preparatory	Competitive	Transition	Minimum	Maximum
Baseball and cricket	20-30	8-10	2-4	900	1,450
Basketball	12-24	4-6	2	450	850
Boxing and martial arts	8-14	3	1	380	500
Cycling	16-22	8-10	2-4	600	950
Downhill skiing	18-36	6-10	2-4	700	1,250
Figure skating	8-12	2-4	2	350	550
Football	30-40	10-12	6	900	1,400
Golf	4-6	2	1	250	300
Gymnastics	10-16	4	4	380	600
High jump	16-28	8-10	2-4	620	1,000
Ice hockey	15-25	6-8	2-4	600	950
Javelin	12-24	4	2	450	800
Jumps	20-30	8-10	2	800	1,200
Kayaking and canoeing	20-40	10-12	4	900	1,200
Lacrosse	14-22	4-8	2-4	500	900
Rowing	30-40	10-12	4	900	1,200
Rugby	10-20	4-6	4	320	600
Shot put	24-40	8-12	4-6	900	1,450
Speedskating	14-26	4-6	2-4	500	930
Sprinting	10-18	4	2	400	600
Squash	8-12	4	4	350	550
Swimming	20	8-10	2-4	700	1,200
Tennis	8-12	2-4	2	350	550
Triathlon	16-20	8-10	2-4	600	1,000
Volleyball	12-20	4	2	450	600
Wrestling	20-30	10	4	800	1,200

Adapted, by permission, from T.O Bompa and M.C. Carrera, 2005, *Periodization training for sports,* 2nd ed. (Champaign, IL: Human Kinetics), 65.

TABLE 10.4 Intensity Zones for Strength Training

Intensity zone	Loading	Intensity (% of 1RM)	Muscle action
1	Supermaximum	>100	Eccentric overload Isometric
2	Maximum	90-100	Concentric/eccentric
3	Heavy	80-90	Concentric/eccentric
4	Medium-heavy	70-80	Concentric/eccentric
5	Medium	50-70	Concentric/eccentric
6	Low	20-50	Concentric/eccentric

Adapted, by permission, from T.O Bompa and M.C. Carrera, 2005, *Periodization training for sports,* 2nd ed. (Champaign, IL: Human Kinetics), 66.

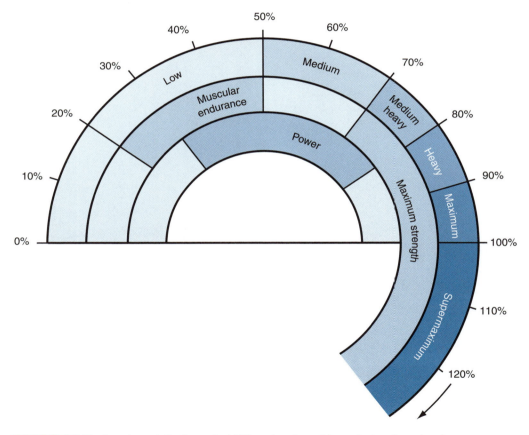

FIGURE 10.7 Load magnitude and abilities developed by using various loads.

cular power appears to be maximized somewhere between 30% and 80% of 1RM depending on the exercise (110).

Intensities between 100% and 125% of 1RM are classified as supermaximum loads; athletes can use these loads when using eccentric overload or forced repetition techniques (42). Although eccentric overload or forced repetition training appears to have a place in strength training, it may not result in significant increases in muscular strength compared with regular training (42). Supermaximum loads should be attempted only by highly strength trained athletes and should be used infrequently.

Training loads that range from 90% to 100% of 1RM are classified as maximum loads. Heavy loads range in intensity from 80% and 90% of 1RM. Loads of 70% to 80% of 1RM can be classified as medium-heavy intensities; loads of 50% to 70% are classified as medium intensity; and loads from 20% to 50% are classified as low intensity. The vast majority of the loading should come from medium and medium-heavy intensities (50% to 80% of 1RM). Support for this can be seen in the training loads undertaken by weightlifters, where the following intensity breakdown can be seen: low = 8%, medium = 59%, heavy = 26%, and maximum = 7% (207). The load encountered in training will vary depending on the training phase and the loading structure used.

Repetitions

The number of repetitions that can be performed is usually a function of the load used (table 10.5). The higher the load, the lower the number of repetitions that can be performed. However, it is difficult to make definitive connections between a percentage of 1RM and the number of repetitions that can be performed because it appears that training status, muscle mass engaged, gender, and type of exercise can change the number of repetitions that can be performed at a given load. For example, Shimano and colleagues (167) reported that at 60% of 1RM, untrained individuals can perform 35.9 ± 13.4 repetitions in the back squat, 21.6 ± 4.2 repetitions in the bench press, and 17.2 ± 3.7 repetitions in the arm curl. Conversely, trained individuals were reported to have performed 29.9 ± 7.4 repetitions in the back squat, 21.7 ± 3.8 repetitions in the bench press, and 19.0 ± 2.9 repetitions in the arm curl at training loads that corresponded to 60% of 1RM. Hoeger and colleagues (88) reported that exercise type, training status, and gender resulted in differences in the number of repetitions that could be performed at various percentages of 1RM. For example, at an intensity of 40% of 1RM, untrained men performed 80.1 ± 47.9 repetitions on the leg press and 34.9 ± 8.8 repetitions on the machine bench press. When the same protocol was repeated with untrained women, 83.6 ± 38.6 repetitions were performed on the leg press; no repetitions were performed on the machine bench press because the load could not be set on the machine. The coach needs to consider the athlete's training status and gender, the muscle mass involved, and the mode of strength training when determining how many repetitions can be performed at various percentages of 1RM. Generally speaking, the higher the neuromuscular efficiency of the subject, the lower the number of possible repetitions at any given percentage of 1RM.

The repetition scheme used results in specific physiological adaptations (27). As illustrated in figure 10.8, low-repetition schemes (1-6 repetitions) are better for the development of maximum muscular strength. Higher numbers of repetitions (>15 repetitions) appear to be more suited for stimulating muscle endurance (15, 27). High-intensity endurance (short duration) appears to be enhanced with repetition schemes of 15 to 30 (27, 49), whereas low-intensity endurance (long duration) is improved with more than 50 repetitions (27). Power-based adaptations are best realized with low-repetition schemes (1-10 repetitions) depending on the phase of training. The repetition scheme should be selected based on the goal of the phase of training and the loading scheme being used. In a periodized training plan, the repetition scheme is manipulated to facilitate specific adaptations.

TABLE 10.5 Load–Repetition Relationship for a Power Athlete

Percentage of 1RM	Number of repetitions
100	1
95	2
90	3
85	5
80	6
75	8-10
70	12-15
65	15-20
60	20-25
50	30-50
40	50-100
30	100+

	Repetitions																																																	
	1	2	3	4	5	6	7	8	9	10	11	12	13	14	15	16	17	18	19	20	21	22	23	24	25	26	27	28	29	30	31	32	33	34	35	36	37	38	39	40	41	42	43	44	45	46	47	48	49	50 50+
Maximum strength	▓	▓	▓	▓	▓	▓																																												
Power							▓	▓	▓	▓																																								
Power endurance																									▓	▓	▓	▓	▓	▓																				
Muscle endurance (short)															▓	▓	▓	▓	▓	▓	▓	▓	▓	▓	▓																									
Muscle endurance (medium)																									▓	▓	▓	▓	▓	▓	▓	▓	▓	▓	▓	▓	▓	▓	▓	▓	▓	▓	▓	▓	▓	▓				
Muscle endurance (long)																																																		▓ ▓

FIGURE 10.8 Number of repetitions required for developing various types of strength.

Buffer

The number of repetitions per set is very much linked to the percentage of 1RM used and the desired buffer. **Buffer** is the difference between the percentage of 1RM necessary to go to failure with the number of repetitions performed in a set, and the percentage of 1RM actually used for that number of repetitions. For example, performing a set of 3 repetitions with 80% of 1RM translates into a buffer of 10%, as 3 repetitions to failure necessitate a percentage of 90% of 1RM. A high buffer allows the athlete to perform more technically correct repetitions (because the load is less challenging) and more explosive concentrics; it also elicits a lower residual fatigue. Thus, sets with a high buffer are used especially for intermuscular coordination work (technique), for power development, and during unloading microcycles.

Throughout a macrocycle, the coach can decrease the buffer by increasing intensity, while maintaining the same number of repetitions. Doing so makes each workout progressively harder, while maintaining the same number of sets and repetitions (a preferred method for maximum strength development, figure 10.9). The coach can also keep the buffer the same while increasing or decreasing one of the other parameters. Usually, the coach would not increase the buffer throughout a macrocycle. During unloading or peaking microcycles, the buffer is increased via a reduction of repetitions per set, while maintaining or only slightly reducing intensity.

As depicted in figure 10.10, buffer 0 means going to concentric failure, a preferred modality for hypertrophy (bodybuilding) training. Doing multiple sets of 1 to 3 repetitions to failure or close to failure (5% buffer) elicits gains in relative strength that represents an increase of strength without an accompanying increase of body weight. Going to failure or getting close to failure with a slightly higher time under tension per set and performing 3 to 6 repetitions will elicit gains in absolute strength that are gains in both strength and muscle size. Performing sets of 1 to 3 reps with a buffer of 10% to 20% will increase both maximum strength and power with high loads (e.g., strength-speed). Performing 3 to 6 reps with a buffer of 25% to 40% will increase both maximum strength, via an improvement of the intermuscular coordination, and power with low loads.

	75%	77.5%	80%	70%	50%	T	82.5%	85%	90%	70%	50%	T
Reps	5	5	5	3	3	1	3	3	2	3	3	1
Buffer	10%	7.5%	5%	20%	40%	0%	7.5%	5%	5%	20%	40%	0%
Week	1	2	3	4			5	6	7	8		
Macrocycle	1						2					
Macrocycle type	3+1						3+1					
Adaptation emphasis	Maximum strength (intermuscular coordination)						Maximum strength (intramuscular coordination)					

FIGURE 10.9 Suggested load progression for an 8-week maximum strength phase (the latter part of the unloading week is devoted to finding the new 1RM on which to base the next cycle).

T = maximum strength testing.

% 1RM	\multicolumn{12}{c}{Buffer}
	\multicolumn{2}{c}{0%}	\multicolumn{2}{c}{5%}	\multicolumn{2}{c}{10%}	\multicolumn{2}{c}{15%}	\multicolumn{2}{c}{20%}	\multicolumn{2}{c}{25-40%}

% 1RM	0% reps	0% effect	5% reps	5% effect	10% reps	10% effect	15% reps	15% effect	20% reps	20% effect	25-40% reps	25-40% effect
Intramuscular coordination												
100	1*	Relative strength										
95	2		1*	Relative strength								
90	3	Absolute/relative strength	2		1*	Maximum strength and power (high load)						
85	5	Absolute strength	3	Absolute/relative strength	2		1*	Maximum strength and power (high load)				
80	6		5	Absolute strength	3	Absolute strength	2		1*	Maximum strength and power (high load)		
75	8	Hypertrophy	6		5		3		2			
70	12						5	Absolute strength	3			
Intermuscular coordination												
65											3*	Intermuscular coordination and power (low load)
60											3-5	
55											3-5	
50											3-6	

*The numbers in this column refer to the number of repetitions.

FIGURE 10.10 The relationship between load (percentage of 1RM), repetitions, buffer, and the resulting training effect.

Reprinted, by permission, from T.O. Bompa and C. Buzzichelli, 2015, *Periodization training for sports*, 3rd ed. (Champaign, IL: Human Kinetics) 115.

Barbell Velocity

Power is the main ingredient for all sports that require a high rate of force, speed, and agility. Sports that are speed and power dominant include sprinting, jumping, and throwing events in track and field; team sports; racket sports; gymnastics; diving; and martial arts. If an athlete desires to increase his level of performance, he has to improve power. Indeed, power is the main ingredient necessary to produce a fast, quick, and agile athlete.

Any increase of power must be the result of improvements in either strength or speed, or a combination of the two. An athlete can be very strong, yet unable to display power because of an inability to contract already strong muscles in a very short time. To overcome this deficiency, the athlete must undergo power training to improve her rate of force development. In the same way, in a sport that requires power endurance or muscle endurance, performance correlates with the ability to maintain the highest power output for the duration of the event.

Today it is possible to conveniently measure the power output of each repetition of a strength training session, thanks to affordable monitoring devices that utilize the technology of an accelerometer with a gyroscope. Such devices measure the peak and mean velocity as well as the peak and mean power output of each repetition of a set. This has been a great advancement in the monitoring of strength training.

Table 10.6 provides the mean velocity suggested for strength lifts (squat, bench press, deadlift, chin-ups), according to the desired training effect. For Olympic lifts, please refer to table 10.7.

TABLE 10.6 Suggested Mean Velocity of Strength Lifts

Mean velocity (m/s)	Suggested utilization
0.1-0.2	One-repetition maximum velocity
0.3-0.4	Maximum strength development (intramuscular coordination)
	Maximum strength maintenance during the competitive phase (heavy load day), at least 2 weeks from competition
0.4-0.5	Maximum strength development (intramuscular coordination)
	Post-activation potentiation training, 6-24 h before competition
0.5-0.6	Maximum strength development (intermuscular coordination)
	Maximum strength maintenance (heavy load day)
0.6-0.7	Maximum strength development (intermuscular coordination)
	Power (high loads) maintenance during the competitive phase
	Maximum strength maintenance (medium load day)
0.8-0.9	Power development
0.9+	Power development
	Strength maintenance, 48-72 h before an important competition (taper)

The accelerometer can be used as a power training monitoring device, allowing the athlete to cut repetitions within sets, and sets of an exercise within a session, whenever a marked drop-off in power output becomes evident. It can be used as a testing tool, too, both for absolute power (peak velocity for ballistic exercises and Olympic lifts, and mean velocity for strength lifts) as well as power output stability for power endurance and

TABLE 10.7 Suggested Peak Velocity of Olympic Lifts

Olympic lift	Peak velocity (m/s)
Clean	1.8-2.0
Snatch	2.4-2.8

muscle endurance purposes. The accelerometer can also be used as an internal load or central nervous system residual fatigue monitoring device; for example, it can be utilized through jump testing before a training session or monitoring the power output during the strength training warm-up sets, and then comparing the data with the best performance of the season.

Sets

Traditionally a set consists of a series of repetitions performed continuously, followed by a rest interval. A single-set training program is insufficient for identifying any visible strength improvements. Rather, a multiple-set protocol is necessary to significantly improve adaptation and, as a result, improve strength in both athletes and nonathletes (144, 151). Peterson and colleagues (144) reported dose–response data that suggested that single-set protocols offer minimal stimulus for strength gains and that between 4 and 8 sets are needed to optimize training-induced strength gains. Rhea and colleagues (151) also reported that a minimum of three sets are needed to maximize strength gains in both trained and untrained individuals. The literature indicates that untrained individuals receive the most benefit from three or four sets, whereas trained individuals will gain the most adaptations from four to eight sets (144, 151). Therefore, when constructing a training program, coaches must consider the training status of the individual; highly trained athletes are able to tolerate and may benefit from higher numbers of sets. The more sets an athlete can tolerate, the greater the stimulus for adaptation and the greater the strength gains.

Regardless of how the set is configured, the phase of training will dictate the makeup of the training set. For example, during the preparation phase of training, when greater numbers of repetitions and exercises are performed, fewer sets may be performed. As the competitive phase approaches, the number of exercises will decrease, whereas the number of sets usually increases. During the competitive phase, everything will decrease, including the number of repetitions and number of sets, so that the athlete has recovered and can focus on technical and tactical training.

A special concern is represented by multiplanar (i.e., acting on multiple planes of movement) sports, such as team sports, contact sports, and martial arts. For these sports, a higher number of exercises and a lower number of sets per exercise has to be employed to address, for instance, the high force demands in the sagittal plane as well as in the frontal and transverse planes.

Interset Rest Intervals

The rest interval between sets is a function of the load being used, the goal of the training plan, the type of strength being developed, and the degree of explosiveness of the training exercise (20). The rest interval must be long enough to allow for the restoration of adenosine triphosphate (ATP) and phosphocreatine (PCr), the clearance of fatigue-inducing substrates, and the restoration of force-generating capacity (199).

The time selected for the interset rest interval may play a distinct role in the replenishment of substrates used during the set. After 30 s of rest, 70% of ATP has been restored, although complete ATP resynthesis does not occur until 3 to 5 min into rest (97). Two minutes of rest is needed to restore approximately 84% of PCr, 4 min of rest is need to restore approximately 89% of the PCr stores, and 8 min of rest is needed for complete restoration of PCr (85, 97, 98). Thus, during high-volume training, rest intervals of less than 1 min may not be long enough to allow for restoration of substrates and may result in inadequate recovery (199). Force- and power-generating capacity have been shown to be almost completely restored after 2 to 5 min of recovery between sets (4, 18, 155). Conversely, when less than 1 min of recovery is allowed between sets, force- and power-generating capacity can be decreased by 12% to 44% (4, 145, 181). These data indicate that short recovery periods (<1 min) should be avoided in favor of longer recovery periods (2 to 5 min) when the athlete is attempting to maximize force- and power-generating capacity.

Clearly, short rest intervals do not allow for enough recovery to sustain training intensities across several sets and are not advantageous when the athlete is attempting to maximize muscular strength and power development (199). However, when the strength training program is designed to emphasize muscle endurance, short rest intervals may be advantageous. It is plausible that when short rest intervals are coupled with high volumes of training, physiological adaptations occur that can facilitate endurance performance. These adaptations may include increases in capillary density, mitochondrial density, and buffer capacity (199).

Short rest interval programs have also been suggested to result in significant hormonal responses that provide a greater stimulus for the improvement of body composition (64, 129, 199). In particular, it appears that when short rest intervals are included in a strength training program that uses higher repetitions (~10 repetitions) with moderate loads, greater levels of **growth hormone** are released (64, 118, 129). Short rest intervals do not allow for complete recovery, and they decrease the total workload that the athlete can accomplish. Frobose and colleagues (52) suggested the work accomplished (i.e., tonnage or volume load) is the primary stimulus for muscular hypertrophy. Thus, depending on the athlete's ability to recover, various rest interval lengths may be used when targeting muscular hypertrophy.

Order of Exercises

The order of exercises in a strength training program can significantly influence the effectiveness of the training session. Large mass, multijoint exercises should be placed early in the training session (8, 165) because these exercises are fundamental to strength development and need to be trained when the athlete has a minimal amount of fatigue. After completing the large mass, multijoint exercises, the athlete can then progress to smaller mass, single-joint exercises (8). Alternatively, it has been suggested that the athlete should alternate between upper body and lower body exercises to facilitate recovery (197).

When an athlete is attempting to maximize strength and power development, it may be advantageous to perform either an explosive exercise (128, 195) or a heavy load, multijoint, large mass exercise (128) before performing an explosive exercise such as a jump or a sprint. This can be termed a postactivation potentiation complex. Postactivation complexes have been shown to significantly increase the rate of force development (RFD), jumping height (206), sprinting performance (128), and sprint cycle performance (171). However, if the initial exercise creates large amounts of fatigue, performance most likely will be impaired during the second exercise of the series (30). The postactivation complex appears to be effective only when used with highly trained individuals (31). There are numerous examples of postactivation complexes in the scientific literature, but some examples that may have significant performance effects can be seen in table 10.8. Potentiation complexes need to

TABLE 10.8 Postactivation Complexes

Study	Postactivation potentiation complex			Results
Chiu et al. (31)	Back squats 5 × 1 at 90% of 1RM	18 1/2 min rest	Jump squats	Power output ↑ with jumps at 30% of 1RM
McBride et al. (128)	Back squat 1 × 3 at 90% of 1RM	4 min rest	40 m sprint	0.87% ↓ in sprint time
Smith et al. (171)	Back squats 10 × 1 at 90% of 1RM	5 min rest	10 s sprint cycle test	4.8% ↑ in average power output
Yetter and Moir (205)	Back squat 3 × at 70% of 1RM	4 min rest	40 m sprint	2.3% ↓ in sprint time
Young et al. (206)	Back squat 1 × 5RM	4 min rest	Loaded countermovement jump	2.8% ↑ in jump height

↓ = decrease; ↑ = increase.

have a heavy-load activity (≥80% of 1RM) such as a back squat for minimal repetitions (one to three repetitions) performed 4 to 5 min prior to an explosive activity, such as jumping or sprinting.

Training Frequency

Training frequency is usually measured as the number of times per week a certain muscle group is trained or how often the athlete trains the whole body. The greater the training frequency, the greater the strength gains. For novice and intermediate weight trainers who are training the whole body during each training session, training 2 or 3 days per week appears to be optimal. As the athlete becomes more developed, the frequency of training may need to be increased.

Support for higher frequencies of training with advanced athletes can be found in the scientific literature. For example, university-level American football players who participated in four or five training sessions per week experienced significantly greater gains in muscular strength than those who participated in fewer training sessions (93). It appears that higher frequencies of training are necessary for maximum muscular strength adaptations (8). It is thought that breaking the training volume into short sessions, followed by periods of recovery in which dietary nutrients and supplements are supplied, will increase training quality. This concept is supported by the work of Häkkinen and Kallinen (72), who demonstrated that increasing the frequency of training to two sessions per day, even when the volume was maintained, results in significantly greater increases in muscle hypertrophy and neuromuscular adaptations, compared with a frequency of one training session per day.

The optimal frequency of training is determined by many factors: training status, the type of strength needed, the phase of the periodized training plan, and the athlete's goal influence the frequency of strength training. For example, most athletes undertake strength training to improve their performance in other activities. Therefore, these athletes may perform two to four strength training sessions per week in conjunction with their other training activities. The phase of training must be considered when selecting a training frequency. For example, during the preparation phase, the frequency of training might be substantially higher than in the later portion of the competition phase. The number of training sessions often is reduced, in order to taper training and dissipate fatigue.

Loading Patterns

The loading pattern used in the training program is particularly important because it will stimulate physiological adaptations. The most effective loading pattern to stimulate maximal strength gains is the flat pyramid (20). In the flat pyramid, the athlete begins with several warm-up sets and works toward a prescribed load at which all of the training sets are performed (table 10.9). The flat portion of the pyramid generally uses an intensity between 70% and 90% of 1RM when the athlete is specifically targeting maximum strength. It appears that performance is maximized when the majority of training is undertaken with intensities of about 70% to 85% of 1RM (63, 207). This is seen in the data presented by Zatsiorsky (207), who reported that 35% of the training volume of Soviet weightlifters was between 70% and 80% of 1RM, 26% of the training volume was between 80% and 90% of 1RM, and only 7% of the training volume was between 90% and 100% of 1RM throughout the training year. Conversely, Häkkinen and colleagues (73) reported that when training volume is increased from 80% to 90% of 1RM and 90% to 100% of 1RM, maximal strength increases significantly. When too much of the training volume is in the 90% to 100% range, performance may not be optimized and overtraining may occur (56).

A second loading pattern is the pyramid loading pattern (20, 169), or an ascending pyramid loading scheme. In this loading scheme, with each set the percentage of 1RM increases and the number of repetitions decreases (table 10.10). The load range of the ascending

TABLE 10.9 — Loading Pattern for a Flat Pyramid Using the Back Squat

	Warm-up				Target sets					
Load (kg)	60	100	140	155	170	170	170	170	170	170
Repetitions	5	5	3	3	2	2	2	2	2	2
Percentage of 1RM	30	50	70	77.5	85	85	85	85	85	85
Buffer (%)	55	35	20	12.5	10	10	10	10	10	10

Note: Loading based on a maximum back squat of 200 kg.

TABLE 10.10 — Loading Pattern for an Ascending Pyramid Using the Back Squat

	Warm-up				Pyramid			
Load (kg)	60	100	140	155	160	165	175	185
Repetitions	5	5	5	5	4	3	2	1
Percentage of 1RM	30	50	70	77.5	80	82.5	87.5	92.5
Buffer (%)	55	35	15	7.5	7.5	7.5	7.5	7.5

Note: Loading based upon a maximum back squat of 200 kg.

pyramid has been suggested to range from 10% to 15% (20). Load ranges greater than 15% are not recommended because the cumulative fatigue that accumulates may impair strength development (20).

A modification of the ascending pyramid loading pattern is what some have termed the double pyramid (20, 65). The traditional loading pattern for the double pyramid would be an increase of resistance up to a maximal attempt followed by a progressive decrease (207, 208). A better approach, which can be utilized to peak strength, is to leave the volume constant, typically at one repetition, and then use an ascending intensity pattern followed by a descending pattern (table 10.11). This pattern elicits a potentiation effect on the descending intensity portion of the pyramid. However, the number of sets must be limited (five to six), and the top intensity must not go beyond 90% of the 1RM; otherwise, the amount of fatigue established in this type of loading structure might result in a lack of potentiation (30).

Another modification to the pyramid loading pattern is the skewed pyramid (20). In this loading pattern, the intensity is increased for a series of sets, and on the last set a down set is performed (table 10.12). Lowering the load in that last set (e.g., the back-off set or down set) and taking it to failure has been proven to retain muscle hypertrophy when the majority of high-intensity, low-repetition sets would only stimulate relative strength (64). This method could be used during the strength maintenance

TABLE 10.11 — Loading Pattern for a Double Pyramid Using the Back Squat

	Double pyramid				
Load (kg)	160	170	180	170	160
Repetitions	1	1	1	1	1
Percentage of 1RM	80	85	90	85	80
Buffer (%)	20	15	10	15	20

Note: Loading based on a maximum back squat of 661.4 lb (200 kg). An appropriate warm-up is required to prepare the athlete for the training bout.

TABLE 10.12 — Loading Pattern for a Skewed Pyramid Using the Squat

	Skewed pyramid						
Load (kg)	100	120	140	160	170	180	160
Repetitions	6	5	4	3	2	1	8 to failure
Percentage of 1RM	50	60	70	80	85	90	80
Buffer (%)	30	25	17.5	10	10	10	0

Note: Loading based on a maximum squat of 200 kg. An appropriate warm-up is required to prepare the athlete for the training bout.

phase of the annual plan. If the last, lighter set is not taken to failure, it can exploit a postactivation potentiation effect to stimulate power development (186). This concept is supported by work by Stone and colleagues (179), who demonstrated that greater barbell velocities are achieved during the back-off set.

Yet another loading pattern is the wave-loading model (182), which is sometimes referred to as segment work (105). In this model the training load increases in an undulating or wavelike fashion (table 10.13). The wave-loading method may be useful because it allows for a potentiating effect, with a light load undertaken after a heavy load.

The traditional format of a set may be modified to change the training stimulus by incorporating a short interrepetition rest interval, creating a **cluster set** (68, 121, 122). During traditional set configurations, with each repetition there is a decrease in repetition velocity, power, and quality. The addition of a 10 to 30 s interrepetition rest interval can allow for partial recovery between each repetition, thus allowing for higher repetition quality (61, 68, 81, 82, 122).

Cluster sets can be structured in several different fashions, depending on the goal of training (table 10.14). Additional variation in the cluster set can be accomplished by changing the loading structure (68). Four distinct repetition schemes can be constructed: a straight cluster set that uses the same intensity across all repetitions, an ascending cluster where the intensity of each repetition is increased, an undulating cluster where loading is implemented in a pyramidal fashion, and a waving cluster where three ascending sets are repeated twice (table 10.15). Contemporary literature suggests that the most effective use of the cluster set is with ballistic or explosive exercise (122) and that traditional sets may be better for the development of muscular hypertrophy or maximum muscular strength (152).

TABLE 10.13 — Wave-Loading Model Using the Deadlift

	Warm-up			Wave segment					
Load (kg)	60	100	140	160	165	170	160	165	170
Repetitions	5	3	2	3	2	1	3	2	1
Percentage of 1RM	30	50	70	80	82.5	85	80	82.5	85
Buffer (%)	55	40	20	10	12.5	15	10	12.5	15

Note: Data calculated for a 1RM deadlift of 200 kg.

Strength and Power Development

TABLE 10.14 Cluster Set Configurations Using Various Configurations for the Clean Pull

	Type of training	Sets × reps	Rest interval (s)	Repetition load (kg)									
Cluster 1	Power training with Olympic lifts	2×(10×1)	30/180	110	110	110	110	110	110	110	110	110	110
Cluster 2	Power training with strength lifts	3×(5×1)	1-3/180	110	110	110	110	10					

2×(10×1) = two sets of 10 repetitions performed with a 30 s rest between each repetition of the set and 3 min between sets; 3×(5×1) = three sets of five repetitions with 1 to 3 s rest and 3 min between sets.

Note: Loads are based on of a 1RM clean of 150 kg and a 1RM back squat of 200 kg.

TABLE 10.15 Intensity Variations for Cluster Set Configurations Using the Clean Pull

	Sets × repetitions	Interrepetition rest interval (s)	Repetition load (kg)					
Straight cluster	3 × 6/1	30	120	120	120	120	120	120
Undulating cluster	3 × 5/1	30	120	130	140	130	120	
Ascending cluster	3 × 5/1	30	120	130	140	150	160	
Waving cluster	3 × 6/1	30	120	130	140	120	130	140

3 × 5/1 = three sets of five repetitions performed with 30 s between each repetition of the set.

Note: Loads are based on of a 1RM clean of 150 kg.

Implementation of a Strength Training Program

Continual monitoring of the training process is an often overlooked but essential part of implementing a periodized strength training plan. Monitoring the athlete's progress allows the coach to determine whether the goals of the training plan are being achieved. The following steps will allow the coach to conceptualize, design, and implement a periodized strength training program.

1. *Determine the phases of training:* Like any other periodized training plan, a strength training program has preparatory, competitive, and transition phases of training. Each

phase is essential to maximize training outcomes. This concept can be considered phase potentiation, which suggests that activities of the general preparatory phase facilitate the athlete's development in both the specific preparatory phase and the competition phase. Thus, the coach must structure the phases of training so the athlete develops the appropriate biomotor abilities.

2. *Determine the training goal:* The most important step in establishing a periodized strength training program is to set separate training objectives for the annual plan as well as for each training phase. This refers not only to performance objectives, but also to the goals for each dominant physical abilities. Remember that performance objectives may be impeded if the goals of the dominant abilities are not achieved.

3. *Determine the athlete's needs:* During the last phase of the annual training program (transition phase), the coach has to analyze whether the objectives for the year have been achieved and, based on this analysis, set realistic objectives for the next annual plan. This is important both for performance, but also for the objectives for each dominant ability. The coach must also analyze the physiological demands needed to achieve superior performance and what the athlete needs in order to achieve it. Remember that the weakest link of a chain always breaks first.

4. *Consider the characteristics of all components of the training plan:* The goals for strength training must be integrated with all of the other components important to the selected sport, including technical, tactical, and physical components (22). Therefore, the coach must consider the strength training program and how it may affect other attributes, such as conditioning agility and technical and tactical training activities (i.e., all of the components that contribute to performance).

5. *Select the exercises:* The training exercises selected must be related to the requirements of the sport. When examining a sport during the needs analysis, the coach can determine the muscles that act as prime movers and match exercises to these activities. For example, analyzing a 100 m sprinter's technique may shows that lower body strength is impeding optimal performance outcomes. Thus, the coach may select exercises such as back squats and kettlebell swings in an attempt to target the prime movers employed during the propulsion phase in sprinting. Support for this idea can be seen in several studies, which suggest that maximum strength capacity in the squat and power clean is significantly related to running performance (13, 24, 36).

   An additional consideration when selecting exercises is the phase of training. Certain exercises are best used at specific times during the periodized plan (22, 84, 146). For example, early in the general preparation phase of training it may be warranted to use general strength exercises. As the athlete moves toward the specific preparation and competitive phases of training, more specific exercises can be used.

6. *Test performance:* After selecting the exercises that are needed to develop the performance

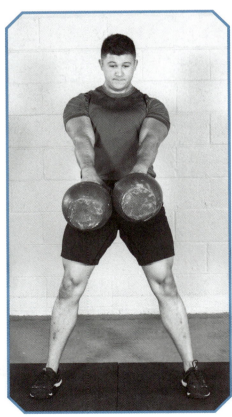

Kettlebell swings work the stretch shortening cycle in a more specific way.

The Specificity of Strength Training Exercises

Under normal conditions an exercise has to be selected based on the needs to target the **prime movers** (the muscles that contract to perform the technical skills). In addition, the muscle contraction has to be performed along the **line of pull** (median direction of contraction of the main muscles involved in the technical skill). In other words, the exercise has to be very specific to the needs of the selected sport.

However, some strength training coaches with a background in Olympic weightlifting (OL) believe that if you want to be as strong as their athletes, you must use the same exercises. This isn't correct: The OL athletes are strong not because of the exercises they do, but rather because of the heavy loads they use (especially in the back squat). In sport training, the OL exercises have far fewer applications than popularly thought because they are not force-vector specific and do not properly target the prime movers employed in many sports. Yet, in many gyms in the United States and the United Kingdom, the only means of training are Olympic lifts. For example, strength coaches can still be seen working with some swimmers and rowers on snatches and military presses.

These exercises are not specific to swimming, where the prime movers are scapular depressors, and shoulder and elbow extensors. The military press and snatches target the shoulder flexors, exactly the opposite muscles used in swimming and other sports. Furthermore, because most sport activities require a fast application of force, in less than 300 ms, once an athlete reaches triple extension (ankle, knee, hip), it does not matter what he does with his arms, if he catches in a clean or snatch position. For this reason, coaches who work in sports that require fast force applied vertically are better off using low or high pulls. Finally, exercises such as plyometrics and kettlebell swings work the stretch shortening cycle in a more specific way and at a greater extent than OL, making them preferable for the sprinting athlete (in track and field and team sports).

In other words, do not allow the athletes to be robots and do just OL moves—it might do a disservice to them.

---

attributes needed by the athlete, the coach must test the athlete's maximum strength. Knowledge of the athlete's 1RM capabilities in at least the primary or dominant exercises will allow the coach to establish the training loads. The 1RM will continually change as the athlete adapts to the physiological stressors of the training program. Therefore, the athlete must be tested at the end of each macrocycle to individualize the loading parameters.

Many coaches wrongly believe that performing a 1RM test is dangerous and will increase the athlete's risk of injury (20, 26, 119, 125, 150). In fact, 1RM testing is very safe for most populations (154, 166) and is considered the gold standard in the assessment of muscular strength (99). Some authors suggest that testing strength with multiple repetition tests is a better way to establish the training intensity (25, 26, 46, 125), but it has been consistently shown that many of the prediction equations misrepresent the 1RM (125). This is a major problem because using an estimate of 1RM capabilities that is too high may increase injury risk during training or induce high-intensity overtraining from consistently training at high intensities (54). Conversely, training with an intensity that is underpredicted will result in inadequate strength development because the athlete will train using suboptimal loads.

7. *Develop the strength training program:* After establishing the athlete's physical performance capabilities, the coach can establish the number of exercises, sets, repetitions, and loading (percentage of 1RM) that will be used during the microcycles within the macrocycle. Throughout the training plan the coach will need to alter volume, intensity, and the exercises selected to allow for continued physiological adaptations that will lead to the maximization of specific strength. As muscular strength increases across the annual plan, the coach will need to periodically retest the 1RM to optimize the training load. It is essential for the coach to test the 1RM before each new macrocycle. A detailed training program will be written down only for one macrocycle at a time.

8. *Record the training plan:* The coach must record the exercises, number of sets, number of repetitions, and training load (table 10.16). The load, number of repetitions, and sets usually are noted as follows:

$$\% \text{ of } 1RM \;/\; \text{number of repetitions} \times \text{sets}$$

Noting the load as a percentage of 1RM is useful when working with many athletes because this allows the coach to calculate the load for every athlete. By using a percentage notation, the coach can individualize the program for each athlete, and athletes can use their own 1RM to establish their training loads.

9. *Create a training log:* One of the most important steps is to record what was done in the training sessions. If the coach and athlete keep detailed records, they will be able to evaluate the athlete's progress and chart her performance. Things to record in the training log include the exercise, the number of repetitions completed, the number of sets performed, the load lifted in lb or kg, and the duration of the training session (figure 10.11). This record will allow the coach to calculate the volume load, tons, and training intensity (volume load divided by total repetitions performed). By using a spreadsheet software program such as Microsoft Excel, the coach can easily calculate the volume load, tons, and training intensity and create figures depicting the volume and intensity of training. Those strength and conditioning coaches who have an accelerometer can record the peak velocity, average velocity, peak power, and average power of the best repetition of each set (figure 10.12). Average velocity during the first sets of a session can be utilized as an indicator of daily internal load, and the training session load or direction can be adjusted accordingly. If the training log is accurate and inclusive, it provides an excellent tool for monitoring training.

TABLE 10.16 Sample Chart of a Strength Training Program for a Sprinter (3+1 Macrocycle)

Exercise number	Exercise	Loading				Rest interval
1	Back squat	80/3 ×3	85/2 ×3	85/2 ×3	70/2 ×3	3 min
2	Bench press	80/3 ×3	85/2 ×3	85/2 ×3	80/2 ×2	3 min
3	Kettlebell swing (48 kg)	3 × 6	4 × 6	4 × 6	2 × 6	3 min
4	Narrow supinated grip lat pulldown	80/3 ×3	85/2 ×3	85/2 ×3	70/2 ×3	3 min
5	Toe raise/ankle press	75/5 ×2	80/5 ×2	85/5 ×2	70/5 ×2	3 min

Loading = % 1RM / repetitions for the number of sets.

Name: _____ Time in: _____

Day: _____ Time out: _____

Date: _____

Exercise		Set 1	Set 2	Set 3	Set 4	Set 5	Set 6	Set 7	Set 8	Set 9	Set 10	Volume load	Training intensity
Back squat	Weight	60	80	110	130	130	130					6,400	106.67
	Repetitions	10	10	10	10	10	10						
1/3 front squat	Weight	160	160	160								4,800	160.00
	Repetitions	10	10	10									
Military press	Weight	60	60	60								1,800	60.00
	Repetitions	10	10	10									
Incline bench press	Weight	70	70	70								2,100	70.00
	Repetitions	10	10	10									
	Weight												
	Repetitions												
	Weight												
	Repetitions												
	Weight												
	Repetitions												

Notes:

Total volume load		15,100
Metric tons		15.1
	Training intensity	99.167

FIGURE 10.11 Training log for a single training session.

Name: _____

Day: _____

Date: _____

Time in: _____

Time out: _____

Exercise		Set 1	Set 2	Set 3	Set 4	Set 5	Set 6	Set 7	Set 8	Set 9	Set 10	Volume load
1/4 squat	100 kg	5 reps	3 min rest interval									2,000
	Peak velocity	1.00	1.19	1.20	1.16							
	Average velocity	0.55	0.70	0.72	0.65							
	Peak power	2,080	2,265	2,588	2,108							
	Average power	902	1,276	1,296	1,154							
Deadlift	100 kg	3 reps	3 min rest interval									1,200
	Peak velocity	1.18	1.31	1.22	1.28							
	Average velocity	0.66	0.83	0.75	0.77							
	Peak power	1,978	2,560	2,026	2,240							
	Average power	989	1,240	1,126	1,190							
Jump squat	40 kg	5 reps	3 min rest interval									800
	Peak Velocity	2.20	2.40	2.55	2.38							
	Average Velocity	1.09	1.15	1.17	1.11							
	Peak Power	7850	8655	9522	8317							
	Average Power	3820	4325	4766	4102							
Notes:									Total volume load			4,000
									Metric tons			4

FIGURE 10.12 Training log for a training session during the power phase.

Testing the One-Repetition Maximum (1RM)

Some coaches believe that testing for 1RM is dangerous and that lifting 100% can result in injury. However, it is not dangerous for trained athletes to lift 100% once every 3 or 4 weeks. Most injuries occur during training and competition, not during testing. Sometimes the body of an athlete is subjected to forces up to five times body weight during the sport activity, so testing maximum strength should not constitute a safety concern. Consider, as well, that testing is performed at the end of the unloading microcycle of a macrocycle, when the athlete has recovered from the fatigue of the previous loading microcycles. However, a test for 1RM must follow a thorough, progressive warm-up, such as the one suggested here for the squat (projected 1RM at 150 kg):

1st set: 20 kg × 10 reps, 30 s rest interval, 13% of 1RM
2nd set: 60 kg × 4 reps, 60 s rest interval, 40% of 1RM
3rd set: 80 kg × 2 reps, 90 s rest interval, 53% of 1RM
4th set: 100 kg × 2 reps, 2 min rest interval, 67% of 1RM
5th set: 120 kg × 1 rep, 2 min rest interval, 80% of 1RM
6th set: 130 kg × 1 rep, 3 min rest interval, 87% of 1RM
7th set: 140 kg × 1 rep, 4 min rest interval, 93% of 1RM
8th set: 145 kg × 1 rep, 5 min rest interval, 97% of 1 RM
9th set: 150 kg × 1 rep, 6 min rest interval, 100% of 1RM

Periodization of Strength

Periodization of strength offers a seven-phase approach that follows the physiological rhythm of the neuromuscular system's response to strength training (table 10.17). The seven phases are anatomical adaptation, hypertrophy, maximum strength, conversion, maintenance, cessation, and compensation. Depending on the physiological demands of the sport, the periodization of strength involves combining, in sequence, at least four of the phases: anatomical adaptation, maximum strength, conversion to specific strength (power or muscle endurance), and maintenance. All models for periodization of strength begin with an anatomical adaptation phase. The seven phases are discussed briefly in the following sections.

TABLE 10.17 — Periodization of Strength and Its Phases

Preparatory				Competitive		Transition
Anatomical adaptation	Hypertrophy (if necessary)	Maximum strength	Conversion to specific strength (power; power endurance; or short, medium, or long muscle endurance)	Maintenance of maximum strength and specific strength	Cessation of strength training	Compensation training

Phase 1: Anatomical Adaptation

The anatomical adaptation phase lays the foundation for the other phases of training. The name of this phase reflects the fact that the main objective of strength training is not to achieve an immediate overload, but to elicit a progressive adaptation of the athlete's anatomy. The anatomical adaptation phase emphasizes prehabilitation in the hope of preventing the need for rehabilitation. The main physiological objectives of this phase are to (1) strengthen the tendons, ligaments, and joints, which is doable through a higher volume of training than in the remainder of the year; and (2) increase bone mineral content and the proliferation of the connective tissue. In addition, regardless of the sport, this phase improves cardiovascular fitness, adequately challenges muscular strength, and tests and assists the athlete with practicing and improving neuromuscular coordination for strength movement patterns. Although this phase does not focus on increasing the cross-sectional area of muscle, some gains in the hypertrophy of some muscles may be visible, especially for novice athletes.

Tendons are strengthened by implementing a time under tension per set that falls between 30 and 70 s (the time under tension that sees the anaerobic lactic system as the main energy system). The hydrogen ions released by lactic acid have been proven to stimulate the release of growth hormone and therefore collagen synthesis, which is also stimulated by eccentric load (10, 35, 40, 112, 113, 120, 131). For this reason, the majority of the time under tension is spent in the eccentric phase of the exercise (3 to 5 s per repetition). Muscular balance is achieved both by using an equal training volume between agonist and antagonist muscles around a joint and by making greater use of unilateral exercises, rather than bilateral ones.

Phase 2: Hypertrophy

Hypertrophy, or the enlargement of muscle size, is one of the most visible signs of adaptation to strength training. The two main physiological objectives of this phase are (1) to increase the muscle cross-sectional area by increasing muscle protein content and (2) to increase storage capacity for high-energy substrates and enzymes. Many principles used in hypertrophy training are similar to those used in bodybuilding, but there are also some differences. In comparison with bodybuilding programs, athletic hypertrophy programs use a lower average number of repetitions per set, a higher average load, and a longer average rest interval between sets.

In addition, athletes should always try to move the weight as fast as possible during the concentric phase of the lift. Bodybuilders train to exhaustion using relatively light to moderate loads, whereas athletes from different sports rely on heavier loads and focus on movement speed and rest between sets. Although hypertrophic changes occur in both fast-twitch and slow-twitch muscle fibers, more changes take place in the fast-twitch fibers (186, 187). This form of hypertrophy is desired for athletes who use strength training to improve their athletic performance. In this manner, muscular adaptations result in a stronger muscular engine that is prepared to receive and apply nervous system signals. When hypertrophy training produces chronic changes, it provides a strong physiological basis for nervous system training.

Hypertrophy training is indicated mostly for athletes who desire an overall increase in body weight (e.g., throwers in track and field) or for tall athletes, specifically those who play in scrums in rugby and American football or who fall in the heavyweight category in combat sports or martial arts. For most other athletes, this strength training phase is not necessary unless the coach is training beginners.

Phase 3: Maximum Strength

In most sports, the development of maximum strength is probably the single most important variable. Maximum strength depends on the diameter of the cross-sectional area of the muscles, the capacity to recruit fast-twitch muscle fibers, the frequency of activation, and the ability to simultaneously call into action all the primary muscles involved in a given movement (96). These factors involve both structural and neural flow changes that occur as a function of training with moderate weights lifted explosively, as well as heavy loads (up to 90% of 1RM or more). These adaptive responses can also be elicited by eccentric training with loads greater than 100% of 1RM, although its practical application is limited to very few situations.

The popularity of maximum strength training is rooted in the positive increase in relative strength. Many sports (e.g., volleyball, gymnastics, combat sports) require greater force generation without a concomitant increase in body weight. In fact, an increase in maximum strength without an associated increase in body weight characterizes the maximum strength phase as central nervous system training (158).

An athlete could benefit from traditional maximum strength training methods, such as performing high loads with maximal rest (3 to 5 min) between sets. However, to increase the weight lifted in an exercise over the long term, the key is intermuscular coordination training (technique training). With time, as the nervous system learns the gesture, fewer motor units are activated by the same weight, thereby leaving more motor units available for activation by higher weights. In addition, the concentric action should be explosive in order to activate the fast-twitch muscle fibers (responsible for the highest and fastest force generation) and to achieve the highest specific hypertrophy.

The most commonly employed methods entail the use of moderately heavy (MxS-I) and heavy (MxS-II) loads, applied in this sequence (see figure 10.13). Improving intermuscular coordination (i.e., coordination of muscle groups) depends strictly on learning (technique), which requires many sets of repetitions of the same exercise using a moderate load (40% to 80% of 1RM) and performed explosively with perfect technique (MxS-I). **Intramuscular coordination**, or the capacity to recruit fast-twitch fibers, depends on training content in which high loads (80% to 90% of 1RM) are moved explosively (MxS-II). Both of these types of strength training, MxS-I and MxS-II, activate the powerful fast-twitch motor units.

The physiological benefits for sport performance lie in an athlete's ability to convert gains in strength, and possibly muscle size, to the specific strength demanded by her particular sport. Building the foundation sets the stage, adding muscle generates force, and adapting the body to use heavy loads improves the capability to voluntarily involve its largest engines (the fast-twitch motor units). Once the mind–muscle connection is made, the physical requirements of the sport determine the next phase.

AA	MxS	MxS	MxS	P	P
3+1	3+1 Intermuscular coordination loads are used (70%-75% of 1RM)	3+1 Intermuscular coordination loads are used (75%-80% of 1RM)	2+1 Intramuscular coordination loads are used (85%-90% of 1RM)	2+1	2+1

FIGURE 10.13 Sequence of MxS-I and MxS-II methods within the maximum strength phase.

Digits (e.g., 3+1) refer to three microcycles of progressive increase of load, followed by one regeneration or recovery cycle. AA = anatomical adaptation; MxS = maximum strength; P = power.

Phase 4: Conversion to Specific Strength

Depending on the sport, a maximum strength phase of training can be followed by one of three fundamental options: conversion to power, power endurance, or muscle endurance. Conversion to power or power endurance is accomplished by using relatively moderate to heavy loads (40% to 80% of 1RM) with the intention of moving the weight as quickly as possible, the difference being the duration of the sets. By engaging the nervous system, methods such as ballistic training and upper or lower body plyometric training improve an athlete's high-velocity strength or ability to recruit and engage the high-powered, fast-twitch motor units. A strong foundation of maximum strength is a must for maximizing the rate of force production. In fact, even maximum strength training with high loads moved at low velocity has been shown to transfer to gains in power if the athlete attempts to move the weight as quickly as possible (16). Depending on the demands of the sport, muscle endurance can be trained for short, medium, or long duration. Short muscle endurance as the main energy system is the anaerobic lactic, whereas medium and long muscle endurance are predominately aerobic. Conversion to muscle endurance requires more than performing 15 to 20 repetitions per set; in fact, it can require as many as 400 repetitions per set, implemented concomitantly with metabolic training. Indeed, metabolic training and muscle endurance training pursue similar physiological training objectives.

Recall that the body replenishes energy for muscular contractions through the combined efforts of three energy systems: anaerobic alactic, anaerobic lactic, and aerobic. Training for conversion to muscle endurance requires heightened adaptation of the aerobic and the anaerobic lactic systems. The main objectives of aerobic training include improvement in physiological parameters, such as heart efficiency; biochemical parameters, such as increased mitochondria and capillary density, which result in greater diffusion and use of oxygen; and metabolic parameters, which result in greater use of fat as energy and an increased rate of removal and reuse of lactic acid. Adapting the neuromuscular and cardiovascular systems physiologically, biochemically, and metabolically provides invaluable benefit to athletes in many endurance sports. To maximize performance in muscle endurance sports, maximum strength training must be followed by a combination of specific metabolic training and specific strength training to prepare the body for the demands of the sport.

Phase 5: Maintenance

Once the neuromuscular system has been adapted for maximum performance, it is time to put the gains to the test. Unfortunately, most athletes and coaches work hard and strategically as the competitive season approaches but cease to train strength once the season begins. In reality, maintaining the strong and stable base formed during precompetitive phases requires the athlete to continue training during the competitive season. Failure to plan at least one weekly session dedicated to strength training results in decreased performance or early onset of fatigue as the season wears on.

Staying up is always easier than falling down and then attempting to get back up. Periodization of strength involves planning phases to optimize physiological adaptation and planning to maintain the benefits for as long as the season lasts. When the season is over, serious athletes can take 2 to 4 weeks off to regenerate their minds and bodies.

Stimulating the body for optimal performance takes time, planning, and persistence. Physiology is helpful in planning the program, but performance improvement is achieved through practical application of the many principles and methods of training inherent in the periodization of strength.

Phase 6: Cessation

As the main competition of the year approaches, most of the athlete's energy must be directed to the main sport-specific biomotor ability or mix of biomotor abilities. Again, the purpose of the cessation phase is to conserve the athlete's energy for competition and peak his or sport-specific biomotor abilities. For this reason, the strength training program should end at least 3 to 14 days before the main competition. The exact timing depends on multiple factors:

- *The athlete's gender:* Female athletes, who retain strength gains less easily than males do, should usually maintain strength training until 3 days before competition.
- *The chosen sport:* A longer cessation phase, 1 to 2 weeks long, may result in improved alactic speed performance due to overshooting of the fast-twitch type IIx muscle fibers. For long endurance sports for which strength is not as important as for anaerobic sports, strength training can be ended 2 weeks before the main competition.

- *Body type:* Heavier athletes tend to retain both adaptations and residual fatigue longer and therefore should end strength training earlier than lighter athletes.

Phase 7: Compensation

Traditionally, the last phase of the annual plan has been inappropriately called the off-season; in reality, it represents a transition from one annual plan to another. The main goal of this phase is to remove fatigue acquired during the training year and replenish the exhausted energy stores by decreasing both volume (through a decrease in frequency) and intensity of training. During the months of training and competition, most athletes are exposed to numerous psychological and social stressors that drain their mental energy. During the transition phase, athletes can relax psychologically by getting involved in various physical and social activities they enjoy.

The transition phase should last no longer than 4 weeks for serious athletes. A longer phase results in detraining effects, such as the loss of most training gains, especially strength gains. The detraining that results from neglecting strength training in the off-season can be detrimental to athletes' rate of performance improvement in the following year. Athletes and coaches should remember that strength is hard to gain and easy to lose. Athletes who perform no strength training at all during the transition phase may experience decreased muscle size and considerable power loss (201). Because power and speed are interdependent, such athletes also lose speed. Some authors claim that the disuse of muscles also reduces the frequency of discharge rate and the pattern of muscle fiber recruitment; thus, strength and power loss may be the result of not activating as many motor units.

Although physical activity volume is reduced by 50% to 60% during the transition phase, athletes should find time to work on the maintenance of strength training. Specifically, it can be beneficial to work on the antagonists, stabilizers, and other muscles that may not necessarily be involved in the performance of the sport-specific skills. Similarly, compensation exercises should be planned for sports in which an imbalance may develop between parts or sides of the body (e.g., pitching, throwing events, archery, soccer, cycling).

Summary of Major Concepts

Strength is one of the most important biomotor abilities for most sports. Strength is the foundation for both generating maximum power and maintaining repetitive muscular contractions (i.e., muscle endurance). A periodized strength training program can be an excellent tool for maximizing performance outcomes. The physiological adaptations to the neuromuscular system that strength training can bring about are very specific to the training program that the athlete uses. Athletic performance can be maximized only if the training program provides appropriate variation. Many methods for inducing training variation are available, and many of them can result in very specific physiological adaptations. Finally, to truly maximize the effectiveness of a strength training program, it must be integrated into the comprehensive periodized training plan developed for the athlete. Simply adding strength training to an athlete's training plan without considering the other training activities will not maximize performance outcomes.

Endurance Training > 11

Endurance can be classified several ways. For example, aerobic endurance, sometimes called low-intensity exercise endurance, allows a person to perform activities continuously for a long duration, whereas anaerobic endurance, or high-intensity exercise endurance, provides the ability to repetitively perform bouts of high-intensity exercise. Although most sports rely on some form of endurance, the type of endurance developed (high or low intensity) can significantly affect performance outcomes. Therefore, the coach and athlete must consider the type of endurance that the athlete needs for the sport and how the appropriate endurance will be targeted within the training plan. The coach and athlete must also consider the athlete's physiological responses to the methods for developing endurance. Once the type of endurance and the physiological responses are understood, the coach can develop a training plan to enhance sport-specific endurance.

Classification of Endurance

The concept of endurance differs distinctly between various sporting activities and thus can be defined in several different ways. For example, the type of endurance that an elite marathon runner needs provides the ability to continuously perform at a specific power output or velocity for a long duration of time. Conversely, an elite ice hockey player needs to repetitively perform periods of high-velocity movements for 30 to 80 s, interspersed with periods of recovery lasting between 4 and 5 min (106). Although some form of endurance affects the performance of both types of athletes, the development of endurance in these athletes will be distinctly different. If the wrong type of endurance training is implemented, the athletes might develop endurance characteristics that do not meet the needs of their sports, and thus performance capacity can be reduced (45, 147). To understand the correct application of endurance training, the coach and athlete must differentiate between the two major types of endurance reported in the contemporary literature: low-intensity exercise endurance (LIEE) and high-intensity exercise endurance (HIEE) (147).

Low-Intensity Exercise Endurance

Activities that are predominated by aerobic energy supply tend to exhibit lower peak powers and thus can be classified as being of lower intensities (29, 148). These activities require the athlete to perform continuously, at a low intensity, for a substantial duration. Thus, this type of endurance is often termed LIEE (148) or aerobic endurance. Many activities rely predominantly on oxidative or aerobic metabolism (see chapter 1 and table 1.2) and require the athlete to develop a high level of LIEE. For such activities, developing LIEE can greatly improve the athlete's performance.

Conversely, the development of LIEE in sports that rely on anaerobic energy supply (e.g., sprinting, American football, ice hockey, volleyball) can result in several maladaptations that reduce the athlete's performance capacity (45). When LIEE is used to improve endurance in athletes who participate in sports that rely predominantly on anaerobic energy supply, marked decreases in power-generating capacity are noted and performance usually is impaired (42, 45, 63, 83). One reason researchers have proposed this explanation of impaired anaerobic performance is that the development of LIEE can reduce the athlete's ability to produce force in the high-velocity region of the force–velocity curve (12). Changes to this region of the force–velocity curve can interfere with the athlete's ability to develop explosive strength, which is required by many anaerobic activities (45). In particular, the ability to achieve high rates of force development and to generate high levels of peak force can be impaired by the implementation of the LIEE program (figure 11.1). There also appears to be a fiber type shift resulting in a decrease in the number of type II muscle fibers and an increase in type I fibers when LIEE is the focus of the endurance development program (154). LIEE training can also impede muscular growth (108), which will impair an athlete's ability to generate high rates of force development (81), maximize peak force-generating capacity (81), and optimize peak power generation (45). The contemporary literature indicates that LIEE training should not be used for athletes in sports that predominantly rely on anaerobic energy supply, require high levels of force production, require high rates of force development, call for fast velocities of movement, or require high levels of power output. LIEE training should be restricted to long-duration activities that rely on aerobic energy supply; other methods for developing endurance should be used by athletes in other types of sports.

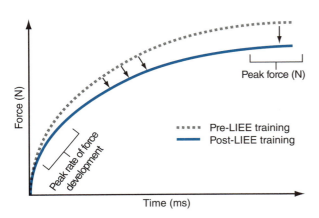

FIGURE 11.1 Force–time curve alterations to the development of low-intensity exercise endurance (LIEE).

Adapted from Häkkinen and Myllyla 1990 (61) and Häkkinen et al. 1989 (60).

High-Intensity Exercise Endurance

Sports that rely on anaerobic metabolism (see chapter 1 and table 1.2) usually require high power outputs or the repetitive performance of high-velocity movements. Because anaerobic activities require higher power outputs than those seen in aerobic activities, anaerobic activities can be classified as being of high intensity (29, 148). Therefore, the ability to sustain and repeat high-intensity exercise bouts is termed high-intensity exercise endurance (HIEE) (147). The development of HIEE does not impair force-generating capacity, as typically occurs when LIEE is developed. One explanation why HIEE does not reduce maximum strength and power development is that HIEE training tends to maintain type II muscle fiber content (45). Because type II fiber content is related to the maximal rate of force development (81, 85), maximal force-generating capacity (81), and the ability to generate peak power outputs (149), it is easy to conclude that HIEE may be more beneficial for sports that rely on these performance factors, especially if high-velocity or high-power movements are performed repetitively. Several authors report that the use of high-intensity intervals can significantly increase markers of both anaerobic and aerobic exercise endurance (95, 126, 152). Therefore, it is recommended that an HIEE or interval training approach be used to develop endurance for sports that require the repetitive performance of high-intensity exercise (e.g., American football, soccer, basketball, ice hockey) (147).

HIEE training should not be limited to the development of anaerobic endurance, because this type of training also has the potential to improve LIEE (87). The development of HIEE with the use of high-intensity interval training appears to have a profound effect on aerobic activities that typically rely on LIEE. For example, it has been shown that 3 km (+3%) and 10 km running performance can be significantly improved with high-intensity interval training (4, 142). Similarly, time-trial performance in the 40 km cycle has been increased significantly (+2.1% to +4.5%) with high-intensity interval training (144, 145, 158). Several authors have suggested that increasing the quantity of traditional LIEE training with elite athletes may not result in the necessary physiological adaptations needed to improve performance (31, 64). Laursen and Jenkins (87) suggested that high-intensity interval training or HIEE training may be warranted for athletes who have established LIEE training as a base. Therefore, it may be beneficial to consider using HIEE training methods for athletes who participate in aerobic sports that require repetitive performance over a long duration of time, especially closer to or during the competitive phase.

Factors Affecting Aerobic Endurance Performance

Several aspects of aerobic endurance are central to determining the athlete's endurance capacity (35, 75). These factors include the athlete's aerobic power, lactate threshold, economy of movement, and muscle fiber type (figure 11.2). Each factor can be improved significantly with appropriate training methods. To develop appropriate aerobic endurance training programs, the coach and athlete must understand the physiological responses associated with endurance performance.

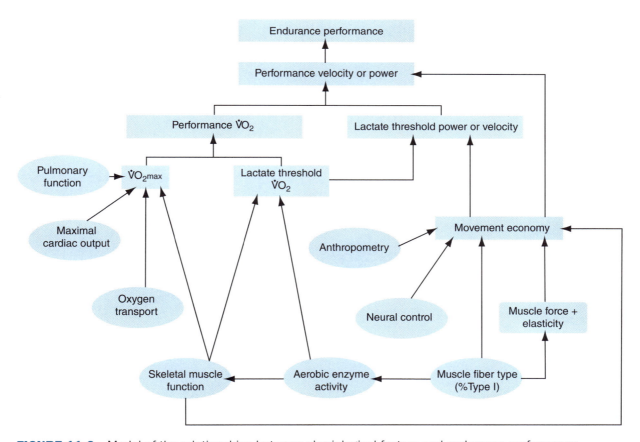

FIGURE 11.2 Model of the relationships between physiological factors and endurance performance.

Adapted from Bassett and Howley 2000 (9), Coyle 1995 (35), Paavolainen et al. 1999 (110), and Joyner and Coyle 2008 (76).

Aerobic Power

Maximal **aerobic power** has long been considered to be a major factor in determining success in endurance sports (33, 131). However, aerobic power is not the only determinant of sport performance. Aerobic power is measured as the highest rate at which oxygen can be taken up and used by the body during maximal exercise (56) and can also be defined as maximal oxygen uptake ($\dot{V}O_2$max) (9, 35). $\dot{V}O_2$max values between 70 and 85 ml·kg^{-1}·min^{-1} have been reported for elite endurance athletes (34, 76). Women exhibit a $\dot{V}O_2$max approximately 10% lower than their male counterparts, as a result of lower hemoglobin concentrations and higher body fat percentages. Regardless of gender, the ability to achieve a high $\dot{V}O_2$max appears to be affected by the functioning of the pulmonary system, maximum cardiac output, oxygen-carrying capacity, and factors associated with the skeletal muscle system (figure 11.3) (9).

Pulmonary System

The **pulmonary system** appears to limit $\dot{V}O_2$max in very specific circumstances (9, 120). For example, oxygen (O_2) desaturation can occur in elite athletes who are performing max-

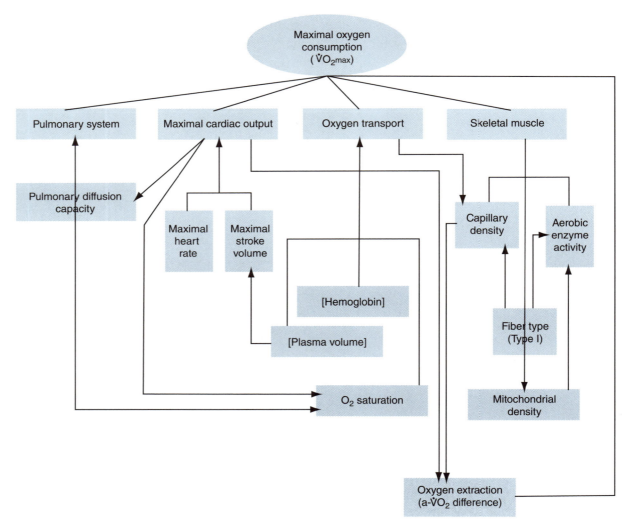

FIGURE 11.3 Factors affecting maximal aerobic power or maximal oxygen consumption.

a-$\dot{V}O_2$ difference = arterial–mixed venous oxygen difference.

Adapted from Bassett and Howley 2000 (9), Coyle 1995 (35), and Joyner and Coyle 2008 (76).

imal work (39), because a high exercise **cardiac output** (Q = stroke volume × heart rate) decreases the red blood cell (RBC) transit time through the pulmonary capillary (9, 39). The decreased transit time for the RBC decreases the time available to saturate the blood with O_2, potentially limiting performance. Support for the contention that the pulmonary system can limit $\dot{V}O_2$max can be seen in studies that have explored the effects of hyperoxia (120). If supplemental O_2 is supplied, there is an increased O_2 "driving force," which elevates $\dot{V}O_2$max as a result of increased oxygen saturation (109, 120).

Similar performance impairments can be seen when exercise is performed at moderately high altitudes (3,000 to 5,000 m) (9, 49). This altitude-induced reduction in performance can be experienced in response to short-term (1 to 3 days) altitude exposure, which can stimulate a reduction in O_2 saturation (23). A similar reduction in performance and oxygen desaturation response can be seen in individuals who have asthma (9). Like athletes, people with asthma who use supplemental O_2 experience an increased driving force for O_2 diffusion (9). These data suggest that pulmonary gas exchange can significantly limit an athlete's ability to express a high $\dot{V}O_2$max (9).

Cardiac Output

Maximal aerobic power is strongly related to maximal cardiac output (Qmax) (75). This relationship can be seen when comparing the typical Qmax and $\dot{V}O_2$max of athletes with those values in untrained individuals (figure 11.4) (164). The Qmax is a function of both the maximal heart rate and the volume of blood (stroke volume) pumped by the heart (92, 164). Lower-level athletes and untrained individuals exhibit a linear increase in both stroke volume and exercise heart rate until approximately 40% of $\dot{V}O_2$max (119, 160, 164), after which stroke volume plateaus or slightly increases, and increases in heart rate determine increases in cardiac output (164). It is believed that the plateau in cardiac output is a direct function of a decreased left ventricular diastolic filling time, which can be seen with increasing exercise intensity (128). Conversely, elite endurance athletes exhibit increases in both heart rate and cardiac output in response to increasing exercise intensity (59, 164). The reason for this discrepancy in stroke volume response between elite endurance athletes and trained or untrained individuals has yet to be determined, but it is generally accepted that elite athletes exhibit higher Qmax values (9).

Because elite athletes exhibit a higher Qmax, it might be speculated that the difference between elite athletes, trained athletes, and untrained individuals rests in either the ability to achieve maximal heart rates or the ability to increase stroke volume (9, 92). Maximal heart rate is slightly lower in elite athletes compared with nonathletes (92, 164); therefore, it is likely that the main factor differentiating the Qmax between athletes and nonathletes is the training-induced alterations in stroke volume (92). The increase in stroke volume seen

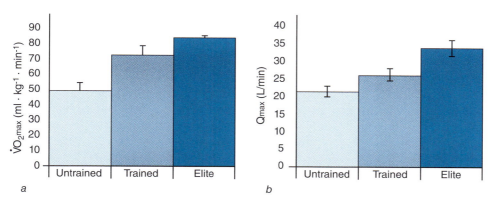

FIGURE 11.4 Comparison of (a) maximal oxygen consumption and (b) maximal cardiac output between untrained, trained, and elite male distance runners.

Adapted from Zhou et al. 2001 (164).

in athletes is likely related to an increase in end-diastolic volume that occurs as a result of improved cardiac chamber compliance or an increase in the distensibility of the pericardium (92). These data indicate that the Qmax partially explains the differences in $\dot{V}O_2$max between athletes and nonathletes.

Oxygen Transport

Another factor that can explain individual differences in $\dot{V}O_2$max is the capacity of the cardiorespiratory system to transport oxygen (9). Alterations to the hemoglobin (Hb) concentration can have a profound effect on O_2 transport to the working muscle (15). For example, if athletes use blood transfusions to artificially increase their Hb concentrations, a concomitant increase in $\dot{V}O_2$max and Qmax is seen (44). These interrelationships of Hb concentration, $\dot{V}O_2$max, and Qmax partially explain why blood doping is effective (15). Although doping appears to exert a profound effect on the body's ability to transport oxygen (15), it also appears that aerobic endurance training can alter this ability (134).

Endurance training appears to reduce Hb concentration, hematocrit (Hct), and RBC count as a result of plasma volume expansion, which can begin to occur after several days of prolonged training (135). Although there is a general decrease in Hct and Hb concentration in response to endurance training, there is an absolute increase in the Hb mass (133). The plasma volume increase noted with endurance training decreases blood viscosity, which increases $\dot{V}O_2$max as a result of an increase in cardiac output that improves oxygen delivery to the working muscles (134).

Skeletal Muscle

Skeletal muscle can play a very important role in determining an athlete's $\dot{V}O_2$max (9). $\dot{V}O_2$max appears to be related to the rate at which O_2 can be delivered to the mitochondria (100). Several factors associated with skeletal muscles can affect their ability to use O_2, including the skeletal muscle fiber type (type I or type II), mitochondrial density, and capillary density.

Muscle Fiber Type Muscle fiber type appears to be significantly related to the $\dot{V}O_2$max of elite athletes (98). Athletes who express higher $\dot{V}O_2$max values also appear to have higher type I fiber content. This phenomenon may be related to the different capillary densities, mitochondrial content, and aerobic enzyme capacities seen between type I and type II fibers. Type I fibers, which have a higher oxidative capacity, have a greater capillary–fiber ratio as a result of being surrounded by more capillaries, compared with type II fibers (165). Type I fibers also display a greater mitochondrial density (127) and a greater reliance on aerobic enzyme activity (51, 70, 156). Finally, there appears to be a general shift from type II to type I fiber content, an increase in mitochondrial content, and an increased reliance on aerobic metabolism in response to endurance training (127, 154). These endurance training–induced adaptations appear to be related to the athlete's training age. Athletes who have trained longer experience greater increases in capillary density and type I fiber content as well as a greater reliance on aerobic enzyme activity (127).

Mitochondrial Density The mitochondria are the sites within the muscle where O_2 is consumed during oxidative metabolism (9). An increase in mitochondrial content of the skeletal muscle may contribute to an increased $\dot{V}O_2$max as a result of a greater extraction of O_2 from the blood (69). Exercise appears to be a powerful stimulator for mitochondrial biogenesis (69, 161), and exercise-induced increases in mitochondrial density may partially explain the improvements in $\dot{V}O_2$max seen with endurance training (69). Theoretically, if the mitochondrial density is increased, a proportional increase in O_2 extraction from the blood should occur (9). However, this does not appear to be the case because only modest increases in $\dot{V}O_2$max occur in response to training (20% to 40%), even though there are marked increases in mitochondrial enzymes (69). It is likely that training induces increases in mitochondrial enzymes, which improves endurance performance (9). These enzymatic adaptations may improve endurance performance via decreased lactate production during exercise and an increase in fat oxidation, which results in a sparing of muscle glycogen and blood glucose (69). Although mitochondrial enzyme adaptations to training result in increases in endurance $\dot{V}O_2$max during whole-body exercise, it appears that performance is most affected by oxygen delivery, not mitochondrial density (9).

Capillary Density Investigators have reported that a greater capillary density or number corresponds to a higher $\dot{V}O_2$max (9, 26, 35, 132). It has been speculated that $\dot{V}O_2$max depends on capillary density, or the number of capillaries per unit of cross-sectional area of muscle (100). An increase in capillary density allows for a maintenance or elongation of the RBC's transient time through the capillary bed (130), which would increase O_2 extraction at the tissue—called the **arteriovenous oxygen difference (a-$\bar{v}O_2$ difference)**—even when blood flow is elevated (9). Investigators also have reported that athletes who possess higher capillary densities are able to exercise for longer durations as a result of being able to tolerate anaerobic metabolism and lactate formation better than athletes with lower capillary densities (76). This suggests that capillary density plays an important role in the delivery of O_2 to working tissue and the removal of waste products created by the muscle.

Capillary density is increased in response to endurance training (36, 71, 130, 136, 151). This increase in capillary density appears to be tightly linked to the training age of the athlete, where a greater training age relates to greater increases in capillary density (127).

Lactate Threshold

It is well accepted that $\dot{V}O_2$max plays a role in endurance performance capabilities. However, with elite athletes there is a narrow range between the $\dot{V}O_2$max of individual athletes (18, 27), which suggests that the $\dot{V}O_2$max does not differentiate between the performances of these athletes (14, 18). If, for example, two elite athletes with different $\dot{V}O_2$max values are competing, the athlete who possesses the lower $\dot{V}O_2$max may be able to compensate for this by working at a higher percentage of her maximal capacity (figure 11.5) (18, 33, 140). The percentage of $\dot{V}O_2$max at which an athlete can work may be a more accurate predictor of performance. This percentage is called the **performance oxygen uptake**, and it is limited by a combination of the individual's lactate threshold and $\dot{V}O_2$max (14, 35).

The performance oxygen uptake can also be considered as the highest amount of work at which an equilibrium between lactate formation and buffering exists. This equilibrium has also been termed the **maximal lactate steady state** (150). The point at which this equilibrium becomes out of balance, and lactate accumulation begins to outweigh buffering capabilities, is the **anaerobic threshold** (150). The anaerobic threshold represents an intensity of exercise at which the body cannot meet its energy demand through aerobic mechanisms and the anaerobic energy supply begins to increase to maintain the intensity of exercise. In this scenario, the increase in lactate production occurs as a result of an increased rate of formation of pyruvate from the glycolytic system, which cannot be incorporated into oxidative metabolism. Instead it is rapidly converted into lactic acid and then lactate (150).

A graded exercise test in which intensity is periodically increased coupled with blood sampling can be used to create a **lactate** accumulation curve (figure 11.6). The lactate accumulation curve shows that breakpoints in the formation of lactate occur as the intensity of exercise increases (148). The intensity of exercise at which a substantial increase in lactate accumulation begins to occur has been termed the lactate threshold (14, 148, 150). The lactate threshold is defined as a 1 mm increase in blood lactate accumulation above resting levels in response to a graded exercise test (35, 162). In untrained subjects the lactate threshold occurs at approximately 50% to 60% of $\dot{V}O_2$max (25, 76, 148), whereas in trained subjects the lactate threshold can occur between 75% and 90% of $\dot{V}O_2$max (76). The power output or velocity of movement that can be maintained at the lactate threshold is a strong predictor of endurance performance (43, 75). Dumke and colleagues (43) reported that the heart rate at lactate threshold is similar to the heart rate during a 60 min cycle time trial performed

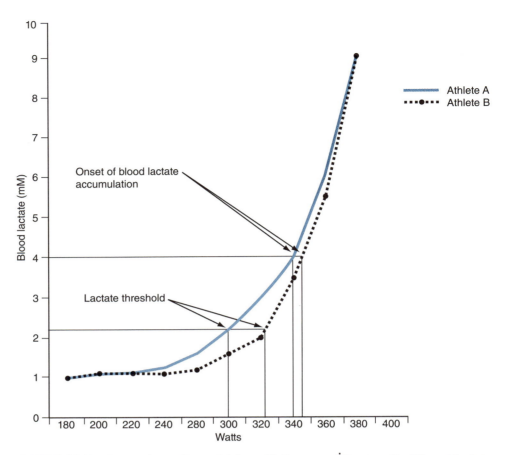

FIGURE 11.5 Comparison of two athletes with the same V̇O₂max with different lactate threshold and onset of blood lactate accumulation (OBLA) values.

Athlete A can produce 300 W at his lactate threshold, whereas athlete B can produce 320 W. Thus, athlete B can work at a 6.7% higher workload. Power at lactate threshold has been strongly correlated to endurance performance capacity (75).

by trained cyclists. Strong evidence exists suggesting that the speed or power output at the lactate threshold explains the vast majority of performance variance seen in distance racing (9, 47, 48). It appears that coaches who work with endurance athletes should quantify the lactate threshold and the heart rate and power or velocity values associated with it.

A second breakpoint on the lactate accumulation curve is called the onset of blood lactate accumulation (OBLA), which occurs at a fixed lactate value of 4 mm (138) (figure 11.6). OBLA is much higher than the lactate threshold and corresponds to an intensity of exercise that is much higher than that seen at the lactate threshold. As with the lactate threshold, OBLA has been suggested to be a strong indicator of endurance performance capabilities (14, 43, 79). Dumke and colleagues (43) reported that the heart rate at OBLA is similar to the heart rate during a 30 min time trial.

Both the lactate threshold and OBLA are sensitive to training (40, 75). Endurance training has been shown to shift the lactate threshold to the right, which suggests that a greater intensity of exercise (power or speed) can be performed without the accumulation of lactate (75). It appears that continuous training at or slightly above the lactate threshold is important to improve endurance performance as a result of shifting OBLA and the lactate threshold (24, 65, 78, 139, 157). Anecdotal evidence suggests that a well-balanced endurance training plan requires periodic training at the lactate threshold via the use of threshold or tempo training to optimize performance (75).

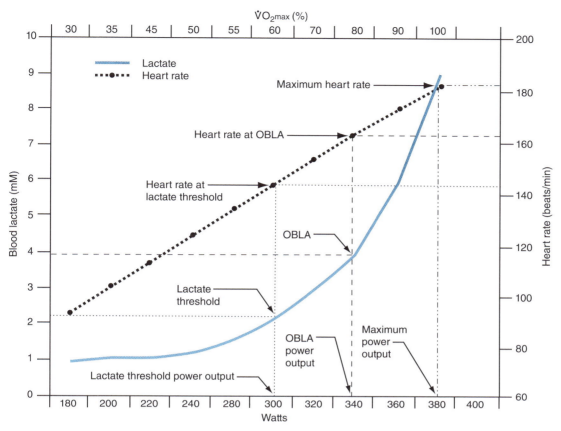

FIGURE 11.6 Lactate threshold and onset of blood lactate accumulation (OBLA) response to a graded cycle ergometer test.

The lactate threshold and OBLA can also be shifted in response to high-intensity interval training performed at intensities that are substantially higher than the lactate threshold power, velocity, or heart rate (40, 65). High-intensity interval training can require multiple high-intensity efforts (>80% of peak aerobic power) of various durations (30 s to 8 min) interspersed with lower-intensity recovery (60 s to 4 1/2 min) (87). The use of strength training in the preparation of endurance athletes also has been shown to improve the lactate threshold (77). The lactate threshold is a primary determinant of endurance performance; understanding what heart rate, power, or velocity corresponds to in the lactate threshold can be very useful in designing endurance training programs.

Exercise Economy

Exercise economy is a key factor dictating endurance exercise performance. Exercise economy, or economy of movement, has been defined as the oxygen uptake required to perform exercise at a given intensity (75), or the ratio of mechanical work done to energy expended (9). The economy of movement and its effect on the energy cost of an exercise bout may partially explain some of the differences in performance noted between athletes who possess similar $\dot{V}O_2$max values (10). Close examination of athletes with similar $\dot{V}O_2$max values suggests that there is a large interindividual variability in the oxygen cost of submaximal exercise (75).

This large interindividual difference is clearly seen when examining the variations among oxygen costs when individuals run at a given submaximal speed (9, 19, 107). These individual differences appear to be affected by training status, because running economy is significantly related to training status (75, 97, 103, 107). Trained individuals express a

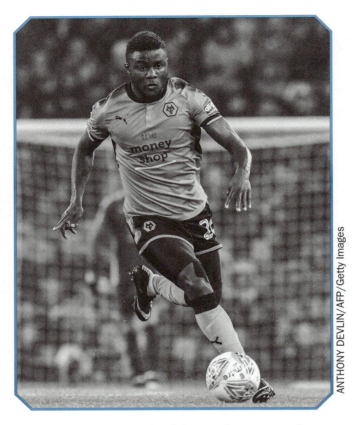

High-intensity interval training can improve running economy, increase $\dot{V}O_2$max, raise the lactate threshold, and improve soccer playing ability.

greater exercise economy compared with their untrained counterparts (107). In fact, the number of training years appears to be significantly correlated ($p < .05$, $r = .62$) with running economy (97). It is speculated that over time, running economy improves as a result of long-term skeletal muscle adaptations, such as the transition of type II fibers to type I (117, 154), and metabolic changes that reduce the energy cost for developing a particular repetitive level of force (103). Long-term training has also been suggested to affect running economy as a result of changes to anthropometric, biomechanical, and technical factors (5).

Training stimulus appears to play a significant role in the development of exercise economy (9, 75, 103). The highest movement economies appear to occur at the speeds or power outputs at which the athlete usually trains (75). It has been suggested that these changes to running economy are related to the athlete's volume of training (75). This is clearly seen by the fact that more experienced athletes or athletes who have accumulated more training miles express higher levels of exercise economy (74, 75).

High-intensity interval training has been suggested to significantly improve running economy and $\dot{V}O_2$max, which are usually associated with improvements in endurance performance (87). Performing interval running with intensities that range between 93% and 106% of $\dot{V}O_2$max has been shown to improve running economy (103). Support for this contention can be found in the work of Franch and colleagues (53); in their study, 6 weeks of long intervals, which consisted of four to six sets of 4 min intervals (4.6 m/s) separated by 2 min of rest, resulted in a 6% increase in $\dot{V}O_2$max and a 3% increase in running economy. In a study of soccer players, 8 weeks of aerobic interval training that consisted of four sets of 4 min high-intensity intervals (90% to 95% of maximum heart rate) separated by 3 min of light jogging performed two times per week resulted in a 6.7% increase in running economy, a 10.7% increase in $\dot{V}O_2$max, a 15.9% increase in the lactate threshold; it also resulted in a 24% increase in involvements with the ball during a game and a 3.5% increase in the ability to perform at a higher average heart rate during a soccer match (62). Although this preliminary data suggest that high-intensity intervals can improve running economy, more research is needed to clarify the types of interval training that are most effective. It does appear that high-intensity interval training should be incorporated into the training plans of both team sport athletes and more traditional endurance athletes.

Another method for improving running economy in distance runners is the addition of strength or low-impact plyometric training (73, 110, 155). These improvements in running economy may occur as a result of an increased mechanical efficiency caused by improved motor unit recruitment patterns, and increased muscular strength (specifically the propulsion phase of running). Although strength training appears to offer a great benefit for the endurance athlete, many athletes worry about gaining weight because of training. This, however, should not be of major concern because the contemporary literature on cell signaling suggests that endurance training blunts the signaling pathways that would need to be activated to induce significant gains in muscle mass (108). This can be clearly seen in the literature exploring the effects of strength training on endurance performance, where athletes typically see less than 1.0% increase in body mass as a result of an increase in lean body mass (68, 110). Therefore, it may be warranted for endurance athletes to include strength and low-impact plyometric training to optimize exercise economy and ultimately endurance performance.

Factors Affecting Anaerobic Endurance Performance

Several factors affect the athlete's ability to repetitively perform high-intensity, anaerobic bouts of exercise (3, 50, 84). These factors include the ability to preferentially activate the anaerobic energy systems, the ability to buffer lactic acid, the functioning of the cardiovascular system, and the ability to maintain neuromuscular characteristics related to performance.

Bioenergetics

HIEE depends on the ability to repetitively perform high-power output activities that preferentially activate the anaerobic energy systems (113). When the athlete incorporates HIEE training into his training plan, he will experience physiological adaptations that increase the concentration or activity of key enzymes of the phosphagen and glycolytic energy systems (3, 50).

Increases in muscular stores of ATP, phosphocreatine (PCr), and muscle glycogen have been reported to occur in response to sprint or interval training (3, 50, 84). These alterations in enzymatic properties appear to allow for a more rapid supply of energy during high-intensity bouts of exercise, thus allowing the athlete to maintain a higher level of performance.

Lactic Acid–Buffering Capacity

One of the most important factors affecting an athlete's ability to develop HIEE is the ability to buffer lactic acid to lactate. The ability to buffer lactic acid or H^+ ions has been suggested to be related to sprint performance ability (93, 159). It is well documented that increases in H^+ ion concentration result in an inhibitory effect on **phosphofructokinase (PFK)** (143). If these H^+ ions are not buffered, the concomitant reduction in PFK activity will reduce the ATP yield from glycolysis, thus reducing the power output that can be maintained during the activity (87).

HIEE training methods such as high-intensity tempo or interval training have been demonstrated to increase the athlete's buffering capacities (101, 159). These increases in buffering capacity enable the body to maintain energetic flux at a rapid rate and thus maintain high-power performance typically seen in sports that rely on HIEE. Therefore, if the bioenergetic profile of the sporting activity indicates a need for HIEE, the training program must include interventions that increase the athlete's ability to buffer lactic acid while maintaining the rate of energetic flux.

LIEE or aerobic training does not allow for the maximal development of the lactic acid–buffering capacity (113). To increase this buffering capacity, the training plan must stimulate the accumulation of H^+ ions, which only occurs if the fast glycolytic system is repetitively stimulated. Because LIEE primarily activates the aerobic energy supply system, especially when undertaken at intensities under the lactate threshold, this training method holds little merit for the athlete who requires HIEE. In fact, it is likely that incorporating LIEE training methods in the training plans of anaerobic athletes will decrease HIEE (125).

Cardiovascular System

Oxidative metabolism and the cardiovascular system play an integral role in recovery from high-intensity interval training, such as resistance or sprint interval training (148). However, athletes who participate in sports that rely on HIEE should not undergo LIEE training, because this training impairs anaerobic performance capacity (45).

Recent evidence clearly demonstrates that high-intensity interval training can increase $\dot{V}O_2$max, stroke volume, and the ability to use oxidative metabolism during recovery from interval training (87, 113). These adaptations appear to play an integral role in the athlete's ability to recover from repetitive bouts of high-intensity exercise. Interestingly, the use of high-intensity interval training does not impair anaerobic energetic supply during exercise or alter the neuromuscular activation patterns typically seen in response to LIEE. Therefore, high-intensity interval training, when implemented correctly, will allow for the cardiovascular system adaptations needed for the development of HIEE. Accordingly, athletes who require HIEE in their sports should not use LIEE training methods, because high-intensity interval training will supply the necessary adaptive stimulus need to optimize performance.

Neuromuscular System

High-intensity interval training does not interfere with the development of high force or power outputs necessary for performance in sports that rely on HIEE. Conversely, LIEE training decreases the athlete's ability to produce force at the high-velocity, low-frequency region of the force–velocity curve (13, 45). The force–time curve can be shifted in response to LIEE training (figure 11.1). The impact of HIEE and LIEE training can be clearly seen in the differences in the force–time curve and electromyographic activation patterns seen in endurance, strength, and power athletes (61).

The rate of force development (RFD) appears to be affected by the type of training used. For example, LIEE methods will substantially decrease the RFD and the ability to generate peak forces (61). The ability to express high RFD appears to depend on the energy system activated, the muscle fiber type, and the neuromuscular recruitment pattern (45, 61).

The ability to rapidly release energy from ATP depends on the activity of adenosine triphosphatase (ATPase), which is related to the myosin heavy chain (MHC) isoforms (fiber type) (163). Muscle fibers that contain MHC type X and IIa are considerably faster than those containing MHC type I (55). Endurance athletes usually contain a higher MHC type I concentration than sprint or strength athletes (163). LIEE training appears to increase MHC type I isoforms (154), which could decrease the rate of ATPase activity. This shift would impair the athlete's ability to produce the high-force and high-velocity movements that are necessary to maintain HIEE capabilities. Conversely, the use of interval training methods will increase MHC type IIa isoforms, which allows the athlete to maintain force- and power-generating capacities (45). The ability to generate force rapidly is an important component of HIEE. Thus, sprints and interval training are the preferred methods of developing endurance for athletes who participate in strength- and power-based sports.

Methods for Developing Endurance

Athletes can develop endurance by using a variety of methods that produce very specific physiological and performance responses. When developing a training plan, the coach must determine the type of endurance that the plan will target because methods of developing endurance are vastly different in their implementation and physiological outcomes. For example, traditional methods to develop LIEE call for continuous training performed at a variety of intensities ranging from 60% to 90% of maximal heart rate (141). The use of high-intensity intervals has been reported to improve LIEE (20, 21, 57, 58, 86-91), thus increasing the training options available to the coach and athlete. Conversely, LIEE training methods appear to decrease HIEE capacity, which would ultimately impede the performance of athletes who must perform repetitive high-intensity or high-power movements during competition. The coach and athlete must be aware of the different methods used to develop both LIEE and HIEE and which kind of endurance is needed for various sports.

Low-Intensity or Aerobic Exercise

Several methods are available to develop endurance, and the choice usually depends on the time of year and the athlete's training goals (table 11.1). The development of LIEE is a

TABLE 11.1 — Methods Used to Develop Low-Intensity Exercise Endurance

Training method	Recommended frequency (times per week)*	Duration of training portion	Intensity — Heart rate (% max)	Intensity — $\dot{V}O_2$max (% max)
Active rest	1 or 2	30-60 min	<60%	<40%
Long slow distance (LSD)	1 or 2	≥30 min (race distance or longer)	60%-70%	42%-56%
Continuous pace or tempo training	1 or 2	20-30 min	At lactate threshold heart rate and $\dot{V}O_2$	
Interval training				
Aerobic intervals	1 or 2	20-40 min total time (depending on structure)	80%-100%	70%-100%
Anaerobic intervals	1 or 2	<2 min work bouts (work rest interval 1:0.5-1:5)	Maximal	Supramaximal
Fartlek	1	>30 min	Varies	Varies

*Other training days contain other training methods or rest and recovery.

function of stimulating physiological adaptations that improve performance. Traditionally, aerobic endurance is developed via the use of long slow distance (LSD) training. However, other methods such as pace or tempo, interval, and resistance training appear can be used to develop LIEE.

Active Rest

Active rest or recovery exercise is often used to stimulate recovery from high-intensity training or competition. This type of activity requires a low exercise heart rate (<65% of maximal heart rate) and lasts around 30 to 60 min (1, 141). This method can be used several times per week, depending on the structure of the microcycle.

Long Slow Distance (LSD) Training

Long slow distance (LSD) training can be considered "conversation" exercise, where the athlete is able to carry on a conversation without undue respiratory stress (118). LSD training involves relatively high training mileages or distances that are performed for a long duration (30 to 120 min or greater depending on the sport) at moderate to low intensities (66% to 80% of maximal heart rate; 50% to 70% of $\dot{V}O_2$max; table 11.2) (103, 118, 129). LSD training has been suggested to improve cardiovascular function, thermoregulatory abilities, mitochondrial energy production, and oxidative capacity of the skeletal muscle (30, 32, 41, 52, 69, 80, 118). These physiological adaptations to LSD training have been consistently demonstrated in untrained individuals (87); however, these physiological changes do not appear to occur as readily in highly trained endurance athletes (31, 64, 87). It is likely that advanced endurance athletes will need higher intensities of training, which may be accomplished via the use of interval training methods (87).

TABLE 11.2 — Relationship Between Heart Rate, Oxygen Consumption, and Ergogenesis

Percentage of FMax	Percentage of V̇O₂max	Ergogenesis	Training modality
50	28	Oxidative/glycolytic aerobic	Active rest
60	42		
66	50		
70	56	Glycolytic aerobic	Extensive training of aerobic capacity
74	60		
77	65		
80	70	Glycolytic anaerobic/aerobic	Intensive training of aerobic capacity or extensive training of aerobic power
85	75		
88	80		
90	83	Glycolytic aerobic/anaerobic	Intensive training of aerobic power
92	85		
96	90	Glycolytic anaerobic/aerobic	Intensive training of aerobic power and extensive training of anaerobic capacity
100	100		

Adapted from M.L. Micheli, E. Castellini, and M. Marella, 2008, "Il condizionamento aerobico," *L'allenatore*, A.I.A.C. (102b), and R. Proietti, 1999, *La corsa: Valutazione e allenamento della potenza aerobica e della resistenza alla velocità nel calcio* (Città di Castello, Italy: Edizioni Nuova Prhomos) (120b).

The intensity of exercise during LSD training is markedly lower than that experienced during competition (118). This suggests that higher-intensity training methods, such as interval and fartlek (speed play, or continuous runs with intensity alternations) training, must be included in the training plan to optimize performance. This is not to say that LSD training should be excluded from the training plan of endurance athletes; this type of training appears to be very important in developing aerobic endurance (46). For example, Esteve-Lanao and colleagues (46) suggested that LSD training should make up a large portion of the training volume, provided that high-intensity training is sufficient.

During the preparatory phase of an endurance training program, the main objective is to establish a physiological base (54, 141). The development of this physiological base is accomplished via the use of LSD and aerobic interval training (steady pace or tempo training) interspersed with active rest, passive rest, and resistance training. A microcycle with an emphasis on establishing a base is presented in table 11.3.

Interval Training

Interval training involves the repeated performance of short to long bouts of exercise usually performed at or above the lactate threshold, or at the maximal lactate steady state, interspersed with periods of low-intensity exercise or complete rest (16). Although interval training is not a new training method (it was made popular in the 1930s by the German middistance runner Rudolf Harbig), contemporary sport science literature (20, 21, 86, 87, 91) has stimulated an increased interest in the concept. This literature has revealed many physiological reasons why interval training should be an integral part of the annual training plan for athletes ranging from novice to elite (87). Interval training can be subdivided into two broad categories: aerobic and **anaerobic intervals**.

TABLE 11.3 — General Preparation Microcycle Emphasizing LSD Training

Day	Monday	Tuesday	Wednesday	Thursday	Friday	Saturday	Sunday
Workout	Rest day						
Endurance training		LSD	Recovery	Aerobic intervals	Recovery	LSD	Fartlek
Strength training			Strength training		Strength training		
Total duration		120 min	60 min	80 min	60 min	150 min	60-120 min
Interval duration		120 min	60 min	15 min	60 min	150 min	—
Recovery		—	—	5 min	—	—	—
Work-to-rest ratio		1:0	1:0	3:1	1:0	1:0	—
Intensity		131-139 beats/min	<131 beats/min	140-146 beats/min	<131 beats/min	131-139 beats/min	—

LSD = long slow distance.

Note: The microcycle example is based on a weekly training volume of 10 h, where the athlete's heart rate at the lactate threshold is 153 beats/min. Based on Friel 2006 (54) and Potteiger 2000 (118).

Aerobic Intervals

Aerobic interval training preferentially stresses the aerobic energy system and involves intensities that are at or slightly above the lactate threshold or those seen during competition. Aerobic interval training has also been termed threshold training or pace or tempo training (118). Pace or tempo training can be performed continuously or intermittently. For example, in a continuous pace or tempo training session, the athlete would maintain a steady pace at or slightly above the lactate threshold for the duration of the exercise bout. Conversely, pace or tempo intervals contain periods of steady-state exercise, as seen in tables 11.4 and 11.5.

When the coach is designing an aerobic interval workout, it is recommended that a graded exercise test be performed to establish the athlete's maximal heart rate, maximal power output or velocity at $\dot{V}O_2$max, and lactate threshold. Integral to this process is determining the time at which $\dot{V}O_2$max power output or velocity can be maintained, which has been termed the **Tmax** (17b, 87, 91). Once the Tmax and the maximal aerobic power output or velocity (i.e., MAS) are established, then the interval durations and intensities can be determined. It has been recommended that the duration of each interval correspond to 50% to 60% of Tmax and be performed at peak power or velocity (17c, 91). The rest interval can be set as the time to reach 65% of the athlete's maximal heart rate, or a lower intensity (usually at 50% of Pmax or MAS) the exercise bout is performed for a duration equal to that of the higher-intensity bout (for example, 3 min at 100% of MAS, followed by 3 min at 50% of MAS) (17c).

Aerobic intervals can also be set by prescribing a heart rate range or power range that is performed for a predetermined duration (145). The rest interval can be preset to specifically target the development of the aerobic system. For example, an athlete may perform eight sets of aerobic intervals that last 5 min and are separated by 1 min of low-intensity active recovery. The intensity for this type of interval would be between 80% and 85% of maximal heart rate or some percentage of the lactate threshold heart rate.

TABLE 11.4 Two Aerobic Interval Workouts

	Aerobic interval format	
	Interval series 1	**Interval series 2**
Warm-up	10-15 min	10-15 min
Number of work intervals	8	8
Intensity	80% peak power* 80%-85% of maximal heart rate	100% peak power output at $\dot{V}O_2$max (413 W)
Duration	5 min	50% of Tmax (~3 min)
Rest interval	1 min	Time to achieve 65% of maximal heart rate (~2-4 min)
Work-to-rest interval	5:1	1:0.5-1:1
Cool-down	10-15 min	10-15 min
Total workout time	67-77 min	66-90 min
Frequency (times per week)	1 or 2	1 or 2

Tmax = time to exhaustion at maximum velocity or power output.
*Peak power at $\dot{V}O_2$max.
Adapted from Stepto et al. 2001 (145) and Laursen et al. 2005 (89).

TABLE 11.5 Pace or Tempo Workouts

	Continuous pace or tempo training	**Intermittent pace or tempo training**
Warm-up	15-20 min	15-20 min
Work bouts		
Number	1	2
Duration	30 min	10 min
Intensity	153-156 beats/min	153-156 beats/min
Recovery bouts		
Number	0	2
Duration	0 min	10 min
Intensity	<131 beats/min	<131 beats/min

Note: Based on a lactate threshold heart rate of 153 beats/min.
Adapted from Potteiger 2000 (118) and USA Cycling 2002 (1).

Regardless of the method used, aerobic intervals can stimulate significant performance gains and concomitant physiological adaptations when performed two times a week for up to 4 weeks (87, 91, 145). Because of the large amount of physiological and psychological stress that can be generated by aerobic interval training, the coach should integrate recovery methods and lower-intensity training into the microcycle to avoid overtraining the athlete. A sample microcycle is presented in table 11.6.

TABLE 11.6 Microcycle With Aerobic Intervals or Pace or Tempo Training

Day	Monday	Tuesday	Wednesday	Thursday	Friday	Saturday	Sunday
Workout	Rest day						
Endurance training		LSD	Pace tempo ride	Recovery	Aerobic intervals	LSD	Fartlek
Resistance training							
Total duration		120 min	80 min	60 min	65 min	150 min	60-120 min
Interval duration		120 min	15 min	60 min	5 min	150 min	—
Recovery		—	5 min	—	1 min	—	—
Work-to-rest ratio		1:0	3:1	1:0	5:1	1:0	—
Intensity		131-139 beats/min	140-146 beats/min	<131 beats/min	80%-85% of maximal heart rate	131-139 beats/min	—

LSD = long slow distance.

Note: This microcycle is based on a weekly training volume of 9 to 10 hours where the athlete's heart rate at the lactate threshold is 153 beats/min.
Adapted from Friel 2006 (54) and Potteiger 2000 (118).

Anaerobic Intervals

Anaerobic interval training for the endurance athlete has recently received a large amount of attention in the scientific literature. In this type of interval training, the work duration is very short (<2 min) and the intensity is supramaximal (all-out or above the power output achieved during the assessment of $\dot{V}O_2$max). Anaerobic interval training bouts that use 4 to 10 sets of 15 to 30 s of all-out work, interspersed with 45 s to 12 min of recovery, have been shown to significantly increase $\dot{V}O_2$max and anaerobic endurance, and stimulate many physiological adaptations that improve performance in as little as 2 weeks (87). These types of training sessions are usually very intense and require the use of recovery methods and appropriate program variations to avoid overtraining. It is likely that this type of training can be very effective when performed one or two times per week and integrated into the training plan. A microcycle that incorporates anaerobic intervals is presented in table 11.8.

Repetition

Another interval training method, characterized by full-recovery rest periods, has been termed the **repetition method**. The distances used with this method can be either longer or shorter than the distance seen in competition. Longer-duration intervals will shift the emphasis toward the development of the aerobic energy systems, similar to aerobic interval training. Conversely, intervals of shorter duration will increase the stress on the anaerobic energy systems, similar to anaerobic interval training. Short bouts of very high intensity will require longer rest intervals (118). The repetition method allows the athlete to improve running speed, running economy, and HIEE.

Fartlek

Fartlek is the Swedish word for "speed play" and is a classic method for developing endurance. This method of training is a rather unscientific combination of interval and continuous training. For example, a runner may intersperse periods of fast running with slow running

Field Test for Maximum Aerobic Speed

Maximum aerobic speed (MAS) is the lowest speed at which maximum oxygen consumption ($\dot{V}O_2$max) occurs. A practical way to assess the maximum aerobic speed is to perform a 6 min running test, possibly on an oval-shaped track. Research suggests 6 min as the time to exhaustion at $\dot{V}O_2$max power output (Tmax) (17d, 17e). The test is self-paced, but it is proposed to request an all-out effort in the last minute (blow a whistle to signal the last minute to the athlete). The distance covered by the athlete is then multiplied by 10 and converted into miles. The resulting value is the maximum aerobic speed.

Example:

Distance covered: 4 laps = 1,600 m

1,600 m × 10 = 16,000 m = 10 mi × 10 mph is the speed at $\dot{V}O_2$max or maximum aerobic speed (MAS).

Use table 11.7 to find the time necessary to cover the most common training distances at the desired speed.

TABLE 11.7 Time Necessary to Cover the Most Common Training Distances, in Relation to the Maximum Aerobic Speed

Maximum aerobic speed (MAS) in mph	Repetitions distance							
	100 m	200 m	300 m	400 m	500 m	600 m	800 m	1000 m
	Time (min/s)							
8.7	0:25.7	-	-	1:43	2:08	2:34	3:25	4:17
9	0:24.8	-	-	1:39	2:04	2:29	3:18	4:08
9.3	0:24	-	1:12	1:36	2:00	2:24	3:12	4:00
9.6	0:23.2	-	1:10	1:33	1:45	2:19	3:06	3:52
10	0:22.5	0:45	1:07	1:30	1:52	2:15	3:00	3:45
10.3	0:21.8	0:43.6	1:05	1:27	1:49	2:11	2:54	3:38
10.6	0:21.2	0:42.3	1:03	1:24	1:46	2:07	2:49	3:32
10.9	0:20.6	0:41.1	1:02	1:22	1:43	2:03	2:44	3:25
11.2	0:20	0:40	1:00	1:20	1:40	2:00	2:40	3:20
11.5	0:19.5	0:38.9	0:58.4	1:18	1:37	1:57	2:35	-
11.8	0:19	0:37.9	0:57	1:16	1:35	1:54	2:31	-
12.1	0:18.5	0:36.9	0:55.4	1:14	1:32	1:51	2:27	-
12.4	0:18	0:36	0:55	1:12	1:30	-	-	-
12.7	0:17.5	0:35.1	0:52.6	1:10	-	-	-	-
13	0:17.1	0:34.3	0:51.4	1:08	-	-	-	-
13.3	0:16.7	0:33.5	-	-	-	-	-	-
13.7	0:16.4	0:32.7	-	-	-	-	-	-
14	0:16	0:32	-	-	-	-	-	-
14.3	0:15.7	-	-	-	-	-	-	-
14.6	0:15.3	-	-	-	-	-	-	-
14.9	0:15	-	-	-	-	-	-	-

TABLE 11.8 — Microcycle for a 10K Runner With Anaerobic Interval Training

Day	Monday	Tuesday	Wednesday	Thursday	Friday	Saturday	Sunday
Workout	Rest day						
Endurance training		Interval	Recovery	LSD	Interval	LSD	Fartlek
Resistance training							
Total duration		30-40 min*	1 hr	2 hr	30-40 min*	45 min	45 min-1 hr
Interval duration		30 s	1 hr	2 hr	30 s	45 min	—
Recovery		60 s	0	0	60 s	0	—
Number of intervals		6			6		
Work-to-rest ratio		1:2	1:0	1:0	1:2	1:0	—
Intensity		Maximal	<131 beats/min	131-139 beats/min	Maximal	131-139 beats/min	—

*Includes 15 min of warm-up and cool-down.

LSD = long slow distance.

Note: This microcycle is based on a weekly training volume of 5-6 h, where the athlete's heart rate at the lactate threshold is 153 beats/min.

Adapted from Friel 2006 (54) and Potteiger 2000 (118).

(98, 118, 141). This type of training can be undertaken on flat ground or up and down hills (141). Fartlek does not call for specific workloads or heart rates. Instead, this type of training relies on the subjective sense of how the bout feels (98). Fartlek training may be most useful during the general conditioning or preparatory phase of the annual training plan because it challenges the physiological systems of the body while eliminating the boredom and monotony associated with daily training (98, 118).

Strength Training

Strength training can enhance the development of endurance. Traditionally, resistance training has not been considered to be a very important part of the development of LIEE (77). However, recent research suggests that strength training has the potential to improve cycling (11, 96), running (73, 110, 153), and Nordic skiing (68, 111) performance. Strength training has been suggested to affect $\dot{V}O_2$max, the lactate threshold, economy of movement, and neuromuscular characteristics of endurance athletes depending on their levels of training (77). For example, untrained individuals can experience improvements in LIEE as a result of improvements in $\dot{V}O_2$max, lactate threshold, and movement economy (77). In highly trained endurance athletes, improvements in LIEE performance are most likely related to changes in the lactate threshold (96), improvements in movement economy (110), and alterations to neuromuscular function (104, 153) (figure 11.7). It appears that incorporating resistance training into the annual training plan for the endurance athlete holds some merit.

Incorporating resistance training into the annual training plan of an endurance athlete appears to produce favorable performance responses (77, 147, 153). However, care must be taken when introducing resistance training in an attempt to improve LIEE performance. When resistance training is simply added to the preexisting endurance training plan, performance usually is not improved (72). It is likely that adding the resistance training load to the overall training load results in excessive training stress, which then elevates fatigue and decreases readiness. Support for this contention can be seen in the work of Jackson and colleagues (72), who reported that the addition of resistance training to a cycling program results in a

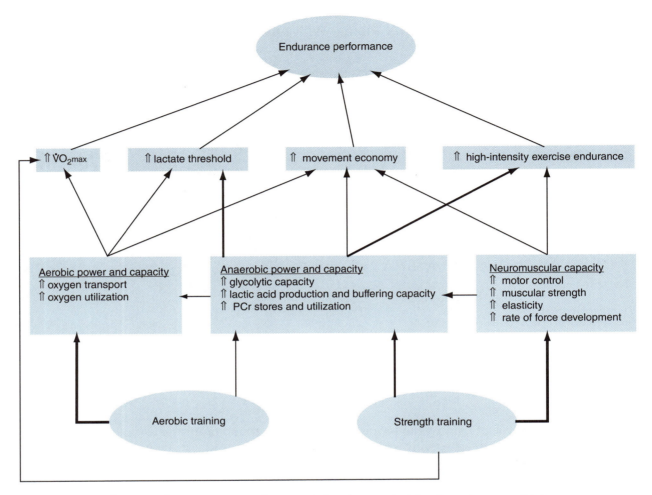

FIGURE 11.7 Structure for concurrent resistance and endurance training in endurance athletes.

PCr = phosphocreatine.

Adapted from Paavolainen et al. 1999 (110) and Stone et al. 2006 (147).

higher sense of fatigue, which corresponds to a lack of performance gains. Investigators who report enhancement of LIEE performance with concurrent resistance and endurance training typically reduce some of the endurance training volume to accommodate the resistance training load (11, 104, 110). It is likely that a 19% to 37% reduction in endurance training load is warranted when adding resistance training to the overall training plan to stimulate performance gains (11, 104, 110).

Methods for Developing High-Intensity Endurance

The use of LIEE techniques will decrease performance capacity for athletes who participate in sports that require the ability to repetitively produce high power outputs (28, 45). Power-based sports fall into two classifications: (1) sports such as American football and baseball, which require brief, intermittent tasks—involving very large power outputs with long rest intervals between them—and derive most of their energy from phosphate energy system; and (2) sports such as soccer, handball, rugby, and basketball, which require repetitive high-intensity activities with short, mostly active, rest intervals, thus tapping both the anaerobic alactic and the anaerobic lactic energy substrates. In both types of sports, oxidative metabolism is important during recovery because the replenishment of phosphocreatine and removal of lactate is an oxidative process (22, 45, 153b). This reliance on oxidative metabolism during recovery is the foundation for the classic argument that LIEE techniques are needed by athletes who participate in anaerobic-based sports (28, 45).

Although LIEE training enhances several physiological factors that may improve the rate of recovery between bouts of exercise, the corresponding decreases in anaerobic abilities and corresponding performance capacities appear to outweigh the benefits of this training intervention (45). Anaerobic athletes should avoid LIEE training and use other strategies that enhance performance and recovery (113, 115). However, the development of HIEE can actually improve LIEE performance, and thus the methods used by anaerobic athletes may benefit the aerobic endurance athlete (87, 147).

One strategy for developing endurance is the use of high-intensity interval training, which allows for improvements in anaerobic power, anaerobic capacity, and also aerobic power (87, 113). Interval training is usually conducted by using sets of repetitions of sprints interspersed with recovery intervals. The duration of these recovery intervals varies depending on the bioenergetic system being targeted (28) (table 11.9). For example, an interval training program with a work-to-rest ratio of 1:1 would target the oxidative system (50), whereas a work-to-rest ratio of 1:20 would target the anaerobic energy systems (28). The use of an interval training program will be dictated by several factors including the bioenergetic demands of the sport, the performance model established for the sport, and the phase of the annual training plan. These factors can be addressed via the manipulation of work-to-rest intervals, interval intensities, interval duration or distance, interval exercise volume, interval training duration, interval training frequency, interval training progression, in-season maintenance, and resistance training.

TABLE 11.9 Bioenergetic Characteristics of Interval Training

Interval ratio (work to rest)	Typical interval format		Sample interval format		Primary energy system used	Maximum power (%)
	Work (s)	Rest (s)	Work (s)	Rest (s)		
1:12-1:20	2-8	60-200	5	60	ATP-PC, fast glycolysis	90-100
1:3-1:5	10-30	45-150	30	90	Fast glycolysis, slow glycolysis	75-90
1:3-1:4	60-180	180-720	60	180	Fast glycolysis, slow glycolysis, and oxidative*	50-75
1:0.5-1:1	>180	>180	240	120	Oxidative metabolism	30-50

*The primary energy system used will vary depending on the length of the interval and the duration of recovery.

Intermittent Runs

This modality of fartlek training is employed in particular for the preparation of team sports in which high intensity bouts are followed by continuous activities of lower intensity, such as soccer, handball, or basketball (i.e., intermittent sports). In this case the combination of high-intensity and low-intensity intervals is structured in a way that will have a specific training effect (table 11.10).

TABLE 11.10	Ergogenesis of Different Durations of Intermittent Runs, in Relation to the Percentage of the Maximum Aerobic Speed
Modality	**Ergogenesis**
Intensity: 100% maximum aerobic speed	
10"-10"	Aerobic
20"-20"	Aerobic
30"-30"	Aerobic
Intensity: 105% maximum aerobic speed	
10"-10"	Slightly anaerobic lactic
20"-20"	Slightly anaerobic lactic
30"-30"	Slightly anaerobic lactic
Intensity: 110% maximum aerobic speed	
10"-10"	Slightly anaerobic lactic
20"-20"	Anaerobic lactic
30"-30"	Predominantly anaerobic lactic
Intensity: 115% maximum aerobic speed	
10"-10"	Anaerobic lactic
20"-20"	Predominantly anaerobic lactic
30"-30"	Predominantly anaerobic lactic

" = seconds

Reprinted, by permission, from G.N. Bisciotti, 2002, "Utilizziamo bene l'intermittente," *Il Nuovo Calcio* 114: 110-114.

Work-to-Rest Intervals

The work-to-rest interval may be dictated by the demands of the sport. It has been reported that the average work-to-rest interval in American football is around 1:6, which is depicted as a work-to-rest (s/s) interval of 4.3:27.9 for rushing plays and 5.8:36.8 for passing plays (115). One study reported that there were 12 to 13 plays per game (3.1-3.3 per quarter) with an average play length of 2 to 12 s (113). The vast majority of the plays lasted between 3 and 6 s (113) for an average play length of around 4 s (112). This information suggests that a series of 10 to 16 sprints, performed with a 3 to 5 s work interval and a 20 to 45 s recovery (1:6 work-to-rest interval), was an ideal interval training program for this population (115).

Soccer provides another example of matching the work-to-rest interval in training. The literature suggests that a work-to-rest ratio of 1:6 is similar to that seen in competition (7, 8) and demonstrates similar speed decrements as seen in a soccer match (94). Soccer demonstrates work-to-rest ratios of approximately 1:7 to 8 with 3 to 4 s of work interspersed with lower-intensity exercise (94). Little and Williams (94) suggested that 40 reps of 15 m sprints performed at a 1:6 work-to-rest ratio simulates the physiological stress seen in soccer match play. The work-to-rest interval should be prescribed based on the individual demands of the sport and in the context of the phase of the training plan.

Once the coach has determined the work-to-rest interval required by a sport, the athlete can choose from several ways to implement an interval session into the training plan. The first method is to use predetermined performance times to calculate the appropriate rest

Sport-Specific Metabolic Test for Intermittent Sports

Among the many fitness tests available are continuous and intermittent tests. Intermittent tests are certainly more specific to intermittent sport such as soccer, handball, basketball, and tennis. The Yo-Yo Intermittent Recovery Test (YYIRT) (figure 11.8) is one of the many beep tests available to test an athlete's ability to repeatedly perform intervals over a prolonged period of time; however, because of the long (10 s) rest interval between reps, the YYIRT mimics more closely the metabolic dynamics of intermittent sports (8b, 83b). Tables 11.11 and 11.12 can be used to evaluate the fitness level of your athletes. A coach can create her own chart, specific to the athlete's sport and competition level, by correlating the competition performance and the YYIRT results of her players.

TABLE 11.11 Grading of Male Professional League Soccer Players' Fitness Levels, According to Their Positions on the Field and Results in the Yo-Yo Intermittent Recovery Test Level 1

	Position		
	Center back, center forward	Center midfielder, winger	Side back, side midfielder
Level	Grade		
<17	Poor	Poor	Poor
17.5-18	Fair	Poor	Poor
18-18.5	Good	Fair	Poor
18.5-19	Very good	Good	Fair
19-19.5	Excellent	Very good	Good
19.5-20	*	Excellent	Very good
20.5-21	*	Excellent	Excellent
>21	*	*	Excellent

*Metabolic training can be kept at maintenance level, while devoting more time to developing the neuromuscular aspects.

TABLE 11.12 Grading of Female Professional League Volleyball Players' Fitness Levels, According to Their Results in the Yo-Yo Intermittent Recovery Test Level 1

Level	Grade
<14	Poor
14-14.5	Below average
14.5-15	Fair
15-15.5	Good
15.5-16	Very good
16-16.5	Excellent
>16.5	*

*Metabolic training can be kept at maintenance level, while devoting more time to developing the neuromuscular aspects.

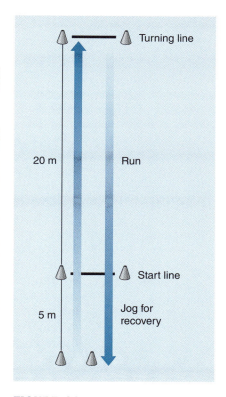

FIGURE 11.8 Setup for the Yo-Yo Recovery Intermittent Test

Adapted, by permission, from M. McGuigan, 2016, Administration, scoring, and interpretation of selected tests. In *Essentials of strength training and conditioning*, 4th ed., edited by G.G. Haff and N.T. Triplett for the National Strength and Conditioning Association (Champaign, IL: Human Kinetics), 278.

TABLE 11.13 — Comparison of Two Athletes' Interval Training Plans

Variable	Athlete A	Athlete B
Intended work-to-rest ratio	1:4	1:4
Maximal 40 m time	5.2 s	6.0 s
Recovery duration	20.8 s	20.8 s
Actual work-to-rest ratio	1:4	1:3

These athletes are performing five sets of 40 m sprints, and the time for recovery is based on the faster athlete. Athlete B is experiencing a harder training session because he has a shorter recovery period.

interval duration (50, 113). Another method for determining the rest interval is to use the time to a specific heart rate, such as 110 to 120 beats/min (116). The rest intervals should be individualized as much as possible to give each athlete the appropriate recovery duration and allow for the training stimulus needed to target the bioenergetic factors specified by the training plan.

A classic mistake that many coaches make is to train all their athletes in one large group and base the recovery duration on the fastest athlete. If this practice is undertaken, the slower athletes will most likely be forced to work at a lower work-to-rest ratio than the fastest athlete, which would result in a harder training session and shift the bioenergetic focus of the training session for these athletes (table 11.13). This practice can increase the chance of overtraining and impedes an athlete's development. It may be warranted to group the athletes based on their maximum aerobic speed, so that the repetitions' duration and work-to-rest ratio are individualized. Then the coach can establish the training volume according to the position played. This practice will ensure that each athlete is using the appropriate work-to-rest ratio and receiving the planned physiological stimulus.

Interval Intensities

The prescription of interval training intensities can significantly affect the performance outcomes stimulated by the training plan. Using heart rate as an indicator of performance intensity during an anaerobic interval training program is not recommended because heart rate is poorly related to intensity in this scenario (113). It is better to set training time goals based on the individual athlete's maximal capacity, which would then allow the coach to manipulate training intensity and determine the rest interval (50, 113). For example, when attempting to develop a fitness base, the athlete may perform a high volume of sprints at 60% to 80% of maximal capacity. Conversely, when shifting to more specific work in the later stages of the preparatory phase of training, the athlete could increase the intensity of interval training to 80% to 90% of maximal or competitive needs (116).

Establishing target times for a specific distance is an excellent tool for individualizing the intensity of the training bout. However, the athlete should be tested periodically so the coach can adjust the intensity of training. When using this method to determine interval intensities, the coach should group athletes of similar capacities (e.g., sprint times) because this will help the coach determine the appropriate work-to-rest intervals and maximize each athlete's physiological and performance gains.

Interval Duration or Distance

The quality of HIEE training is more important than the quantity (113). The duration and distance of the work portion of the interval training plan will depend on the tactical model established for the individual sport (114). For example, Plisk (114) reported that three sets of six or seven 43.7 yd (40 m) sprints with a work-to-rest ratio of 1:6 would meet the metabolic demands of American football. It appears that this intensity targets the phosphagen and glycolytic energy supply mechanisms better than does the duration (148), so extending the duration or distance beyond that required by the sport would be impractical and would likely induce maladaptive responses (113). Therefore, the distance or duration of the interval should be matched to the competitive model established for the sporting activity.

Interval Exercise Volume

The interval training volume will be dictated by the phase of the annual training plan, the targeted physiological adaptations, and the sport. The volume of interval training will be higher during the early preparatory phase and decrease during the competitive phase of the annual training plan. The scientific literature provides limited information about the optimal volume of interval training needed to induce physiological and performance adaptations.

Investigators have explored interval training volume schemes that require between 2 and 24 repetitions (87, 94) and as high as 40 repetitions (94). Some empirical evidence has suggested that sprinters need between 6 and 12 repetitions per workout, whereas middle-distance runners may need between 1.5 and 2 repetitions when performing fast intervals and 2 to 3 repetitions when performing slow interval workouts (113). Not enough scientific evidence is available regarding the effects of different interval training volumes on performance to make volume-based recommendations. Therefore, decisions about how to manipulate the training volume should be based on the athlete's needs and response to training-induced stress.

Duration of Interval Training Phase

Anaerobic interval training has been shown to stimulate significant physiological adaptations in 2 to 15 weeks in previously untrained individuals depending on the frequency, duration, and intensity of the interval program used (37b). Elite cyclists have demonstrated significant physiological adaptations and performance gains in as little as 2 weeks of using a high-intensity interval training plan (86, 87, 144). Although the literature has shown significant performance enhancement in both cyclists and runners as a result of as little as 2 weeks of high-intensity interval training, further research is needed to establish guidelines for the duration of training needed to optimize performance. However, both research and practice suggest use of higher-intensity interval training after a period of moderate-intensity endurance training (4, 46b, 135b, 162b).

Interval Training Frequency

The scientific literature on high-intensity interval training has explored a variety of training frequencies ranging from 2 to 7 days per week (16, 87). According to a research study by Billat and colleagues, when athletes have passed from six running sessions (using the steady state method at low to moderate intensity) to four sessions, plus an anaerobic threshold training session and a high-intensity interval training session, both the speed at $\dot{V}O_2$max and running economy have improved (but not the $\dot{V}O_2$max). When athletes increase the high-intensity interval training sessions to three, there is no further improvement of performance, while the overtraining markers increase (17c). In another study, 2 to 8 weeks with frequent high-intensity interval training sessions (3 to 4 times per week) also resulted in a worsening of the performance and an increase of overtraining markers (61b).

Thus, both empirical and scientific evidence suggest that it may be practical to limit HIEE training to 1 or 2 days per week (17c, 141b, 142). This general recommendation is warranted because HIEE training increases the risk of overtraining, as it is inherently intense and research showed an increase in stress markers at the increase of HIEE weekly frequency (17c); HIEE training must be considered in conjunction with the other training modalities (e.g., strength, plyometric, agility, tactical, technical training) that are included in the training program. If integrated appropriately, HIEE can be addressed with skill, technique, or agility drills that can also stimulate improvements in endurance (113). The coach should modulate the training stimulus to allow for appropriate restoration while continuing to stimulate physiological and performance-based adaptations across the microcycle.

Interval Training Progression

Creating an HIEE training plan involves integrating several training factors (e.g., tactical, technical, strength, power, endurance) into the periodized program. The coach can establish the basic progression of training after determining the work-to-rest interval and endurance demands of the sport (114). The intensities and volumes used in the interval training plan depend on the phase of the annual training plan and the method being used to develop HIEE. When the athlete is attempting to develop a fitness base during the early portion of the preparatory phase of training, the interval intensities should be lower and contain more extensive methods (table 11.9) (113). As the athlete progresses toward the season, she can use higher intensities and lower volumes of training (table 11.14) (113, 114). In the later stages of the preparatory phase and the early part of the competition phase of the annual training plan, the athlete will begin to incorporate elements from the competitive trial method of developing HIEE, which has also been termed special endurance (114, 116) (table 11.15). As the competitive phase of the season progresses, the athlete uses specific strategies, including various interval training and competitive trial methods, to maintain HIEE capacity across the season.

TABLE 11.14 Interval Characteristics for the Development of Speed Endurance

Interval method	Variable	Novice athlete	Advanced athlete
Extensive	Relative intensity	60%-80% of competitive speed	60%-80% of competitive speed
	Intensity classification	Low to medium	Low to medium
	Duration or distance	20-100 s or 100-400 m	14-180 s or 100-1,000 m
	Volume	5-12 repetitions	8-20 repetitions
	Target recovery heart rate	110-120 beats/min	125-130 beats/min
	Recovery duration	60-120 s	45-90 s
Intensive	Relative intensity	80%-90% of competitive speed	80%-90% of competitive speed
	Intensity classification	High	High
	Duration or distance	14-95 s or 100-400 m	13-180 s or 100-1,000 m
	Volume	4-8 repetitions	4-12 repetitions
	Target recovery heart rate	110-120 beats/min	125-130 beats/min
	Recovery duration	120-240 s	90-180 s

Adapted from Plisk and Stone 2003 (116).

TABLE 11.15 Competitive Trial Methods of Developing High-Intensity Exercise Endurance

Method	Intensity	Duration or distance	Example for a 400 m sprinter
Supramaximal training	Competition	< Competition	100-200 m sprint intervals
Maximal training	> Competition	= Competition	200-400 m sprint intervals
Submaximal training	< Competition	≥ Competition	400-600 m sprint intervals

Interval Training During the Competitive Phase

Over the course of the competitive phase, the athlete can fall into a state of deconditioning if special attention is not paid to integrating conditioning activities into his competitive training schedule (84, 105, 113, 137). Support for this contention can be found in the scientific literature, which suggests that when the volume of anaerobic interval training (e.g., sprint and agility training) is significantly reduced or when this training is eliminated altogether during the competitive season, there is a concomitant reduction in markers of fitness and muscle mass (105). The magnitude of these decreases is likely to be different when comparing starters and nonstarters (84). Thus, specific HIEE conditioning strategies must be implemented in the in-season training plan.

When examining in-season responses, the coach must first consider what happened in the 6 to 8 weeks before the initiation of the season. If acute overtraining is induced during this time, a general catabolic state will predominate during the season and performance capacity will decline (84). Even if the preseason training plan is implemented appropriately, performance can decline during the season if the HIEE is not appropriately incorporated into the in-season training plan (105). The best approach is to include a combination of sport-specific practices, strength training, and HIEE-based conditioning (49b, 137). When the frequency of competition is more than once a week, though, those players that are going to play three games within 7 days would be better off training in LIEE modality, to avoid overtraining and foster recovery.

HIEE can be trained in conjunction with sport-specific skills to maximize training time. In soccer, for example, soccer-specific drills can be used as a conditioning tool (121). Rampinini and colleagues (121) reported that using a three-sided training game on a large pitch can increase the exercise intensity to a level similar to that seen in actual game play. Using this type of strategy will allow the athlete to develop specific endurance that is closely related to the demands of a soccer game. The training stimulus can be modified by manipulating the field dimensions, number of players, duration of plays, and skills used during a small-sided soccer game (table 11.16), in an attempt to target conditioning goals while still practicing sport-specific skills in an environment that models game play (121).

Although skill-based conditioning drills are important, it is equally important to include strength training (105) in conjunction with HIEE and sprint agility training to avoid the

TABLE 11.16 How Manipulation of Loading Parameters Changes the Training Effect of Small-Sided Games for Soccer

Rules		Training effect
Number of players per team	+	Less frequency of play per player
	−	More frequency of play per player
Field dimensions	+	Less frequency of play per player
	−	More frequency of play per player
Ball touches	+	More reasoning time and lower speed of play
	−	Less reasoning time and more speed of play
Duration of play	+	Lower mean play intensity
	−	Higher mean play intensity
Duration of rest intervals	+	Higher mean play intensity
	−	Lower mean play intensity

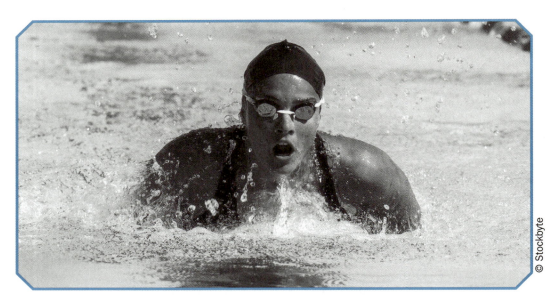

The competitive phase is an important part of any training plan. Do not let deconditioning occur during the competitive season.

typical losses in performance capacity seen across a season (137). Different training factors (e.g., HIEE, drills, and strength training) should be integrated to avoid overtraining, because overtraining would only compound the typical degradation in performance seen across the season. The coach must allow for recovery between training sessions and competitive events. The coach must perform a balancing act by providing an adequate training stimulus to maintain fitness and performance while avoiding overtraining.

Monitoring Team Sport Players Using an Accelerometer With Gyroscope and GPS

In the early 2000s, motion video analysis was used to monitor the performance of players during training and, especially, games. At that time, each player's performance was categorized into speed brackets (figure 11.9). Although it was an advance in sport science, the speed bracket categorization was insufficient in its depiction of a player's performance during a game, because intermittent sports are characterized by numerous accelerations and decelerations which do not necessarily lead to high speed, yet constitute high-intensity efforts (figure 11.10).

In 2005, Di Prampero and colleagues conducted a research study in which they demonstrated that "sprint running on flat terrain, during the acceleration phase is biomechanically equivalent to uphill running at constant speed, the slope being dictated by the forward acceleration and that, conversely, during the deceleration phase, it is biomechanically equivalent to running downhill (40c)." This allowed the creation of an algorithm to measure the metabolic power of each action during an intermittent activity, typical of team sports (109b). Accelerometer devices with GPS and gyroscope became more practical and cheaper than video analysis tools, accessed in order to represent the performance of team sports' players. The performance could then be categorized in power output brackets: minimum power (0 to 10 $W \cdot Kg^{-1}$), low power (10 to 20 $W \cdot Kg^{-1}$), intermediate power (20 to 35 $W \cdot Kg^{-1}$), high power (35 to 55 $W \cdot Kg^{-1}$), and maximum power (55 $W \cdot Kg^{-1}$ and higher) (figure 11.11). These devices allow for a better depiction of the physical demands of match play (4b, 56b); they also allow strength and conditioning coaches to quantify the work performed by each player during the ever-increasing utilization of game-based training activities (i.e., small-sided games), as a means of improving the skill and physical fitness levels of team sport athletes (56b, 56c).

As of today, scientific literature indicating training standards according to such performance monitoring devices is quite scarce; thus, strength and conditioning coaches using this technology are building their own database and performing data analysis to estimate the workload profile of specific drills and the individual players' readiness fluctuation. This process is, in fact, paramount when substituting general training means (e.g., runs) with specific drills (e.g., small-sided games) and increasing the load over time. Furthermore, a good technical level of the team is required for the specific drills to reach a high enough intensity, which, in certain cases, is easier to reach with general means.

Strength Training

Investigators have repeatedly shown that strength training improves HIEE (66, 67, 99, 125, 147) and that gains in HIEE performance are likely related to increases in muscular strength, morphological adaptations, or metabolic adaptations that increase buffering capacity (102, 125).

HIEE performance is improved when the training plan includes resistance training with 12 or more repetitions per set (125). This improvement in performance is most noted as the intensity of exercise is increased (66). Higher repetitions per set (more than eight repetitions) performed for multiple

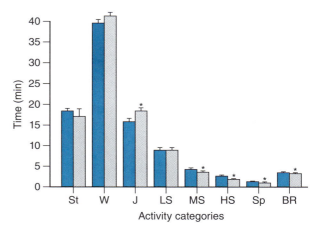

FIGURE 11.9 Locomotor categories of top-level players (black columns) and mid-level players (white columns) during a soccer game.

St = standing; W = walking; J = jogging; LS, MS, and HS = running at a low, moderate, and high speed, respectively; Sp = sprinting; BR = backwards running; *= significant difference ($P < 0.05$) between groups.

From M. Mohr, P. Krustrup, and J. Bangsbo, 2003, "Match performance of high-standard soccer players with special reference to development of fatigue," *Journal of Sports Sciences* 21(7): 519-528. Reprinted by permission of the publisher (Taylor & Francis Ltd., www.tandfonline.com).

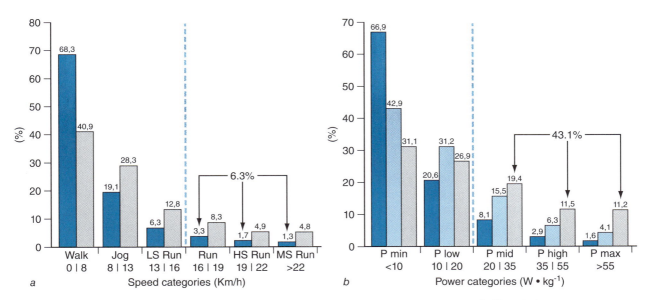

FIGURE 11.10 (a) Power output categorization gives a better depiction of the level of effort during a soccer game, compared to (b) speed categorization.

LS, MS, and HS = running at a low, moderate, and high speed, respectively; P = power.

Data from C. Osgnach, S. Poser, R. Bernardini, R. Rinaldo, and P.E. di Prampero, 2010, "Energy cost and metabolic power in elite soccer: A new match analysis approach," *Medicine & Science in Sports & Exercise* 42: 170-178. Used courtesy of P.E. di Prampero, C. Osgnach, and S. Poser.

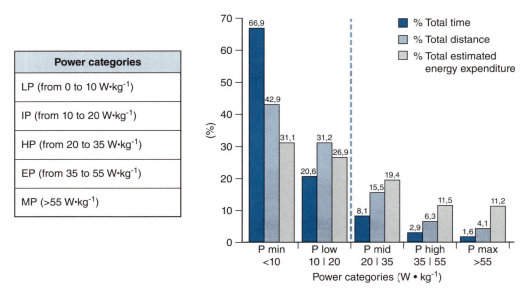

FIGURE 11.11 Mean data on match play power output during 56 games of professional soccer in Italy.

Reprinted, by permission, from C. Osgnach, S. Poser, R. Bernardini, R. Rinaldo, and P.E. di Prampero, 2010, "Energy cost and metabolic power in elite soccer: A new match analysis approach," *Medicine & Science in Sports & Exercise* 42(1): 170-178.

sets appear to improve HIEE more than do lower-repetition protocols or single-set protocols (51, 99, 146). HIEE performance seems to be improved to a greater extent with high volumes (volume loads) of resistance training.

Several authors have suggested that short rest intervals between sets of resistance training can increase HIEE capacity (51, 146). This theory was recently supported by Hill-Haas and colleagues (67), who demonstrated that a resistance training program that includes short rest intervals (20 s) results in significantly greater HIEE performance gains (+12.5%) compared with a resistance training program that uses longer rest intervals (80 s). It is likely that the program that includes short rest intervals increases the lactate-buffering capacity in response to resistance training due to repeated exposure to high lactate levels that allows for a greater HIEE performance. Conversely, Robinson and colleagues (125) reported that short rest intervals (30 s) do not result in greater improvements in HIEE performance compared with longer rest intervals (180 s). Their findings suggest that simply increasing the volume of resistance training is more effective at improving HIEE without compromising other training-induced adaptations.

Both studies found muted strength gains in response to short rest intervals (67, 125). Because sprinting speed is highly correlated with muscular strength (6, 37), the validity of decreasing the rest interval between sets may be questionable because increasing volume and intensity of training appears to improve HIEE (99, 125). Therefore, the coach and the athlete should be cautious when manipulating rest interval lengths because drastic decreases in interset rest intervals appear to impair the development of strength.

Periodization of Endurance

Although the methodology for developing biomotor abilities for sport has been improving constantly, some antiquated methods are still in use, especially in the area of developing endurance. In speed- and power-based sports, the role of aerobic endurance is less important (except for some team sports, such as soccer, lacrosse, and water polo). Yet, in sports such as American football, cricket, baseball, hockey, and basketball, long-distance jogging is still prescribed to develop aerobic endurance, although this work does not correspond to sport-specific performance demands and the energy systems dominant in these sports. During a game, for instance, an American football linebacker performs 40 to 60 short accelerations of 3 to 6 s each with rest intervals of 1 to 3 min. This performance will not be improved by running 5 miles. For these power sports, the first macrocycle of the general preparation can consist of tempo training (400-600 m) in sets of repetitions of the same distance or descending ladders (varying intensity according to the distance of each repetition; figure 11.12) or lower-intensity intermittent runs. In both cases, there is a weekly variation of distances and intensities, from general to more specific training parameters. Distances can be broken down to perform more sport-specific shuttle runs, too.

The progression from aerobic-dominant types of training (intensity zones 5 to 3) to anaerobic lactic system training (zone 2) should follow the natural progression of the annual plan, beginning with the preparatory phase and moving into the competitive phase (see the example in figure 11.13).

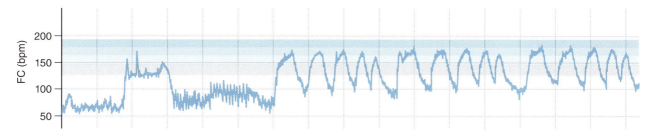

FIGURE 11.12 Heart rate variations during an aerobic power training session in ladder fashion, consisting of three sets of 600-500-400-300-200 m repetitions, at 95%-95%-100%-100%-100% of maximum aerobic speed, with a 1:1 rest interval between reps.

Endurance Training Programming With Six Intensity Values

In all athletic programs, the coach must alter the intensity of training throughout a microcycle to enhance the athletes' physiological adaptation to training and regeneration after a demanding training session. Such alternation of intensities depends, however, on the ergogenesis of the event and the characteristics of the training phase.

As most sports use fuel produced by all of the energy systems, training has to be more complex, exposing athletes to all energy systems, especially during the last part of the preparatory and throughout the competitive phases.

We propose six intensity values in table 11.17, to assist coaches in achieving scientific and well-planned training that considers the physiological profile and the energy requirements of a sport. These intensities are listed in order of magnitude of power output, with number 1 being the energy system with the highest power output and 6 being the system with the lowest power output.

Zone 1: Alactic System Training (AST)

The intent of AST is to increase an athlete's ability to be faster with less effort. AST should improve the start and acceleration. This is possible by applying

TABLE 11.17 Six Intensity Zones of Endurance Training

Intensity zone	Type of training
1	Alactic System Training (AST)
2	Lactic Acid Training (LAT)
3	Maximum Oxygen Consumption Training ($\dot{V}O_2maxT$)
4	Anaerobic Threshold Training (AnTT)
5	Aerobic Threshold Training (ATT)
6	Aerobic Compensation Training (CoT)

Chart of the Annual Plan

Type: Coach:

Date											
Month	October	November	December	January	February	March	April	May	June	July	August
Phases	Preparation						Competition				Transition
Subphases	General			Specific		Pre-competition	Competitive				Transition
Macrocycles	1	2	3	4	5	6	7	8	9	10	11	12	13	14	15
Microcycles	1 2 3 4	5 6 7 8	9 10 11	12 13 14	15 16 17	18 19 20	21 22 23	24 25 26	27 28 29	30 31 32	33 34 35	36 37 38	39 40	41 42 43	44 45 46
Periodization of endurance — Endurance	Tempo	Aerobic intervals		Anaerobic intervals		Specific endurance	Maintenance				LSD
Intensity (% $\dot{V}O_2$max)	70 75 80 75	80 85 85 90	90 95 90	95 90 100	90 100+ 90	100+ 90	100/60 95/60 100/60	95/60 100/60	95/60 100/60	95/60 100/60	95/60 100/60 90/60	60 65 60 65 70 65

FIGURE 11.13 Hypothetical periodization of endurance annual plan for a team sport with a 20-week preparation phase.

LSD = long slow distance training.

short work periods of 2 to 8 s, with a speed in excess of 95% of maximum. Such a training program employs the phosphate energy system; the outcome is an increase in the quantity of creatine phosphate (CP) stored in the muscle and increased activity of the enzymes that release energy through the ATP-CP system.

Long recovery intervals between work periods (work to recovery interval ratio = 1:50-1:100) are necessary to completely refill the muscles' CP supply. If the rest interval is short, the restoration of CP will be incomplete; as a result, anaerobic glycolysis will become the major source of energy, rather than the phosphate reaction. This in turn will produce lactic acid that will reduce speed, and the athlete will not realize the desired training effect. AST or sprint training should not, therefore, cause muscle acidosis because this is a sign of anaerobic glycolysis.

Zone 2: Lactic Acid Training (LAT)

LAT increases an athlete's ability to perform during lactic efforts and tolerate lactic acid buildup; it is useful for fast repetitions of 15 to 90 s. Very high levels of lactic acid buildup can result from high-intensity reps of 40 to 50 s, although the fastest rate of lactic acid accumulation happens with maximum effort between 12 and 16 s. Power output during lactic efforts is improved via the increase of the lactic energy system's metabolic enzymes, as well as adaptations of the nervous system. In fact, performance in lactic power events (10 to 20 s in duration) seems to be subject to a major limitation involving the nervous system's ability to maintain the frequency of discharge to the muscles rather than any metabolic reasons (155b).

On the other hand, lactic acid tolerance increases as a result of skeletal muscles repeatedly removing lactic acid from the bloodstream. Studies have demonstrated that lactate transporters increase in number as a function of high-intensity training (17g). The ability to clear lactic acid from the bloodstream and transport it to slow-twitch muscle fibers for energy usage is an adaptive response that delays fatigue and inevitably improves performance in sports that require lactic acid tolerance.

An athlete can perform better for longer if his nervous system is trained to maintain the frequency of discharge for the duration of a lactic effort or if he can tolerate the pain of acidosis (high lactic acid concentrations in the blood). Therefore, the purposes of training in intensity zone 2 are to adapt to the nervous strain of longer maximum-intensity efforts, to resist the acidic effect of lactic acid buildup, to buffer the effects of lactic acid, to increase lactic acid removal from the working muscles, and to increase the athlete's physiological and psychological tolerance of the pain of training and of challenging competitions.

Training for intensity zone 2 comes in the following variations:

1. *Lactic power short:* Organize a series of shorter, near-maximum and maximum-intensity repetitions or drills (3 to 10 s) with shorter rest intervals (15 s to 4 min, depending on duration of effort, number of repetitions, and relative intensity) that result in only partial removal of lactic acid from the system. The physiological consequence of this type of training is that the athlete tolerates increased amounts of lactic acid while producing high levels of anaerobic power under the condition of extreme acidosis. This method is often used as the competitive season approaches and the athlete's system is challenged to the maximum capacity.

2. *Lactic power long:* Organize near-maximum and maximum-intensity repetitions of longer duration (10 to 20 s) that make the lactic acid energy system work at its maximum rate of energy production. This method is one of the highest possible stressors for the neuromuscular system. Therefore, to repeat the same quality of work, the athlete needs very long rest intervals (12 to 30 min, depending on the athlete's performance level and the number of repetitions) to facilitate an almost complete removal of lactic acid and the recovery of the central nervous system. If the rest interval is not long enough, recovery is incomplete and injury risk is high.

3. *Lactic capacity:* Organize high-intensity repetitions of longer duration (20 to 60 s) that result in increased amounts (well over 12 mmol) of lactic acid. To repeat the same quality of work, the athlete needs moderate rest intervals (4 to 8 min, depending on duration of effort, number of repetitions, and relative intensity) to facilitate near-complete removal of lactic acid. If the rest interval is not long enough, removal is incomplete and acidosis is severe. Under these conditions, the athlete is forced to slow the speed of a repetition or drill below the intended level. Consequently, the athlete does not achieve the planned training effect, which is to increase her ability to tolerate lactic acid buildup. Rather, the athlete will end up training the aerobic system.

Psychologically, the purpose of lactic tolerance training is to push the athlete beyond the pain threshold. However, this type of training should not be used more than two times per week, because it exposes the athlete to critical levels of fatigue. Overdoing it may bring the athlete closer to the undesirable effects of injury, overreaching, and overtraining.

Zone 3: Maximum Oxygen Consumption Training ($\dot{V}O_2maxT$)

During training and competition, both parts of the oxygen transport system—central (heart) and peripheral (capillaries at the level of the working muscle)—are heavily taxed to supply the required oxygen. Because the supply of oxygen at the working muscle level represents a limiting factor in performance and because athletes with large $\dot{V}O_2$ capacity have demonstrated better performances in endurance events, $\dot{V}O_2maxT$ must be an important concern for both coaches and athletes.

Increased $\dot{V}O_2max$ results from improved transportation of oxygen by the circulatory system, and increased extraction and use of O_2 by the muscular system. Consequently, you must dedicate a large portion of the training program to developing $\dot{V}O_2max$. Achieving these effects requires training periods of 1 to 6 min at 90% to 100% of maximum oxygen consumption (higher intensity for shorter repetitions and slightly lower intensity for longer repetitions). The number of repetitions performed in a training session depends on the specific duration of the sporting event: the longer the duration, the lower the number of (longer) repetitions. Therefore, in a given training session, an athlete might derive similar benefits from performing, say, six repetitions of 3 min each at 100% of $\dot{V}O_2max$ or eight repetitions of 5 min each at 95 % of $\dot{V}O_2max$, with a 1:1 rest interval.

Athletes can improve $\dot{V}O_2max$ through shorter work periods (30 s to 2 min), provided the rest interval is short as well (10-30 s) and the intensity above the $\dot{V}O_2max$. Under such conditions, training effect will result through the accumulative effect of several repetitions (4 to 12) that will reach $\dot{V}O_2max$ and not from one or two repetitions, which may primarily solicit the anaerobic system.

Zone 4: Anaerobic Threshold Training (AnTT)

AnTT refers to the intensity of an exercise at such a level that the rate of lactic acid diffusion in the bloodstream equals the rate of its removal (AnTT = 4-6 mmol). The lactic acid produced in the muscles diffuses into adjacent resting muscles, thus lowering its concentration level. It is metabolized in the working muscle and is removed from the blood by the heart, liver, and muscles at the rate it is accumulated.

This training can use shorter repetitions of 1 to 6 min with an intensity between 85% and 90% of $\dot{V}O_2max$ or 92% to 96% of maximum heart rate, but with slightly longer rests between bouts (work-to-rest ratio between 1:0.5 and 1:1). Such training can stimulate both the aerobic and the anaerobic metabolism without a significant rise in lactic acid production. This effect can also be achieved through longer repetitions: five to seven repetitions of 8 to 15 min at 80% to 85% of $\dot{V}O_2max$ or 87% to 92% of maximum heart rate with a work-to-rest ratio between 1:0.3 and 1:0.5. During such training programs, the subjective feeling of the athlete should be mild distress, with the speed slightly faster than what is comfortable.

Zone 5: Aerobic Threshold Training (ATT)

High aerobic capacity is a decisive factor for all events of medium and long duration. Similarly, it is a determinant for all sports in which the oxygen supply represents a limiting factor. Using ATT is beneficial for most sports because it enhances quick recovery following training and competition; develops the functional efficiency of the cardiorespiratory and nervous systems; and enhances the economical functioning of the metabolic system. It also increases the capacity to tolerate stress for long periods.

ATT is performed mostly through a high volume of work without interruption (uniform pace), or interval training using repetitions longer than 10 min. The duration of an ATT session could be between 1 and 2 h. The athlete achieves the intended training effect only when the lactic acid concentration is between 2 and 3 mmol, with a heart rate of 130 to 150 beats/min. If the figures are less than this, the training effect is questionable.

During the competition phase, you can plan ATT one or two times per week as a method of maintaining aerobic capacity and as a recovery session to reduce intensity but maintain the general fitness level.

Zone 6: Aerobic Compensation Training (CoT)

CoT facilitates athletes' recovery following competitions and the high-intensity training sessions characteristic of intensity zones 2 and 3. Specifically, to eliminate metabolites from the system and speed recovery and regeneration, workouts must be planned using very light intensity (45% to 60% of $\dot{V}O_2max$).

High-intensity endurance training is a necessary component of adaptation and performance enhancement. However, strenuous exercise often negatively affects the body before it can recover and strengthen. Recovery and regeneration can be aided by active recovery methods such as cycling or running for 5 to 20 min at about 50% of maximum capacity.

In contrast, following strenuous endurance-type training with static rest (such as lying or sitting down) can delay regeneration of the body's systems and removal of the by-products of training. Recovery and regeneration are slowed by elevated levels of plasma cortisol and adrenaline, and by decreased levels of white blood cells and low levels of immune system catalysts (e.g., neutrophils and monocytes) (66b, 72b, 159b).

On the other hand, active recovery (along with proper postworkout nutrition) has been shown to counteract the increase in cortisol and adrenaline, override the drop in white blood cell count, and eliminate the drop in neutrophil and monocyte count (66b, 72b, 159b). In other words, active recovery reignites immune system function following strenuous training, which in turn allows the body to regenerate faster.

Therefore, by the end of the training session, the difficult part of the workout is complete, but athletes who are willing to live with the sacrifice needed for improvement and adaptation should devote another 15 to 20 min to foster healing and regeneration. Choosing not to do so slows the recovery process and may negatively affect the next training session; it also leads to overtraining and injury. During very demanding weeks of training, intensity zone 6 may be used one to three times, sometimes in combination with other intensities (in that case, at the end of a workout).

Designing the Weekly Program

Now that we have illustrated the six intensities of training, the critical question is how to incorporate them within a training program. Traditionally, a coach designs a training program by assigning certain physical, technical, or tactical objectives to certain days of a microcycle. Yet the critical element is training the energy systems, which represent the foundation of good performance. The coach must do this in conjunction with the technical and tactical elements, based on knowledge of the physiological profile prevailing in an event. When planning a microcycle, the coach does not need to write down the training content, but the mathematical values of the intensities needed in the cycle. This will suggest the components of the energy systems to emphasize in that training session. The distribution per microcycle of the six intensities depends on the phase of training, the athlete's needs, and whether a competition is planned at the end of the cycle.

A major training concern for distributing intensity values in a microcycle is the athlete's physiological reaction to training and the level of fatigue a given intensity generates. An intensity from the top of the intensity scale will constantly generate higher levels of fatigue. Such a training session can be followed, therefore, by one session at intensity five, which facilitates supercompensation by being less demanding. This is the principle of alternation of intensity and energy systems within the microcycle. On the other hand, for a purely aerobic sport (marathon running, cross-country skiing), you will plan just the alternation of intensities, as almost all sessions will be of aerobic ergogenesis.

Combinations of various intensities in a training session are often a necessity. For instance, a combination of intensities one and three or two and six suggests that after working an anaerobic component (i.e., intensities one and two), which are the most taxing and fatiguing, the coach can plan a less demanding intensity (i.e., intensity six). Such a combination will enhance the development or maintenance of aerobic endurance and will especially facilitate the recovery rate between training sessions.

Physiological adaptation to the profile of an event may result in other possible combinations as well. One such possibility could be 1 + 3 + 2. Such a combination models a race in which the beginning (an aggressive start) relies on the energy produced by the phosphate system (1); the body of the race uses the energy produced by the lactic and oxygen systems (3); and the finish, in which the athlete can tolerate the increased levels of lactic acid (2), makes the difference between winning and losing.

It is necessary to incorporate a scientific basis in the methodology of planning if a coach expects high efficiency from the time invested in planning the training. Applying the six intensities to the training plan incorporates the entire spectrum of energy systems necessary in all endurance-dominant or endurance-related sports—from the phosphate, to the lactic acid, to the aerobic system. In this method, the coach plans numerical values, which he rations and distributes in a microcycle depending on the ergogenesis of the sport, the phase of training, and the athlete's needs.

To avoid the undesirable effects of overtraining, consider the sequence and frequency of the intensity symbols while strictly adhering to the concept of supercompensation. Under such circumstances, planning becomes more scientific, has a logical sequence, and observes the important training requirement of alternating high-intensity and low-intensity stimuli so that fatigue is constantly succeeded by regeneration.

Summary of Major Concepts

All sports require some level of endurance. The coach must determine the type of endurance needed to optimize performance in a given sport. Endurance is classified as low-intensity exercise endurance (LIEE) and high-intensity exercise endurance (HIEE). LIEE is typically needed in aerobic sports that require work to be continuously performed for a long duration. Conversely, HIEE requires the repetitive performance of high-intensity activities interspersed with periods of recovery. Sports that rely on HIEE also appear to rely on the ability to express high power outputs or generate high levels of force. Interestingly, HIEE training methods appear to improve LIEE performance, but LIEE training methods can reduce HIEE performance. When training in a team sport setting, the coach must tailor the endurance program according to the played position—its dominant energy system, its match running volume at different speeds or power outputs, and ultimately, the player's maximum aerobic speed—to adjust intensity and rest intervals. Only an individualized training program can maximize the development of the sport-specific endurance of an athlete.

Speed and Agility Training   12

Speed, agility, and speed endurance are crucial abilities that can affect performance in a variety of sports. These abilities are related and depend in large part on the athlete's muscular strength. Integrating speed, agility, and speed endurance training into the annual training plan and manipulating specific training variables can optimize performance capacity. Therefore, understanding the factors that affect speed, agility, and speed endurance enables coaches to develop sport-specific training plans that maximize performance.

Speed Training

Speed is the ability to cover a distance quickly. The ability to move quickly in a straight line or in different directions (changes of direction) is an integral component of successful performance in a wide variety of sports. Straight-line sprinting can be broken down into three phases: acceleration, attainment of maximum speed, and maintenance of maximum speed (27, 75).

Acceleration is the ability to increase maximum velocity in a minimum amount of time. Acceleration determines sprint performance abilities over short distances (e.g., 5 m and 20 m) and is usually measured in m/s or simply as a unit of time (e.g., s). The ability to accelerate differentiates between athletes for a variety of sports. For example, during a 100 m race, untrained sprinters achieve maximum speed within 20 to 30 m (27), whereas highly trained sprinters do not attain maximum speed until around 50 to 60 m (65). It is likely that maximum strength levels for the knee extensors, hip extensors, and plantar flexors (calf muscles) explains the acceleratory abilities of various athletes because strength is strongly related to sprinting ability. Support for this contention can be garnered from the literature, which reports that faster sprinters are significantly stronger and are able to accelerate at faster rates than their slower counterparts (6, 24, 69, 110).

In many sports, such as soccer, the ability to accelerate underlies successful game play. During soccer game play, the average sprint length is around 17 m (9) and ranges from 5 to 50 or 60 m. Often, these sprints are initiated while the athlete is moving at slower speeds (110) or when the athlete is making a breakaway or initiating a tackle. Therefore, the ability to accelerate rapidly in the first few steps is essential to effective game play. These data reveal that a sprint training program that targets the acceleration phase should develop specific strength (maximum strength and power) characteristics and mechanical skills (110).

After completing the acceleration phase of a sprint, the athlete achieves maximum running velocity. Athletes may have great acceleratory capacity but lack the ability to achieve high velocities in this phase of a sprint, which suggests that acceleration and the maximum speed of running are very specific sprinting qualities (26). Differences in the kinematics of the acceleratory and maximum velocity portions of a sprint support this observation and suggest that running mechanics (78, 110) and specific strength qualities (69) play a role in developing maximum running speed.

The final phase of a straight-line sprint requires the athlete to maintain maximum speed, described among sprinters as **speed endurance**. Although the athlete is moving at maximum

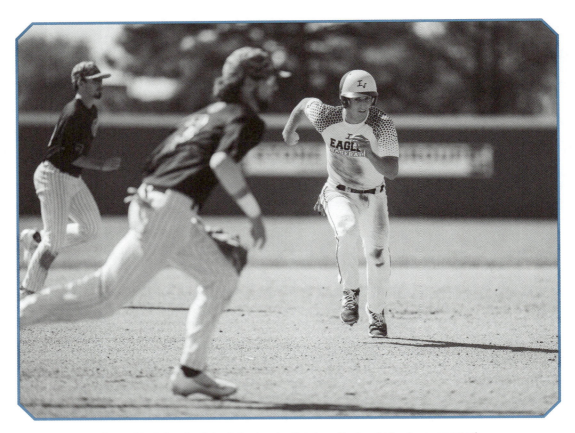

Speed training isn't just for track athletes; it should be incorporated into training plans for athletes in all sports.

speed, the development of fatigue begins to affect the athlete's ability to maintain force output, effective running mechanics, and thus speed. During a bout of maximum sprinting, insufficient rest intervals can lead to depletion of phosphocreatine and accumulation of lactic acid, which is formed in response to the rapid glycolytic rate (91). As phosphocreatine levels decrease, there is a higher reliance on the anaerobic lactic system; as **lactic acid** increases, there is an accumulation of hydrogen ions (H^+), which can reduce the athlete's capacity to exert force (99) and lead to a breakdown in running mechanics and mechanical efficiency. Both short-repetitions sprinting programs with incomplete rest intervals and long-repetitions sprinting programs with complete rest intervals appear effective in improving muscle buffering capacity and reducing fatigue (25, 57, 91). Maximum speed, on the other hand, should be trained with short repetitions and complete rest intervals.

Speed is the expression of a set of skills and abilities that allow for high movement velocities. Although it is often suggested that skills and abilities are unrelated, they are highly related and thus can be developed with specific training practices (91, 92). The application of appropriate sprint training methods in conjunction with a periodized training plan can improve sprint performance (e.g., acceleration, achievement of maximum velocity, and maintenance of high velocities) and thereby improve competitive performance.

Factors Affecting the Development of Speed

To develop speed, the coach and athlete must understand the factors that affect an athlete's ability to generate high movement speeds. Several physiological and performance factors affect sprinting ability, as described in the following paragraphs.

Energy Systems

Sprinting involves a rapid release of energy that allows for a high rate of cross-bridge cycling within the muscle and a rapid and repetitive production of muscular force. The body meets the energy demands of muscle under sprinting conditions by (1) altering the enzymatic activity of specific energy-producing pathways, (2) increasing the amount of energy stored within the muscle, and (3) increasing the muscles' ability to overcome the accumulation of fatigue-inducing metabolites (91).

Enzymatic Activity All three of the body's energy systems (phosphagen, glycolytic, and oxidative) contribute to energy supply (67). However, the phosphagen and glycolytic systems predominate during most sprinting activities. The degree of contribution of the oxidative energy system depends on the duration, length, and number of sprints performed as well as the rest interval between repetitions. For example, if the sprinting activity is long (≥30 s in duration) and repeated several times with short rest intervals between bouts, the contribution of the oxidative energy system will progressively increase (67). Therefore, the enzymatic adaptations will be very specific to the sprinting tasks performed in training (91).

The response of the phosphagen system (ATP-PC) to sprinting activities shows that muscular stores of adenosine triphosphate (ATP) and phosphocreatine (PCr) can be significantly reduced in response to bouts of sprint training (45). The rate of PCr breakdown is significantly higher in the fastest sprinters (45), which may occur as a result of an increased rate of **creatine phosphokinase (CPK)** activity in response to sprint training (78, 83, 102). To meet the increased demand for ATP during sprint training, an increased **myokinase (MK)** enzyme activity is stimulated, which may increase the rate of ATP resynthesis (25, 93). This increase in MK activity has been reported to occur in response to training with both short- and long-duration sprints (25, 83).

Several key enzymes associated with the glycolytic system also are affected by various forms of sprint training (91). For example, glycogen **phosphorylase (PHOS),** the enzyme responsible for stimulating muscle glycogen breakdown, is increased in response to both short (<10 s) and long (>10 s) bouts of sprinting (25, 51, 66, 83, 91). Phosphofructokinase (PFK) activity (the enzyme that regulates the rate of the glycolytic system) appears to increase in response to short-duration, long-duration, or combination sprinting activities. Changes in PFK activity may be of particular importance because the rate of PFK activity has been related to performance in high-intensity exercise such as sprinting (101). Finally, **lactate dehydrogenase** (LDH) activity has been shown to increase in response to both short- and long-duration sprinting (19, 47, 66, 79, 90, 91).

The contribution of the oxidative system to an acute 10 s bout of sprinting is considered to be minimal (~13%) (11). However, during multiple sprints of a longer duration (≥30 s) there is a significant decrease in the glycolytic energetic supply and a concomitant decrease in maximum power output and speed (10). This may occur in response to elevated H^+ concentrations slowing the glycolytic rate and allowing for a decreased production of lactate. To meet the energy demands of the exercising muscle, the contribution of oxidative metabolism increases (8, 10, 97). However, the contribution of oxidative metabolism to the energy supply is affected largely by the duration of the sprint (8, 97) and the rest interval between bouts (7). For example, longer sprints performed multiple times with short rest intervals will increase the contribution of the oxidative systems to energy supply. With this increased energy supply from oxidative metabolism, it is not surprising that there are increases in succinate dehydrogenase and citrate synthase activity (key enzymes of the oxidative system) in response to sprinting (19, 47, 66).

Short and long sprint interval training bouts can significantly increase the athlete's aerobic power ($\dot{V}O_2$max) (57, 97). Thus, high-intensity interval training is an important tool for the development of sport-specific fitness for sports dominated by both anaerobic (e.g., soccer, American football, basketball) and aerobic (e.g., long-distance running, cycling, skiing) energy supplies. Although repetitive sprint bouts, similar to those seen in competition, may have a large aerobic contribution, this does not mean that long-distance aerobic training is the best way to develop fitness (44, 46). For example, Helgerud and colleagues (44) reported that high-intensity interval training resulted in significantly greater increases in $\dot{V}O_2$max than traditional aerobic training. This interval-based training increase in $\dot{V}O_2$max was related to significant increases in running economy, distances covered, number of involvements with the ball, and average work intensity during a soccer game (43).

The enzymatic alterations stimulated by sprint training may play an integral role in facilitating rapid muscular contractions by allowing for a faster rate of ATP supply from the glycolytic systems. Adaptation to multiple bouts of high-intensity sprint intervals seems to produce a superior training stimulus, which appears to translate to team sports play better than does traditional endurance training. High-intensity interval training should be, then, the preferred endurance training modality for team sports, especially during the specific preparation phase.

Energy Substrate Storage   An increased availability of metabolic substrates (PCr, ATP, and glycogen) prior to the initiation of an exercise bout may enhance the athlete's ability to perform or maintain high-intensity exercise (91, 106). Parra and colleagues (83) reported that a short sprint protocol elevated resting PCr and glycogen levels, whereas a long protocol elevated only resting glycogen levels. This suggests that the sprint training program may alter the energy substrates stored in the muscle. These changes to energy substrate storage may have contributed to the increases in sprint performance noted in the investigation (83).

Accumulation of Fatigue-Inducing Metabolites   Lactic acid accumulation as a result of multiple sprint bouts appears to contribute to impaired sprinting performance (62, 107). With an increase in lactic acid accumulation, there is an increase in H^+ ion concentration (which can inhibit PFK activity) (41), a decrease in the Ca^+ transport rate (59), and a decrease in the rate of cross bridge cycling within the skeletal muscle (100). If the H^+ ions are not buffered, the ability to sprint, and more importantly to repetitively sprint, will be impaired (57).

The use of high-intensity interval training has been demonstrated to result in an increased buffering capacity (70, 107). With this increased buffering capacity, there is an increased ability to maintain energetic flux and thus to maintain high power output performance, such as sprinting. Therefore, when developing a physiological base for sprint and agility performance, it is important to include high-intensity interval training in the overall training plan as it has the ability to increase buffering capacity, which allows the body to deal with the accumulation of metabolic fatigue inducing factors (e.g., lactic acid or H^+). For more information on the increasing endurance and buffering capacity, refer to chapter 11.

Neuromuscular Systems

The morphological characteristics of the muscle as well as adaptations to neural activation patterns can play a significant role in the expression of high-velocity movements. Late 20th century literature has suggested that performance in sprinting activities depends largely on genetic factors, yet recent literature suggests that muscle fiber characteristics as well as neural activation patterns can be altered in response to various training stimuli (92, 103-105, 108, 109).

Muscle Composition   Muscle fiber type or composition appears to play a role in determining sprint performance abilities. A higher percentage of type IIb or IIx myosin heavy chain (MHC) isoforms (fast-twitch) is advantageous for activities that require the expression of high power outputs or forces (17, 84), such as those seen in sprinting. A continuum of muscle fiber MHC isoforms ranging from type I (slow-twitch) to type IIa, IIb, or IIx can be delineated, along with specific hybrids that exist as transitional states (e.g., I/IIa, I/IIa/IIx, IIa/IIx) between the major subtypes (5, 85, 108). Within this continuum of individual MHC isoforms, a spectrum of force- and power-generating capacity can be created (figure 12.1). In this spectrum, type I fibers exhibit the lowest force- and power-generating capacity, whereas type IIb or IIx MHC isoforms are associated with the highest

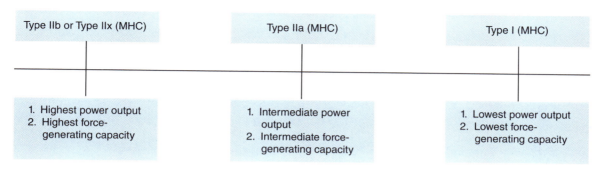

FIGURE 12.1 Power output and force-generating capacity by the myosin heavy chain (MHC) muscle fiber subtype.

power- and force-generating capacity (16, 17).

Because of the interrelationships of power, force, and fiber type, it appears that sprinting performance capacity may be partially explained by the athlete's fiber type. Support for this contention can be seen in the scientific literature, which suggests that sprint performance is significantly correlated with the athlete's percentage of type II fibers (25, 32, 73). Sprint-trained athletes appear to exhibit greater rates of force development and force output than either untrained or endurance-trained individuals (39, 68), which may be related to a higher percentage of type II fibers. In fact, sprinters have been shown to have a high percentage of type II fibers (23). Thus, a potential explanation for improved sprinting performance may center on specific training-induced adaptations to the muscle fiber composition.

The ability of sprint training to alter the muscle fiber depends partially on individual differences and genetic predisposition to different types of training (31, 59, 61, 91). Prolonged endurance training usually induces a shift from type II to a type I fiber composition (e.g., IIx or IIb → IIa → I), which is disadvantageous for sprinting performance (104). Conversely, sprint training can increase type II fiber content (25, 31, 47, 48). A sprint training program that entails a frequent exposure to lactic bouts induces a bidirectional shift toward type IIa fibers (I → IIa → IIb or IIx) (3, 4, 91). However, it appears that this favorable adaptation to the muscle fiber composition can be muted if endurance training is included in the training plan (91). Providing insufficient rest between repetitions or sets of sprinting efforts (42, 60, 91) and including only long-duration sprints (19, 58, 91, 96) results in a fiber type transition similar to that seen with endurance training. Given this information, coaches must carefully consider the content of the periodized training program. The first program concern is that traditional endurance training, such as long slow distance (LSD) work, should be avoided by athletes who must express high levels of sprinting speed. Second, depending on the needs of the athlete and the sport being trained for, the use of short rest intervals and longer sprinting bouts should be reserved for the general preparatory phase of the annual training plan. As the athlete progresses through the specific preparatory phase and into the competitive phase, the use of shorter sprints with longer rest intervals will help the athlete produce higher speeds of movement.

Neural Factors High-velocity training, such as maximum intensity sprints, requires a high level of neural activation (29, 52, 81, 92). Several neural factors influence sprinting ability, include the sequencing of muscle activation, the stretch reflex, and the development of neural fatigue (92).

Muscle Activation When performing a sprinting motion, a multitude of different muscles are activated at specific times and intensities to optimize movement speed (92). It appears that training results in a refinement of neural innervations' patterns and a more developed and efficient motor program (72, 92). It appears that the ratio of contribution of co-agonist muscles is altered with changes in muscle contraction speed (20, 92). Alterations to the stretch shortening cycle (SSC) have also been reported (92) and appear to contribute to propulsive forces during running (29). Finally, the ability to fully or selectively recruit type II muscle fibers may be important when optimizing sprint performance capacity (92). Engaging in training practices that use ballistic or explosive activities (e.g., sprinting, weightlifting, plyometrics) may alter the motor unit recruitment pattern so that type II fibers are recruited sooner (38).

Stretch Reflex Short latency stretch reflexes appear to influence sprint running performance (92). In particular, the **stretch reflex** appears to enhance force production when the athlete is sprinting. During the nonsupport phase of sprinting (discussed further in the section titled Technique), the numerous muscles involved in the development of force are activated (35), and there is an increase in muscle spindle sensitivity (36, 40, 92). Training-induced adaptations to muscle spindle sensitivity may occur in response to sprint training (55, 56) and can improve muscle stiffness upon ground contact (92). Increases in muscle stiffness appear to be related to both maximum running velocity and speed maintenance (21, 64). Increases in stiffness also appear to decrease contact time during the support phase of sprinting by increasing the rate of force development and the peak forces generated during this time (92).

Neural Fatigue Neural fatigue can affect sprint performance by reducing voluntary force-generating capacity (90). As fatigue manifests itself during a maximum 100 m sprint there is a slight decline in speed, especially in the later stages of the race, which corresponds to a decrease in stride rate (2, 92). Ross and colleagues (92) suggested that this reduction in stride rate is the result of neural fatigue, whereby motor unit recruitment patterns are altered and change the motor-unit firing rate.

During sprinting, such as the 100 m dash, there is a preferential recruitment of type II (fast-twitch) muscle fibers, which are particularly susceptible to acute neural fatigue as a result of their short contraction times and high axial conduction velocities (74). As the 100 m dash progresses, there is a progressive reduction in recruitment that probably occurs as a result of a less-than-optimal output from the motor cortex (92). A 4.9% to 8.7% reduction in muscle activation has been noted once maximum velocity has been achieved during a 100 m dash. This reduction in recruitment may occur as a result of fatigue of the neuromuscular junction, a decreased firing rate, or a reduction in the recruitment of higher threshold motor units (type IIb or IIx) (92).

Ross and colleagues (92) postulated that acute neural fatigue may decrease reflex sensitivity. Even though it has yet to be demonstrated in response to sprint exercise, it is possible that large volumes of traumatic stretch shortening can reduce reflex sensitivity, which could reduce force output during running (92). This reduction in force output could impair sprint performance.

Technique

Sprinting is a ballistic activity in which a series of running strides launch the body forward with maximum velocity over some distance. Sprinting contains two major phases: a nonsupport (or flight) phase and a support phase. The nonsupport phase contains recovery and ground preparations, whereas the support phase includes both landing or eccentric breaking and concentric propulsion subphases (1). As an athlete sprints, she alternates between the nonsupport and support phases. As the athlete enters the support phase, a force-absorbing eccentric action precedes an explosive concentric contraction (propulsion phase). With increasing running speed, the time spent in the nonsupport phase generally increases and the time spent in the support phase decreases (1). As the time spent in the support phase decreases, it becomes particularly important that the athlete demonstrate a high rate of force development (RFD) to maintain or continue to elevate running speed. The decrease in duration of the supporting phase is essential for success in any high-velocity activities and directly depends on the improvement of the athlete's maximum strength and power capabilities. This is why we can say that:

- Nobody can be fast before being strong (strength training makes you fast).
- If you want to be fast you have to shorten the duration of contact phase. Only gains in

maximum strength and power will decrease the duration of the contact (supporting) phase. To achieve that, you have to improve maximum strength and power of the quadriceps, gastrocnemius, and soleus muscles.

The speed at which an athlete runs or sprints depends largely on an interaction between stride rate and stride length. As the athlete accelerates and approaches maximum velocity, stride rate increases to a greater extent than stride length. Stride length is related to both body height and the force exerted during the propulsion phase. However, elite sprinters tend to achieve a greater stride rate and stride length in a shorter amount of time, which suggests that both stride rate and length can be optimized with appropriate training interventions. The phases of a sprint are the start, acceleration, and maximum velocity.

Start The optimal starting position is a medium heel-to-toe stance, regardless of whether the athlete is in a two-point (standing) or three- or four-point (crouching) stance. Initiating a sprint from the starting stance is then accomplished by overcoming inertia through the explosive application of force against the ground with both legs. The front leg extends while the rear leg swings forward with what is called a low heel recovery, which will be maintained for at least two steps before gradually raising (figure 12.2). As the rear leg comes forward, the hip is flexed to at least 90° and the ankle is dorsiflexed, preparing the foot to apply force down to the ground. At the same time, the arm opposite the leg initiates starting actions by swinging forward and up, with the elbow flexed at approximately 90°, and the hand moves past the head. As the front leg moves through the support phase and extends, the opposite arm should swing backward with the elbow fully extended. When the start is performed correctly, the body is at an angle of 45° or less from horizontal, the head is aligned with the back, and the push-off is performed with perfect alignment from the tip of the foot to the

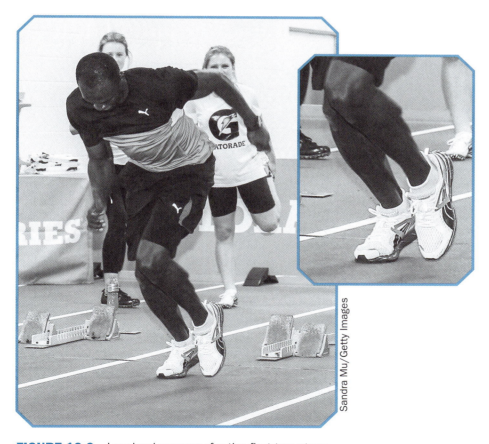

FIGURE 12.2 Low heel recovery for the first two steps.

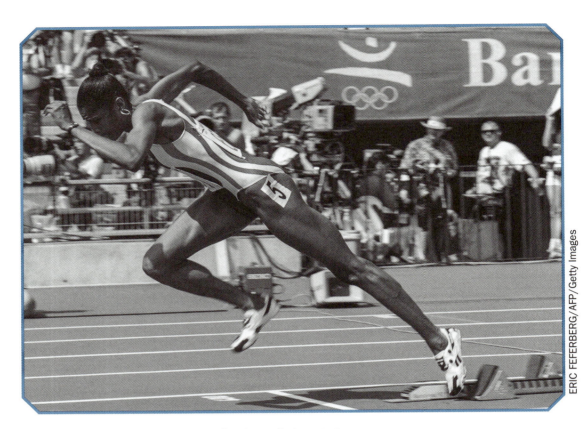

FIGURE 12.3 The optimal angles for the sprinting start.

shoulder. Figure 12.3 shows the sprinting technique for the starting position.

Acceleration During the initial acceleration period from a static start, both stride rate and length will increase during the first 15 to 20 m or 9 to 12 strides. Analysis of elite sprinters show that stride length increases more than stride frequency during the first 20 m of a 100 m dash (65). However, it appears that stride frequency is the performance discriminant among fast and slow team sports athletes (78). During the preliminary portion of the acceleration period, the body will have a forward lean (≤45°), which will progressively move to a more upright position as the athlete approaches maximum velocity. The forward lean position allows the athlete to have the vertical projection of the center of gravity ahead of the supporting legs, a technical position that is favorable to higher acceleration. During the whole acceleration phase, the leg is fully extended and in line with the body's longitudinal axis at push-off. From this position, the recovery of the leg is performed by passing the foot progressively higher at each step, always ending with the thigh perpendicular to the trunk. As the leg enters the support phase, it extends downward and back; at the same time, the elbow angle of the arm simultaneously swinging backward will close a little more with each step, finally staying at 90° for the whole cycle when the athlete is in the upright position typical of the maximum speed phase.

The arm motion should always originate from the shoulder and move backward and forward. These arm motions offset the axial momentum generated by the contralateral leg and hip. During the support phase, the athlete will transition between an eccentric and concentric subphase with the use of a stretch shortening cycle (SSC) action (87). As the athlete accelerates, greater ground reaction forces must be developed to continue to accelerate (54, 77). These data seem to suggest that strength training, especially activities that improve the rate of force development, is an essential component of a training program designed to enhance sprinting performance. Horizontal ground reaction forces, in particular, seem

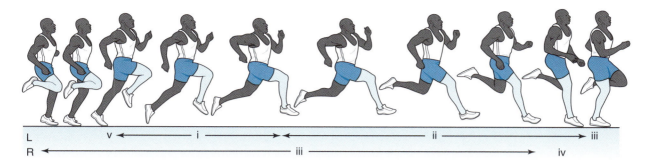

FIGURE 12.4 Technique for sprinting at maximum velocity.

i = early nonsupport; ii = mid nonsupport; iii = late nonsupport; iv = early support; v = late support.

Reprinted, by permission, from G. Schmolinsky, ed., 1993, *Track and field: The East German textbook of athletics* (Toronto: Sport Books).

to be the discriminant between slower and faster sprinters (18, 18b, 53, 71, 77, 82), which suggests that more emphasis should be granted to training means with anteroposterior force vector (kettlebell swing versus Olympic lifts, hip thrust versus squat [22]) or requiring more horizontal force application (horizontal jumps versus vertical jumps) than traditionally used.

Maximum Velocity When maximum velocity is achieved (within 30 to 60 m, depending on the athlete), the trunk position will be more upright (figure 12.4), and the stride rate and length will both contribute to the velocity of movement. During this phase, the time spent in the nonsupport phase will be maximized by the application of vertical ground reaction forces during the initial support phase, allowing sufficient time for the swinging leg to be repositioned in preparation for the transition into the next support phase. Athletes who are able to apply higher horizontal ground reaction forces during the support phase of the maximum velocity portion of a sprint, though, are able to reach and maintain higher velocities of movement (18, 18b, 53, 71, 77, 82). This further strengthens the contention that strength and power training are essential components of a periodized training plan that emphasizes speed development.

As the athlete enters the support phase, he will contact the ground directly beneath his center of gravity. While moving into the support phase, the athlete will transition from an eccentric braking action into a concentric action with the use of an SSC action. During the concentric phase, the athlete will perform a "triple extension" of the hip, knee, and ankle to properly apply forces against the ground. After the triple extension is performed, the athlete will then initiate a triple flexion of the ankle, knee, and hip, which will place the heel close to the buttocks. At this point, the heel of the recovery leg will pass above the knee (figure 12.5). This triple flexion motion allows the athlete to rapidly move the knee to a position in front of the hip, effectively positioning the leg on the front side of the body. This movement prepares the foot for a rapid descent and allows the athlete to maximize ground reaction forces as the foot moves down and back during ground strike (87).

Fatigue

During sprint training, the athlete should be conscious of fatigue because the development of fatigue can reduce sprint performance capacity. As

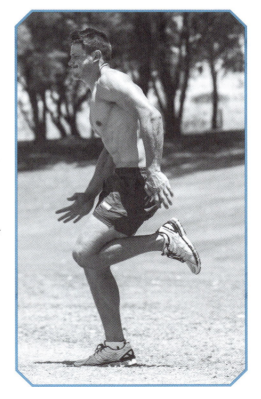

FIGURE 12.5 Over the knee heel recovery and upright position at maximum speed.

fatigue is manifested, stride rate can be decreased, while stride length increases and the duration of the ground support phase can increase. These events effectively decrease the effectiveness of the SSC that is applied between the eccentric and concentric subphases of the support phase. High levels of fatigue may also reduce ranges of leg extension (87). These breakdowns in running mechanics may be partially explained by the occurrence of metabolic fatigue (91).

Fatigue can reduce sprinting capacity, especially when a series of maximum sprints are performed (92). This type of fatigue may occur as a result of supraspinal failure, segmental afferent inhibition, depression of motor neuron excitability, loss of excitation branch points, and a decreased ability of the neuromuscular junction to fully activate the muscle (92). Neuromuscular fatigue can play a large role in reducing sprinting speed.

Methods for Developing Speed and Speed Endurance

Speed and speed endurance can be developed by manipulating a multitude of training factors. For example, the acceleration phase can be developed by targeting the ATP-PC system and performing short sprints (10 to 40 m) at 95% to 100% of maximum speed with longer recovery periods between repetitions and sets. Conversely, extensive tempo work in which longer distances (>200 m) are covered and lower intensities (<70% of maximum) are interspersed with short rest intervals (<60 s) will develop the athlete's aerobic capacity (33). Table 12.1 gives examples of manipulations for the development of several different aspects of speed and speed endurance.

TABLE 12.1 Methods for Developing Speed and Speed Endurance

Type of training		Target energy system		Objectives	Distance (m)	% of Best	Recovery time	
		Global	Specific				Repetitions	Sets
Speed		Anaerobic	ATP-PC	Acceleration	10-40	95-100	1 min per 10 m/yd	—
				Maximum speed	50-60	95-100	1 min per 10 m/yd	—
Speed endurance		Anaerobic	ATP-PC and glycolytic	Short speed endurance	5-30	95-100	0.5-1.5 min	3-5 min
			Glycolytic	Short speed endurance	60-100	90-95	1-3 min	3-6 min
				Long speed endurance	120-200	90-95	3-5 min	6-10 min
						95-100	12-30 min	—
		Anaerobic/ aerobic	Glycolytic and oxidative	Special endurance	250-400	90-95	5-6 min	8-12 min
						95-100	10-20 min	—
Tempo	Intensive	Anaerobic/ aerobic	Glycolytic and oxidative	Anaerobic capacity	80	80-90	30 s-5 min	3-5 min
	Extensive	Aerobic	Oxidative metabolism	Aerobic power	100	50-70	<1 min	<3 min

Agility Training

Straight-line sprinting ability is important for track and field athletes and athletes who participate in other field-based sports (e.g., soccer, American football, baseball); but the ability to rapidly accelerate, decelerate, and change direction is quite determinant for court-based and team sports. Often these athletes have to quickly decelerate, stop, and reaccelerate in other directions in response to external cues. These abilities are usually considered an expression of agility. Some literature uses the term quickness synonymously with agility or change-of-direction speed (76, 94). However, Sheppard and Young (94) suggested that the definition of quickness does not consider deceleration or a change of direction and that quickness in and of itself contributes to agility. The term cutting has been used to describe change-of-direction capabilities (94) and is sometimes falsely used to describe agility. This term only considers the change of direction initiated by the foot's ground contact (94) overlooking the determinant role played by the extensors' eccentric strength.

Agility is a complex set of interdependent skills that converge for the athlete to respond to an external stimulus with a rapid deceleration, change of direction, and reacceleration. Young and colleagues (111) and Sheppard and Young (94) suggested that agility is affected by the athlete's perceptual and decision-making ability and her ability to quickly change direction (figure 12.6).

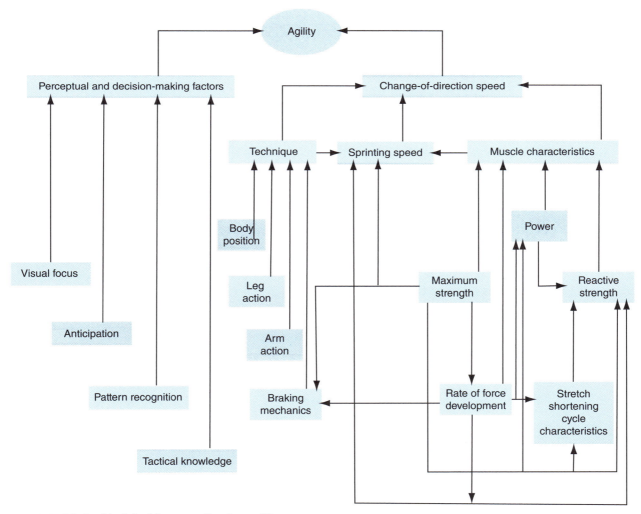

FIGURE 12.6 Model of factors affecting agility.

Adapted from Young, James, and Montgomery 2002 (111) and Sheppard and Young 2006 (94).

Perceptual and Decision-Making Factors

During competition, the athlete must be able to perceive a situation, make a decision, and then change his direction of movement and speed in response to some external stimulus. The ability to engage in this process involves a complex interaction of visual interpretation, anticipation, recognition of patterns, and knowledge of tactical situations (94, 111).

The ability to visually scan or focus while performing multidirectional tasks appears to positively influence performance (86). The ability to visually recognize a specific action, process the ramifications of that action, and respond with the appropriate change of direction or movement pattern differentiates between athletes. Knowledge of the tactical situation and the ability to anticipate the potential movements of the opponent also affect the athlete's ability to change direction appropriately (94). Although it appears that perceptual decision-making factors can affect competition agility, there is a paucity of scientific data on this relationship.

Because there appears to be a relationship between visual interpretation and changes in direction, it may be warranted to include activities or drills that require the athlete to perform a specific movement in response to a visual or auditory stimulus (58). These activities can be integrated into both speed and agility training and may translate into competitive play. However, research exploring the efficacy of such training practices is limited.

Change-of-Direction Speed

Three key factors affect the athlete's ability to perform change-of-direction tasks: technique, sprinting speed, and muscle characteristics (94, 111).

Technique

Leg action, arm action, and braking mechanics can all affect an athlete's ability to express agility in movements. When the athlete is accelerating or decelerating, the body lean must increase to allow the base of support to move away from the athlete's center of gravity (87) while the center of gravity is lowered. These actions allow the athlete to maintain dynamic stability and change direction rapidly (94). When initiating the deceleration action prior to the change of direction, the athlete will decrease her stride length (93). Upon reacceleration, the athlete will progressively increase both stride length and rate while the body position becomes more vertical or incline in the new direction of movement. It may be warranted for the athlete to run with a lower center of gravity and a more pronounced forward lean when participating in sports that require frequent changes in direction (93, 94).

Powerful arm actions are a fundamental component of multidirectional movements, since the arm's drive directly affects the athlete's leg frequency during acceleration or reacceleration. This is not true during deceleration, when the arms' frequency and radius are visibly reduced, effects that favor a quick deceleration and change of direction. Force is essential for both acceleration and deceleration. In the case of acceleration, propulsion force is performed concentrically, while during deceleration force is expressed eccentrically. The latter requires more force since the athlete has to also overcome inertia (12).

For successful deceleration, the athlete has to contact the ground with the full foot to maximize the surface area that is contacting the ground and reducing the eccentric load by engaging the entire lower extremity (86).

Sprinting Speed

Some coaches believe that straight-line sprint training directly affects the athlete's ability to change direction (94). This is far from being the case in field and court-related sports. Straight-line sprinting ability explains only a small amount of the variance seen with change-of-direction activities (94, 111, 112). When only straight-line sprinting is used, there is very little improvement in performance of multidirectional change-of-direction tasks. The addition of the ball (e.g., a soccer ball or basketball) and agility drills can significantly improves the athlete's ability to perform multidirectional tasks such as change-of-direction movements (94, 112). Therefore, both straight-line sprinting and change-of-direction tasks with and without implements must be incorporated at various stages of the athlete's development and preparation for competition.

Muscle Characteristics

For many years it was commonly accepted that muscular strength and power characteristics determined the athlete's ability to sprint. There appears to be a relationship between muscular strength and power and change-of-direction performance. The literature indicates that this relationship may be stronger with distinct change-of-direction movements than with directional changes performed at speed over longer durations (as is often the case for a soccer forward) (94). The athlete should always strive to become stronger and more powerful because this will translate into change-of-direction ability.

Reactive strength, or the ability to engage the stretch shortening cycle (SSC), also appears to contribute to the athlete's ability to change direction (34, 111). The ability to engage the SSC in response to eccentric loading allows for greater forces to be generated during the concentric phase of a change-of-direction task (56). The ability to engage this mechanism may allow for a more rapid acceleration when changing direction. Therefore, it is strongly recommend to incorporate plyometric activities into training, given their strong relationship to change-of-direction performance (111).

Program Design

Developing a training plan involves planning at several distinct levels. These include the microcycle, macrocycle and annual training plan. At each level of planning, the coach must consider the principles of developing speed and agility and understand the physiological and performance responses to specific training variables.

Principles of Speed and Agility Development

When considering the development of speed, several principles must be considered (28).

Quality Over Quantity

Speed training places a large physiological stress on the athlete. To maximize training effects, speed training needs to be meticulously dosed and incorporate low training volumes interspersed with long periods of restoration. Excessive use of sprint activities will eventually result in overtraining. It is not wise to perform sprint and agility training under conditions of fatigue or with excessively short rest intervals.

Proper Technique at All Times

To develop the appropriate movement patterns, the coach must emphasize proper technique in all training activities. If the athlete performs drills with inadequate technique, she will stabilize inappropriate movement patterns that will hinder the development of speed and the expression of agility. Focus on proper technique should begin during the warm-up and continue into the main body of the training session. If fatigue causes technical breakdowns, it may be warranted to reduce the training volume of that session.

Specificity of Speed and Agility Development

When developing speed and agility, the athlete should develop skills in relationship to the demands of his sport. For example, it may be warranted for soccer players to perform some speed and agility activities with a ball because this will be a major component of competitive performance. Coaches also should consider the bioenergetics, the work-to-rest ratio, and the dynamics of the targeted sport when designing specific sprint and agility sessions. The coach should develop specific sprint and agility activities based on the needs of the sport. For example, the coach can use short side games or the dribble track (see figure 5.14 in chapter 5) in soccer because these activities will more closely model what occurs in competition (45).

Development of Supporting Characteristics

Many factors can contribute to the athlete's ability to exhibit speed and effectively perform change-of-direction movements. Coaches must understand the bioenergetic demands of different sprint and agility training activities and how they relate to the athlete's targeted sport. Additional aspects to consider are the role of strength training in the expression of speed and the development of change-of-direction abilities.

Feedback

It is important to record the athlete's objective and subjective feedback throughout the training process. Objective feedback can include recorded times and video analysis of performance; subjective feedback may include the concept of perceived maximum speed (28). With novice athletes or when the skill set is complex, the coach should provide constant feedback and reinforcement. This feedback appears to be essential during the early stages of skill development; as the athlete develops, less feedback is necessary. Consider providing information on proper performance and methods for correcting errors. Try to address one or two technical corrections per session, following a priority sequence. As the skill develops, feedback should be less frequent and should progress from qualitative to quantitative.

Motivation

To develop speed or agility, the athlete must be highly motivated. High power output activities always require a high level of motivation and maximum concentration. Furthermore, sprint and agility training produces a large amount of fatigue, especially when targeting **speed endurance** (86). A motivated athlete is more likely to tolerate this type of training. Motivation can be cultivated by providing feedback, especially feedback that emphasizes the positive aspects of the athlete's training, and by including the athlete in the planning process. If the plan is implemented correctly, the athlete will be more likely to push himself to higher levels.

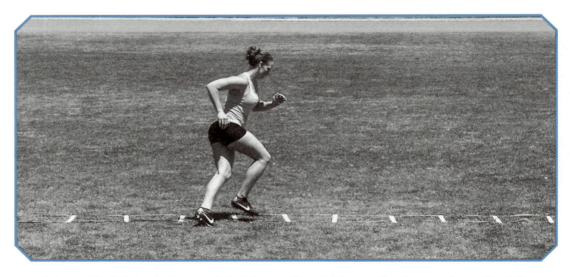

Cater agility training to the sport. In this way, the athlete can develop sport-specific skills at the same time that she develops speed and agility.

Variables Associated With Training for Speed or Agility

When integrating speed or agility training into the annual periodized training plan, the coach should consider manipulating several training variables (87).

Density

The density of training is the amount of training that occurs within a given time period (training session). When considering a sprint, sprint endurance, or agility session, the density is a ratio of the interval of exercise and rest within a set or series of sprints. If quality of work is expected, longer rest intervals are necessary to facilitate good recovery between sets of sprints or agility drills. This is why density of training for both sprinting and agility training has to be low.

Duration and Distance

A run can be calculated in either seconds or minutes to determine the duration of exercise. The distance traveled can also be quantified in meters or yards. For example, if an athlete sprints 100 m (distance) in 12 s (duration), both distance and duration have been determined and can be used to calculate an intensity factor.

The duration or distance of an activity determines the bioenergetic pathway and the specific quality targeted. Short-duration or short-distance activities tend to target the phosphagen system and the development of acceleration or speed. For example, acceleration is emphasized when the athlete runs short sprints (10 to 40 m), whereas maximum speed is targeted with longer sprints (50 to 60 m). If, on the other hand, the objective is to train speed endurance, the distance is increased from 80 to 150 meters. Elite sprinters appear to reach maximum velocities after 5 to 6 s in about 50 to 60 m, whereas novice sprinters attain top speeds by 20 to 30 m (65, 87). If the sprint is extended, reliance on the oxidative energy system will increase. Therefore, the distance and duration of the sprint are important considerations when an athlete is targeting acceleration, maximum speed, or endurance characteristics.

In the case of agility training, duration has to be selected depending on the energy systems dominant in the selected sport and should be position-specific. In most cases the type and duration of an agility drill is relatively short and very intensive (between 5 and 10 s). This might be advisable for some but sports, such as volleyball and American football, where the dominant energy system is the phosphagen system. However, in other team sports where the oxidative system is the main supplier of the energy (e.g., soccer, rugby), the total duration of the agility drills can be much longer or the short agility drills can be separated by very short rest intervals.

A similar discrepancy has to be envisioned for specific positions in team sports. For instance the duration of agility drills for full or central back players in soccer has to be shorter (10 to 15 s), very intense, and to incorporate reaction time and movement time exercises. On the other hand, for midfielders, for whom the dominant energy system is aerobic, the coach has to create an agility drill of longer duration, such as 20 to 40 s or longer.

Exercise Order

The exercise order is the sequence in which specific training tasks are performed. When prescribing the order of exercises in a speed, speed endurance, or agility session, the coach must consider both the management of fatigue and the development of fitness. Because sprint and agility training activities impose large metabolic, neuromuscular, and coordinative demands, they should be conducted when the athlete has a minimal level of fatigue.

A multitude of factors that can contribute to the generation of fatigue should be considered when sequencing a training session. The activities are best undertaken after a dynamic

Duration of Agility Drills

An agility drill must not be of standard duration (i.e., the same for every athlete). On the contrary, agility drills have to be created based on the dominant energy system in the selected sport and should also be position-specific. Therefore the duration and intensity of agility drills is directly dependent on the desired sport-specific adaptation. The same is true for the position an athlete plays.

warm-up that primes that athlete for the training bout and before more fatiguing bouts of training are undertaken. It may be advisable to separate the training session into specific segments within the daily training plan. For example, the morning session (9:00 a.m.) after a recovery day may focus on speed training, and the afternoon session (4:00 p.m.) may target speed endurance or strength training. However, sessions in which maximum speed or high-intensity agility is the goal are best performed in the afternoon, especially they follow a restful morning.

Ideally, the athletes should be in a state of supercompensation, since maximum speed is a determinant quality in speed training. It is also recommended that speed and agility training sessions are best structured with brief work periods separated by frequent rest intervals that last between 3 and 5 min. An effective method for performing this type of activity is the repetition method, which contains very short, high-intensity work bouts performed for low volumes and long rest intervals that maximize recovery and the development of speed and technical proficiency (table 12.1). It is possible to create sessions that target speed and speed endurance, but the coach must take care in ordering the exercises in these sessions.

Intensity

When an athlete is training for speed, speed endurance, or agility, the intensity is often quantified in relation to maximum velocity or speed of movement.

$$\text{Intensity}(m/s) = \frac{\text{Distance}(m)}{\text{Time}(s)}$$

According to this equation, if an athlete runs 100 m in 12 s, she would have an intensity of 8.33 m/s. Additional examples of the calculation of intensity for individual sprints are presented in tables 12.2 and 12.3. The coach must consider that short sprints performed at high velocities provide a higher-intensity bout of exercise.

When designing the training plan, the coach can establish intensity zones based on the athlete's best times in a prescribed distance (table 12.3). To create the intensity zones, the coach can use the following formula to determine the percentage maximum intensity (velocity):

$$\text{Percentage maximum velocity (m/s)} = \text{Maximum intensity} \times \text{Percentage}$$

If the athlete ran a maximum 100 m in a time of 11 s, his maximum intensity of 90% would be represented by the following equation:

$$90\% \text{ maximum velocity} = 9.1 \text{ m/s} \times 0.90 = 8.2 \text{ m/s}$$

TABLE 12.2 Determination of Volume Load and Average Intensity for a Sprint Training Session

Workout 1				Workout 2			
Distance (m)	Time (s)	Intensity (m/s)	Volume load	Distance (m)	Time (s)	Intensity (m/s)	Volume load
200	48	4.17	833.33	400	79	5.06	2,025.32
200	35	5.71	1,142.86	400	89	4.49	1,797.75
200	36	5.56	1,111.11	200	42	4.76	952.38
200	39	5.13	1,025.64	200	40	5.00	1,000.00
Training intensity =		5.14		Training intensity =		4.83	
Training session volume load =			**4,112.94**	**Training session volume load =**			**5,775.45**

Note: Volume load is in arbitrary units. Training intensity is the average velocity of the workout. This concept is based on methods presented by Plisk (87).

TABLE 12.3 Training Zone Intensities for Sprint Training

Zone	Percentage maximal	Velocity (m/s)	Time (s)	Intensity
1	>100	>9	<11.0	Maximum
2	95-100	8.6-9	11.6-11.0	High
3	90-95	8.1-8.5	12.2-11.7	Medium-high
4	85-90	7.6-8	12.8-12.3	Medium
5	80-85	7.1-7.5	13.4-12.9	Low

Note: Times are based on a best 100 m time of 11 s.

If the training zone were set at 90% to 100% of maximum, the limits for time would be calculated with the following equations:

Training time (s) = Distance (m) / Percentage maximum velocity (m/s)

Training time at 90% intensity = 100 m / 8.2 m/s = 12.2 s

Therefore, in a 4-week macrocycle, the three loading microcycles could progress from 90% to 92.5% to 95%, requiring this athlete to run 100 m at 12.2 s, 11.9 s, and 11.6 s respectively. Further examples of the training zones can be found in table 12.3.

Rest Intervals

Manipulation of the interrepetition and interset rest interval can significantly affect the physiological stress and performance outcomes of a speed, speed endurance, or agility training session. Long rest intervals (work/rest = 1:50-1:100) should be used when targeting the development of absolute speed because they allow for a greater replenishment of stored phosphagens and allow for the expression of maximal power outputs. When targeting high-intensity interval endurance, the coach should use shorter rest intervals (work/rest = 1:4-1:24).

Finally, short rest intervals (work/rest = 1:0.3-1:1) are used when targeting the oxidative system (aerobic) (13). A summary of the effect of manipulating rest intervals can be found in chapter 11 and in tables 11.9, 11.13, and 11.14.

When establishing the work-to-rest ratio, the coach can examine the work-to-rest ratios that occur in the sporting event. For example, the work-to-rest ratio in rugby games is between 1:1-1.9 and 1-1.9:1 (30), whereas American football generally has a work-to-rest ratio of 1:6 (88) and soccer exhibits a 1:7 to 1:8 work-to-rest ratio (63). By determining these ratios, the coach can design the training program to target the metabolic demands of the sport while also developing the appropriate speed characteristics required for successful performance.

Training Intensity

The training intensity is associated with the rate of performing work or the rate at which energy is expended (100). The higher the training intensity, the higher the rate of performing work, which corresponds to higher energy expenditures. The training intensity during sprint and agility training can be calculated as follows:

$$\text{Training intensity}(\text{m/s}) = \frac{\text{Training session volume load}}{\text{Total distance covered in training}}$$

In table 12.2, an example training series is presented in which an athlete's volume load is 4,112.94 and the total distance covered during the training session is 800 m.

$$\text{Training intensity}(\text{m/s}) = \frac{4{,}192.94}{800} = 5.14 \text{ m/s}$$

Therefore, the training intensity of this session is 5.14 m/s. Note that as the volume load increases, there is a general trend for the intensity or velocity of movement to decrease.

Volume

The volume of training represents the amount of work performed in a training session or training phase and is often expressed as the total repetitions of a prescribed workload or task assignment. The most accurate method for determining the volume of workload completed in a training session is the **volume load**, which is a product of the intensity and distance completed per repetition (87).

Volume Load

When looking at the interactive effects of intensity and volume, coaches and athletes must have a quantifiable method for estimating training stress (87). Volume load is an excellent indicator of training stress and is generally calculated as a product of work volume and intensity (87, 100). In the context of sprint or agility training, the volume load of training can be determined using running speeds (intensity) and distances covered (87), as in the following formula:

$$\text{Sprint or agility training volume load} = \text{Velocity (m/s)} \times \text{Distance (m)}$$

As with resistance training (see chapter 10), when the intensity (speed) of the session decreases, the volume load can be increased. An example calculation of volume load can be found in table 12.2.

When the coach is designing the training plan, it may be warranted to predict the volume load fluctuations for sprint training and integrate the volume loads with those established for resistance training activities. If done appropriately, the integration of the training loads will allow for a superior management of fatigue while maximizing fitness and preparedness for competition.

Periodization of Speed and Agility Training

A key aspect of implementing a speed and agility training plan is ensuring that the training factors are integrated to allow the athlete to attain the training goals. Developing a sprint program for a track athlete is somewhat easier than developing a plan for a team sport athlete that must include agility, technical skills, and tactics. Please note the periodization of the main biomotor abilities in each annual plan, exemplified below.

Annual Training Plan

Developing a plan for speed and agility training begins with the development of the annual training plan. As noted in chapter 6, key information needed when developing the annual plan includes dates of important competitions and the individual preparation, competition, and transition phases. The annual training plan will be structured based on the sport's characteristics. For example, a sprinter will typically use a bi-cycle annual training plan, whereas a team sport athlete may not, depending on league requirements.

The annual training plan for an elite sprinter uses a tri-cycle model in which three major peaks are planned, whereas a monocycle structure may be warranted for less developed sprinters. In the tri-cycle model presented in figure 12.7, the first peak (for the indoor season) occurs on March 20; the second peak (for the National Trials) is planned for July 7; and the final peak (for the Olympics) is planned for August 17.

The dynamics of the annual plan structure for team sports can be vastly different compared with an individual sports athlete, such as a sprinter. The competitive phase is generally dictated by the league or conference in which the athlete's team competes, and it entails weekly competitions.

Figure 12.8 is an example of an annual training plan for a collegiate soccer program. The annual training plan presented in figure 12.8 has a bi-cycle structure in which major competitive emphasis occurs in competition phase 1. Note that as with traditional annual training plans, the year is broken into preparatory, competition, and transition phases.

Macrocycle

In the annual training plan presented for a sprinter in figure 12.7, preparatory phase 1 is substantially longer than preparatory phase 2. Preparatory phase 1 contains two subphases, which are classified as general and specific preparation. The general preparation phase targets conditioning with an emphasis on anatomical adaptation, or what is also referred to as strength endurance. A secondary emphasis is placed on tempo work, which targets both anaerobic and aerobic development. In the early part of the general preparation work, long tempo work or aerobic intervals are completed; in the later stages of the phase, short-duration tempo work (anaerobic intervals) is used. As the athlete transitions into the specific preparation subphase, a greater emphasis is placed on the development of maximum strength and the use of anaerobic interval work. Anaerobic interval work is then used to develop repetitive speed endurance. As the athlete transitions into the competitive phase, the focus shifts to developing maximum speed while increasing power-generating capacity and maintaining speed endurance.

The annual training plan can be structured to target aspects of the athlete's development, depending on the phase of training. For example, during the general preparation phase, the primary emphasis is developing strength and general endurance, whereas in the specific preparation phase anaerobic endurance as well as short speed endurance is emphasized. When structuring the phases of the annual training plan, the coach must consider the goals of each phase because this will dictate which factors associated with sprinting are targeted. For example, in the general preparation phase, aerobic capacity and power development is a secondary development emphasis. Selecting extensive tempo work early in the phase would

Date	Months	Oct.				Nov.				Dec.				Jan.				Feb.				Mar.				Apr.				May				June				July				Aug.			
	Weekends (Sunday)	11	18	25		1	8	15	22	29	6	13	20	27	3	10	17	24	31	7	14	21	28	6	13	20	27	3	10	17	24	1	8	15	22	29	5	12	19	26	3	10	17	24	31
Competitions	International																										Birmingham	Portland WIC								Albuquerque				Eugene Trials			London DL		Rio OG		
	National																			Torun	Glasgow				X	X											X					X			X		
	Location																			X	X															X							X		
Phases		Preparatory 1																		Competition 1								Preparatory 2								Competition 2							Competition 3			
Subphases		GP									SP								PC	C					T	T			SP								C			T	T		C	T	T
Macrocycles		1				2					3				4				5	6					9			10	11				12				13	14		15	16		17	18	
Microcycles		1	2	3	4	5	6	7	8	9	10	11	12	13	14	15	16	17	18	19	20	21	22	23	24	25	26	27	28	29	30	31	32	33	34	35	36	37	38	39	40	41	42	43	44	45	46	47
Periodization of biomotor abilities	Strength	AA				MxS					MxS				P				Maintenance						Co			MxS				P-E				Maintenance				Co	Maintenance				Co
	Speed	Uphill sprints and technique				Acceleration					Acceleration/maximum speed								Maintenance						—			Acceleration/maximum speed								Maintenance				—	Maintenance				—
	Endurance	Ext. tempo				Int. tempo					Special endurance				Special endurance				Maintenance						ET			Speed endurance								Maintenance				IT	Maintenance				ET

FIGURE 12.7 Periodization model for an Olympic-level sprinter.

X = secondary important tournament; T = transition; GP = general preparation; SP = specific preparation; PC = precompetition; C = competition; AA = anatomical adaptation; MxS = maximum strength; P = power; Co = compensation; P-E = power endurance; ET = extensive tempo; IT = intensive tempo.

FIGURE 12.8 Annual training plan for an American university soccer team.

T = transition; GP = general preparation; SP = specific preparation; PC = precompetition; C = competition; AA = anatomical adaptation; MxS = maximum strength; P = power; Co = compensation; COD = change of direction; ET = extensive tempo; IT = intensive tempo.

accomplish this goal. As the athlete progresses through the phase, the distance covered can be shortened and intensive tempo work can be used to tap both aerobic and anaerobic energy supply. Once the athlete shifts into the specific preparation phase, speed endurance activities (e.g., short speed activities) can be selected.

One important factor to consider is that the use of long slow distance (LSD) to develop aerobic capacity is detrimental to the development of speed (88). It is best to develop aerobic capacity and power or speed endurance by using extensive and intensive tempo methods, which may also be termed aerobic and anaerobic intervals (87,88). Recent research suggests that these methods result in physiological adaptations that improve speed endurance performance (57).

The dynamics of working with team sports creates additional issues at the macrocycle level; this is because the training plan must include both technical and tactical activities in conjunction with activities that are designed to develop endurance, strength, and sprint and agility capabilities. In the team sport example presented in figure 12.8, preparatory phases one and two have an equal length, whereas competition phase one is longer than competition phase two due to the specifics of the schedule of games. As it happens in most team sports today, preparatory phase one contains a shorter general preparation subphase, with greater emphasis placed on specific preparation. Each subphase is broken into macrocycles of training that have specific emphasis in figure 12.8. For example, in macrocycle one, the primary emphasis is placed on anatomical adaptation, linear speed, and aerobic endurance. Macrocycle two focuses primarily on maximum strength, linear speed and agility, and aerobic or anaerobic endurance. Macrocycles three and four focus primarily on power, agility, and specific endurance.

Microcycle

Once the characteristics of the macrocycle are established, the individual microcycles can be constructed. One of the main factors dictating the construction of the microcycles contained in a speed, agility, or speed endurance portion of an annual training plan is the management of fatigue (87). The management of fatigue is important because high levels of fatigue can affect the athlete's ability to effectively perform speed- and agility-based drills with appropriate technique and power output. In fact, it is advisable that the athlete perform speed- and agility-based activities under a minimal amount of fatigue to maximize technical proficiency, allow for the mastery of skills, and maintain a high power output. This requires that the athlete perform these activities after completing an appropriate warm-up that emphasizes a combination of general and specific warm-up activities (50); in addition, the coach must incorporate adequate rest between repetitions or sets. It may be warranted to organize the different training components into multiple sessions within the training day (figure 12.9).

Unlike speed and agility training, speed endurance training is designed to increase the athlete's ability to resist and tolerate fatigue. This is accomplished by specifically taxing the metabolic systems by manipulating training variables, such as the work-to-rest interval, duration, and intensity of the sprint bout. Increasing the volume of multiple bouts of sprinting can result in very specific metabolic adaptations that can aid in the development of speed endurance.

Month	Macrocycle	Weeks	Emphasis	Monday	Tuesday	Wednesday	Thursday	Friday	Saturday	Sunday
May	1	1-3	Strength training	ST	ST		ST	ST		
			Speed and agility	SA			SA			
			Speed endurance		SE			SE		
June	2	4-7	Strength training	ST		ST		ST		
			Speed and agility	SA				SA		
			Speed endurance		SE		SE		SE	
July	3	8-10	Strength training	ST	ST		ST	ST		
			Speed and agility	SA			SA			
			Speed endurance							
August	4 (deload)	11-14	Strength training	ST			ST			
			Speed and agility	SA						
			Speed endurance				SE			

FIGURE 12.9 Microcycle structure for a 14-week sequenced preparation phase of training plan for university or professional American football.

ST = strength training; SA= speed agility; SE= speed endurance.

Note: On days when multiple activities are scheduled, the activities must be separated so that one factor is addressed in a morning session and the other at least 4 h later. If time constraints dictate that both factors must be trained in the same session, the priority item should be addressed first. On days when SA and ST occur, the ST generally is performed afterward.

Summary of Major Concepts

The development of speed, agility, and speed endurance is important for the majority of sports. It must reflect the physiological characteristics of the selected sport or position, and ultimately it must be integrated into the periodized training plan. Long-distance training methods will impede the development of both speed and agility and should be avoided when attempting to maximize these performance abilities. Both maximum strength and power are important characteristics, which emphasizes the need for an integrated strength training program for athletes who are attempting to maximize speed performance.

Some very specific movement mechanics are essential to maximizing an athlete's speed of movement and facilitate change-of-direction activities. Although speed plays a role in change-of-direction performance, agility activities must also be included in the training plan. In several sports, speed is considered a straight-line running activity (as with track or wide receivers in American football). In other sports (e.g., racquet sports), quickness or swift movement is, in fact, agility. Many athletes spend large amounts of time performing straight-line training tasks, but it may be warranted to use more change-of-direction tasks that emphasize acceleration, deceleration, changes in direction, and reacceleration activities. It also may be warranted to include the implements used in competition (e.g., a soccer ball or basketball).

Glossary

absolute density—The ratio between the effective work an athlete performs and the absolute volume (duration) of the training session.

absolute strength—The amount of force that can be generated regardless of body size.

absolute volume—The total volume or duration of the work that the individual performs in a session, including rest intervals.

acceleration—The ability to increase movement velocity in a minimum amount of time.

acidosis—A condition in which an accumulation of H^+ increases muscles acidity.

acyclic combined skills—Cyclic skills followed by an acyclic skill.

acyclic skills—Integral functions performed in one action.

adenosine diphosphate (ADP)—A high-energy phosphate compound that can be used to form ATP.

adenosine triphosphate (ATP)—A high-energy phosphate compound that allows for the release of energy when its phosphate bounds are broken.

aerobic intervals—Intervals that are designed to stress the aerobic system and are also referred to as pace-tempo training. Aerobic intervals can be performed in a continuous or intermittent fashion.

aerobic power—Maximum rate of ATP production via the aerobic energy system.

agility—Ability to rapidly change direction and accelerate or decelerate in response to an external cue.

anabolic—An environment in which building of tissue can occur.

anaerobic intervals—A form of interval training in which very high-intensity bouts are retentively performed for short periods of time, with periods of rest interspersed between efforts.

anaerobic threshold—The intensity of exercise at which the body cannot meet its energy demand with aerobic means; the point at which lactate production outweighs buffering capacities.

annual training plan—A long-term training plan that typically lasts for 1 year.

arteriovenous oxygen difference (a-$\dot{V}O_2$ difference)—The oxygen difference between the arterial and mixed venous blood. This reflects the amount of oxygen used by the tissue.

asynchronous—Asynchronous motor unit firing occurs as a result of one motor unit deactivating while another activates.

athletic shape--See *readiness*.

bi-cycle plan—An annual training plan with two major peaks.

bioenergetics—The process by which the body converts foods such as carbohydrates, proteins, and fats into a biologically useable form of energy.

bioenergetic specificity—Training the specific bioenergetic characteristics of a specified sport or activity.

biological age—An indication of age based upon sexual maturation.

biomotor abilities—Abilities whereby the body can perform a range of activities, such as strength, speed, and endurance. Biomotor abilities are influenced by training and may be genetically determined.

block—A period of training that usually last 4 weeks and is sometimes referred to as a mesocycle.

block training—A sequential approach to structuring training in which individual blocks of training (which contain a distinct focus) are linked together.

bodybuilding—A sport in which muscle size, definition, and symmetry determine the winner.

buffer—The difference between the percentage of 1RM necessary to go to failure with the number of repetitions performed in a set, and the percentage of 1RM actually used for that number of repetitions.

capillarization—An increase in the capillary networks that bring oxygen and nutrients to the tissues of the body.

carbohydrate—A compound composed of carbon, hydrogen, and oxygen.

cardiac output (Q)—The volume of blood pumped by the heart per minute. Calculated as stroke volume multiplied by heart rate.

chronological age—The age of the individual.

cluster set—A series of repetitions interspersed with a short rest interval.

complexity—Degree of sophistication and biomechanical difficulty of a skill.

concentrated loading—A short-term period in which training loads are increased dramatically.

conjugated sequence—A method of sequencing training to take advantage of training residuals developed with periods of concentrated loading; also called the coupled successive system.

cortisol—A corticosteroid hormone released from the adrenal cortex that stimulates the catabolism of proteins, the sparing of glucose utilization, an increase in gluconeogenesis, and an increase in free fatty acid mobilization.

creatine phosphokinase (CPK)—An enzyme contained in the phosphagen system that adds a phosphate to taken from phosphocreatine to and adenosine diphosphate to create ATP.

cross-bridges—Projections around the myosin filament that latch onto the binding site on actin.

cross-over concept—Lower-intensity exercise receives its ATP primarily from the oxidation of fat and some carbohydrates.

cyclic skills—Sporting activities that contain repetitive movements of the same motor skill.

degree of training—See *preparedness*.

delayed-onset muscle soreness (DOMS)—Muscle soreness or pain that occurs 24 to 48 hr after a heavy bout of exercise.

density of training—The frequency at which an athlete performs a series of repetitions of work per unit of time.

detraining—Reversal of the adaptations stimulated by training. The effects of detraining can occur very rapidly when workloads are significantly reduced.

detraining syndrome—A syndrome that occurs when training is intentionally or unintentionally stopped and results in several maladaptations including insomnia, anxiety, depression, and alterations to the cardiovascular system; also known as relaxation syndrome, exercise abstinence, or exercise dependency syndrome.

differentiation—The process of dissecting skill into subunits and determining where errors are.

discharge rate—The average number of action potentials per unit of time.

enzyme—A protein compound that speeds a chemical reaction.

ergogenesis—Literally translated as "energy creation," it indicates the dominant energy systems of an activity.

excess postexercise oxygen consumption (EPOC)—The oxygen debt; an oxygen consumption that is elevated above resting after exercise.

exhaustion—Training to the point of momentary muscular failure.

fartlek—The Swedish word for "speed play;" a classic method for developing endurance.

fast glycolysis—One of the two ways in which glycolysis proceeds. Fast glycolysis results in the formation of lactic acid from the breakdown of glucose and has a faster rate of energy supply when compared to slow glycolysis.

fatigue—A general sense of tiredness that is often accompanied by a decrease in muscular performance.

fitness–fatigue relationship—The relationship between fitness and fatigue and how they modulate athlete preparedness. This concept is a major factor associated with periodization.

flexibility—The range of motion of a joint or set of joints, dependent on the length of the muscles crossing the joints.

force–velocity curve—A graphic representation of the relationship between force and velocity.

frequency of training—The number of training sessions within a given time frame.

general adaptation syndrome (GAS)—A syndrome conceptualized by Hans Selye that explains the body's response to stressors, including physiological and psychological stress. The GAS is often cited as being a foundational component of periodization theory.

general strength—The strength of the whole muscular system.

glucose—The most common mechanism for transporting carbohydrates in the body; primarily broken down by the glycolytic energy system.

glucose transporter-4 (GLUT4)—A contraction-sensitive glucose transport protein that aids in the uptake of glucose by working skeletal muscle.

glycogen—A storage form of carbohydrate that is found in the skeletal muscle and liver.

glycolytic system—The energy system that provides energy via the breakdown of glucose; also known as glycolysis. It generally supplies energy for higher-intensity activities lasting 20 s to 2 min.

Golgi tendon organ—A sensory receptor that monitors tension and is located in the muscle tendon.

growth hormone—An anabolic hormone that can enhance cellular amino acid uptake and stimulate protein synthesis; also known as somatotropin.

hemoglobin (Hb)—The iron-containing compound in blood that binds oxygen.

Henneman size principle—A principle which suggests that the size of the motor unit dictates its activation.

high-intensity exercise endurance (HIEE)—A type of endurance that requires the athlete to sustain or repeat high-intensity or high-power movements with exercise durations lasting 2 min or less.

hypertrophy—Index indicating the systemic impact of a training session.

index of overall demand (IOD)—Index indicating the systematic impact of a training session.

inflammation—A local cellular response that is marked by leukocytic infiltration, pain, swelling, and often loss of function.

insulin—An anabolic hormone that facilitates the uptake of glucose and can stimulate protein synthesis.

integration—A process of constructing whole skills.

intensity—The qualitative element of training such as speed, maximum strength, and power. In strength training, intensity is often expressed in load related to the 1RM.

interexercise recovery—The form of recovery that occurs during the exercise bout and relates to the bioenergetics of the activity being performed.

intermuscular coordination—The strategy of the nervous system in the organization of a kinetic chain, in terms of timing of activation and deactivation of agonist and antagonist muscles.

interval training—The repeated performance of short to long bouts of exercise usually performed at or above the lactate threshold interspersed with periods of rest or low-intensity exercise.

intramuscular coordination—The strategy of the nervous system in the recruitment of a muscle group.

involution—Also known as a decay or detraining.

lactate—A salt formed from lactic acid. Lactate is not believed to be associated with fatigue but can be used to create energy.

lactate dehydrogenase—An enzyme contained in the glycolytic energy system that converts pyruvate to lactate.

lactate threshold (LT)—The point at which lactate formation begins to abruptly increase above baseline.

lactic acid—The end product of the fast glycolytic system that is often associated with fatigue because it can inhibit calcium binding to troponin or interfere with cross-bridge formation.

line of pull—Median direction of contraction of the main muscles involved in the technical skill.

long slow distance (LSD)—Endurance training that can be classified as conversational exercise, where the athlete can carry on a conversation without respiratory stress.

low-intensity exercise endurance (LIEE)—A form of endurance that relates to the ability to continuously perform work for a long duration of time.

macrocycle—A medium-term training cycle that lasts between 2 and 6 weeks.

maximal aerobic capacity—The maximal capacity for oxygen consumption; also known as the $\dot{V}O_2$max, maximal oxygen uptake, or maximal aerobic power.

maximal lactate steady state—A balance between lactate production and lactate buffering.

maximum strength—The highest force that the neuromuscular system can generate during a maximal voluntary contraction.

metabolism—The sum of the anabolic and catabolic reactions occurring in the body.

metric ton—A tonne, which is equivalent to 1,000 kg.

microcycle—A short training cycle that lasts 3 to 7 days.

mitochondria—Specialized cell organelles in which oxidative production of ATP occurs.

monocycle—An annual training plan with one major peak.

monotonous program overtraining—A form of overtraining that occurs in response to a lack of training variation and results in a reduction or stagnation of performance gains.

motor unit—The motor nerve and all of the muscle fibers it innervates.

movement time—The athlete's ability to quickly move a limb in the desired direction.

multipeak plan—An annual plan with multiple competition phases.

muscle endurance—The ability of the neuromuscular system to produce force in a repetitive manner.

myoglobin—A compound found in muscle that carries oxygen from the cell membrane to the mitochondria.

myokinase (MK)—An enzyme of the phosphagen system that takes a phosphate from an adenosine diphosphate and adds the phosphate and adenosine diphosphate to make adenosine triphosphate.

myosin heavy chain (MHC)—MHC consists primarily of the head of the cross-bridge and is typically associated with the fiber type of the muscle.

nonprogressive taper—A taper that is marked by standardized reductions in training load; also known as a step taper.

onset of blood lactate accumulation (OBLA)—Point at which the blood lactate concentration reaches 4 mmol/L.

overreaching—A short-term period during which the athlete intentionally overtrains.

overtraining—A long-term decrement in performance that occurs in response to accumulation of training and non-training stressors.

oxidative metabolism—The metabolism that occurs during the aerobic (oxidative) energy system.

oxidative system—The primary source of ATP at rest and during low-intensity exercise, also known as the aerobic system. The system is active in the mitochondria and requires oxygen to make energy.

oxygen deficit—The anaerobic contribution to the total energy cost of an exercise.

peaking—An athlete's high physiological and psychological state of competitiveness prior to an important competition, characterized by no residual fatigue and maximum adaptations to the previous training phases.

peaking curve—The line depicting the dynamic of the athlete's athletic shape throughout the annual plan.

performance oxygen uptake—The highest value of oxygen consumption during the performance of an exercise without the accumulation of lactate.

periodization—The logical and systematic sequencing of training factors in an integrative fashion in order to optimize specific training outcomes at pre-determined time points.

phosphagen system (ATP-PC)—An anaerobic energy system that primarily provides energy for short-term, high-intensity activities and contains three major enzymatic reactions including the ATPase, creatine kinase, and myokinase reactions.

phosphocreatine (PCr)—A component of the ATP-PC system that provides energy for muscle actions by maintaining ATP stores.

phosphofructokinase (PFK)—The rate-limiting enzyme of the glycolytic system.

phosphorylase (PHOS)—The enzyme responsible for stimulating muscle glycogen breakdown.

postactivation potentiation complex—Performing a heavy or an explosive exercise to excite the neuromuscular system before jumping or sprinting, thus obtaining a short-term performance improvement.

postexercise recovery—A form of recovery that occurs after the cessation of exercise.

power—The quick application of force against resistance. This unit of work is expressed per unit of time (i.e., power = work/time) and is often considered a factor of intensity. It may also be calculated by multiplying force $\times$ displacement.

power clean—A weightlifting movement in which the barbell is lifted from the ground to the shoulders in one movement.

power snatch—A weightlifting movement in which the barbell is lifted from the ground to a position an arms-length over the head in one movement.

preparedness—The stable component of the athlete's athletic shape, representing his physical preparation, as well as the acquisition of skills and tactical maneuvers. For this reason, it is the foundation on which to base other training states.

prime movers—The muscles that contract to perform the technical skills.

progressive overloading—A progressive increase in the training load (i.e., intensity, volume) above a normal magnitude.

progressive taper—A systematic reduction in training load.

proteins—Combinations of linked amino acids, all of which contain nitrogen.

pulmonary system—A series of structures that work together to ventilate the body.

quadrennial plan—A 4-year training plan, typically used with high school, collegiate, and Olympic athletes.

rate coding—The firing rate of a motor unit.

rate of force development (RFD)—The rate at which force is developed; it is calculated by dividing the change in force by the change in time.

reactive agility—Agility training where reactive exercises predominate.

readiness—The ability of the athlete to display his preparation level in the specific performance.

recovery—Process of returning to preexercise state.

recruited—Activated.

relative density—The percentage of work volume the athlete performs compared with total volume in the training session.

relative strength—The ratio between the athlete's maximum strength and his body weight or lean body mass.

repetitions—The number of work intervals within a set.

repetition maximum (RM)—The heaviest weight that can be lifted for a predetermined number of repetitions. A 1RM is the heaviest weight that can be lifted one time, whereas a 10RM is the heaviest weight that can be lifted 10 times.

repetition method—A higher intensity, longer rest interval type of interval training.

sarcoplasmic reticulum—An extensive, lattice-like, longitudinal network of tubules and structures that store Ca^{2+}.

sequenced training—See *block training*.

set—The total number of repetitions an athlete performs before taking a rest.

short ton—The unit that equals 907.2 kg.

slow glycolysis—One of the two ways in which glycolysis proceeds. Slow glycolysis results in the formation of pyruvate from the breakdown of glucose and proceeds with a rate slower than fast glycolysis.

specific strength—The strength that is related to the movement patterns of a specific sport.

speed—The ability to cover a distance in the fastest time possible.

speed-endurance—The ability to maintain speed or repetitively express high speeds of movements.

speed-strength—The ability to develop force rapidly and at high velocities.

stability (of training stimuli)—The body needs a certain number of exposures to a training stimulus for an adaptation to be induced; the repetitiveness of the training stimulus defines its stability.

step taper—See *nonprogressive taper*.

strength—The maximal force or torque a muscle or muscle group can generate.

stretch reflex—The contraction of a muscle in response to a stretch; also known as the myototic reflex.

stretch shortening cycle (SSC)—A combination of eccentric and concentric muscle actions.

stroke volume (SV)—The amount of blood ejected from the left ventricle during contraction.

supercompensation—See *general adaptation syndrome (GAS)*.

sympathetic nervous system—The part of the automatic nervous system that affects, among other things, the cardiovascular system. This system releases norepinephrine from its postganglionic nerve endings.

synchronization—The simultaneous activation of numerous motor units.

taper—An unloading phase of training prior to a major competition that generally lasts between 8 and 14 days.

testosterone—The predominant male sex hormone, which is produced in the testes in men and the adrenal cortex and ovaries in women. Testosterone is often used as an index of anabolism or the anabolic status of the body.

testosterone/cortisol ratio (T:C ratio)—An indicator of the anabolic-to-catabolic balance.

Tmax—The duration at which maximal velocity or power can be maintained during an endurance bout.

tonnage—A method for quantifying volume in resistance training; it is calculated by multiplying the number of repetitions performed by the number of sets and the resistance in kilograms used.

tonne—See *metric ton*.

torque—The rotational force a muscle or muscle group can generate.

total training demand—A summation of all the training factors contained in the plan.

training—A structured exercise program that is designed to develop specific performance characteristics related to sports performance.

training age—The number of years an individual has been training.

training effect—A physiological, performance, or psychological response to a training program.

training intensity—The intensity determined by dividing the total volume load by the total number of repetitions.

training log—A document used to record training information.

tri-cycle plan—An annual training plan that contains three major peaks.

type I muscle fiber—Fibers that have a low force-generating capacity; also known as slow-twitch fibers. These fibers tend to be smaller, have higher concentrations of oxidative enzymes, and be more fatigue resistant than type II fibers.

type II muscle fiber—Fibers that have a high force-generating capacity; also known as fast-twitch fibers. These fibers tend to be larger, have higher concentrations of anaerobic enzymes, and be more fatigue sensitive than type I fibers.

$\dot{V}O_2max$—See *maximal aerobic capacity*.

variability—Changes or variations in training volume, intensity (load), and frequency in order to stimulate an athlete's improvement.

velocity—The speed of movement of the body or an object.

volume—A quantitative element of training that can be measured as time or duration of training, the distance covered, the volume load of resistance training, or the number of repetitions performed.

volume load—A method for quantifying volume in speed and agility training; it is calculated by the intensity and distance completed per repetition.

work—This unit is calculated by multiplying force by displacement.

References

Chapter 1

1. ABERNETHY, P.J., J. JURIMAE, P.A. LOGAN, A.W. TAYLOR, and R.E. THAYER. Acute and chronic response of skeletal muscle to resistance exercise. *Sports Med* 17:22-38, 1994.
2. ABERNETHY, P.J., R. THAYER, and A.W. TAYLOR. Acute and chronic responses of skeletal muscle to endurance and sprint exercise: a review. *Sports Med* 10:365-389, 1990.
3. AHTIAINEN, J.P., A. PAKARINEN, W.J. KRAEMER, and K. HÄKKINEN. Acute hormonal and neuromuscular responses and recovery to forced vs maximum repetitions multiple resistance exercises. *Int J Sports Med* 24:410-418, 2003.
4. Alpine Canada Alpin. *Physiological Profile of Skiing Events*. Alpine Canada News Letter 32, Calgary, Alberta, Canada, 1990.
5. BAAR, K. Training for endurance and strength: lessons from cell signaling. *Med Sci Sports Exerc* 38:1939-1944, 2006.
6. BALOG, E.M., B.R. FRUEN, P.K. KANE, and C.F. LOUIS. Mechanisms of P(i) regulation of the skeletal muscle SR Ca(2+) release channel. *Am J Physiol Cell Physiol* 278:C601-611, 2000.
7. BANGSBO, J. The physiology of soccer—with special reference to intense intermittent exercise. *Acta Physiol Scand Suppl* 619:1-155, 1994.
8. BISHOP, D., and M. SPENCER. Determinants of repeated-sprint ability in well-trained team-sport athletes and endurance-trained athletes. *J Sports Med Phys Fitness* 44:1-7, 2004.
9. BONDARCHUK, A.P. Constructing a Training System. *Track Tech*. 102:254-269, 1988.
10. BROOKS, G.A., T.D. FAHEY, T.P. WHITE, and K.M. BALDWIN. *Exercise Physiology: Human Bioenergetics and Its Application*. 3rd ed. Mountain View, CA: Mayfield, 2000.
11. BURGOMASTER, K.A., G.J. HEIGENHAUSER, and M.J. GIBALA. Effect of short-term sprint interval training on human skeletal muscle carbohydrate metabolism during exercise and time-trial performance. *J Appl Physiol* 100:2041-2047, 2006.
12. BURKE, L.M. Nutrition for post-exercise recovery. *Aus J Sci Med Sport* 29:3-10, 1996.
13. BURKE, L., and V. DEAKIN. *Clinical Sports Nutrition*. Roseville, Australia: McGraw-Hill Australia, 2000.
14. BURLESON, M.A., Jr., H.S. O'BRYANT, M.H. STONE, M.A. COLLINS, and T. TRIPLETT-MCBRIDE. Effect of weight training exercise and treadmill exercise on post-exercise oxygen consumption. *Med Sci Sports Exerc* 30:518-522, 1998.
15. CAREY, D.G., M.M. DRAKE, G.J. PLIEGO, and R.L. RAYMOND. Do hockey players need aerobic fitness? Relation between VO2max and fatigue during high-intensity intermittent ice skating. *J Strength Cond Res* 21:963-966, 2007.
16. CERRETELLI, P., G. AMBROSOLI, and M. FUMAGALLI. Anaerobic recovery in man. *Eur J Appl Physiol Occup Physiol* 34:141-148, 1975.
17. CHESLEY, A., J.D. MACDOUGALL, M.A. TARNOPOLSKY, S.A. ATKINSON, and K. SMITH. Changes in human muscle protein synthesis after resistance exercise. *J Appl Physiol* 73:1383-1388, 1992.
18. CLOSE, G.L., T. ASHTON, A. MCARDLE, and D.P. MACLAREN. The emerging role of free radicals in delayed onset muscle soreness and contraction-induced muscle injury. *Comp Biochem Physiol* 142:257-266, 2005.
19. COFFEY, V.G., and J.A. HAWLEY. The molecular bases of training adaptation. *Sports Med* 37:737-763, 2007.
20. CONLEY, M. Bioenergetics of exercise training. In: *Essentials of Strength Training and Conditioning*. T.R. Baechle and R.W. Earle, eds. Champaign, IL: Human Kinetics, 2000, pp. 73-90.
21. COOKE, S.R., S.R. PETERSEN, and H.A. QUINNEY. The influence of maximal aerobic power on recovery of skeletal muscle following anaerobic exercise. *Eur J Appl Physiol Occup Physiol* 75:512-519, 1997.
22a. COOPER, K.H. *Aerobics*. New York, NY: Bantam Books, 1968.
22b. COOPER, K.H. *The New Aerobics*. New York, NY: M. Evans and Company, 1970.
23. COSTILL, D.L., P.D. GOLLNICK, E.D. JANSSON, B. SALTIN, and E.M. STEIN. Glycogen depletion pattern in human muscle fibres during distance running. *Acta Physiol Scand* 89:374-383, 1973.

24. COSTILL, D.L., and J.M. MILLER. Nutrition for endurance sport: carbohydrate and fluid balance. *Int J Sports Med* 1:2-14, 1980.
25. COSTILL, D.L., D.D. PASCOE, W.J. FINK, R.A. ROBERGS, S.I. BARR, and D. PEARSON. Impaired muscle glycogen resynthesis after eccentric exercise. *J Appl Physiol* 69:46-50, 1990.
26. COSTILL, D.L., W.M. SHERMAN, W.J. FINK, C. MARESH, M. WITTEN, and J.M. MILLER. The role of dietary carbohydrates in muscle glycogen resynthesis after strenuous running. *Am J Clin Nutr* 34:1831-1836, 1981.
27. COYLE, E.F. Physical activity as a metabolic stressor. *Am J Clin Nutr* 72:512S-520S, 2000.
28. COYLE, E.F. Substrate utilization during exercise in active people. *Am J Clin Nutr* 61:968S-979S, 1995.
29. COYLE, E.F. Timing and method of increased carbohydrate intake to cope with heavy training, competition and recovery. *J Sports Sci* 9(Spec No):29-51, discussion 51-22, 1991.
30. DAHLSTEDT, A.J., A. KATZ, B. WIERINGA, and H. WESTERBLAD. Is creatine kinase responsible for fatigue? Studies of isolated skeletal muscle deficient in creatine kinase. *FASEB J* 14:982-990, 2000.
31. DAL MONTE, A. *The functional values of sport*. Firente: Sansoni, 1983.
32. DAVIS, J.M. Central and peripheral factors in fatigue. *J Sports Sci* 13(Spec No):S49-S53, 1995.
33. DAVIS, J.M., Z. ZHAO, H.S. STOCK, K.A. MEHL, J. BUGGY, and G.A. HAND. Central nervous system effects of caffeine and adenosine on fatigue. *Am J Physiol Regul Integr Comp Physiol* 284:R399-R404, 2003.
34. DI PRAMPERO, P.E., L. PEETERS, and R. MARGARIA. Alactic O_2 debt and lactic acid production after exhausting exercise in man. *J Appl Physiol* 34:628-632, 1973.
35. DUMKE, C.L., D.W. BROCK, B.H. HELMS, and G.G. HAFF. Heart rate at lactate threshold and cycling time trials. *J Strength Cond Res* 20:601-607, 2006.
36. DUNLAVY, J.K., W.A. SANDS, J.R. MCNEAL, M.H. STONE, S.A. SMITH, M. JEMNI, and G.G. HAFF. Strength performance assessment in a simulated men's gymnastics still rings cross. *J. Sports. Sci. Medicine* 6:93-97, 2007.
37. EDGE, J., D. BISHOP, C. GOODMAN, and B. DAWSON. Effects of high- and moderate-intensity training on metabolism and repeated sprints. *Med Sci Sports Exerc* 37:1975-1982, 2005.
38. ENDEMANN, F. Teaching Throwing Events. In: *The Throws: Contemporary Theory, Technique, and Training*. J. Jarver, ed. Mountain View, CA: Tafnews Press, 2000. pp. 11-14.
39. ESFARJANI, F., and P.B. LAURSEN. Manipulating high-intensity interval training: effects on VO_{2max}, the lactate threshold and 3000 m running performance in moderately trained males. *J Sci Med Sport* 10:27-35, 2007.
40. FEBBRAIO, M.A., and J. DANCEY. Skeletal muscle energy metabolism during prolonged, fatiguing exercise. *J Appl Physiol* 87:2341-2347, 1999.
41. FRY, A.C. The role of training intensity in resistance exercise overtraining and overreaching. In: *Overtraining in Sport*. R.B. Kreider, A.C. Fry, and M.L. O'Toole, eds. Champaign, IL: Human Kinetics, 1998, pp. 107-127.
42. FRY, A.C., and W.J. KRAEMER. Resistance exercise overtraining and overreaching: neuroendocrine responses. *Sports Med* 23:106-129, 1997.
43. FRY, A.C., W.J. KRAEMER, M.H. STONE, B.J. WARREN, S.J. FLECK, J.T. KEARNEY, and S.E. GORDON. Endocrine responses to overreaching before and after 1 year of weightlifting. *Can J Appl Physiol* 19:400-410, 1994.
44. FRY, A.C., W.J. KRAEMER, F. VAN BORSELEN, J.M. LYNCH, J.L. MARSIT, E.P. ROY, N.T. TRIPLETT, and H.G. KNUTTGEN. Performance decrements with high-intensity resistance exercise overtraining. *Med Sci Sports Exerc* 26:1165-1173, 1994.
45. FRY, A.C., B.K. SCHILLING, L.W. WEISS, and L.Z. CHIU. Beta2-Adrenergic receptor down-regulation and performance decrements during high-intensity resistance exercise overtraining. *J Appl Physiol* 101:1664-1672, 2006.
46. GALLIVEN, E.A., A. SINGH, D. MICHELSON, S. BINA, P.W. GOLD, and P.A. DEUSTER. Hormonal and metabolic responses to exercise across time of day and menstrual cycle phase. *J Appl Physiol* 83:1822-1831, 1997.
47. GARCIA-LOPEZ, D., J.A. DE PAZ, R. JIMENEZ-JIMENEZ, G. BRESCIANI, F. DE SOUZA-TEIXEIRA, J.A. HERRERO, I. ALVEAR-ORDENES, and J. GONZALEZ-GALLEGO. Early explosive force reduction associated with exercise-induced muscle damage. *J Physiol Biochem* 62:163-169, 2006.
48. GARRANDES, F., S.S. COLSON, M. PENSINI, and P. LEGROS. Time course of mechanical and neuromuscular characteristics of cyclists and triathletes during a fatiguing exercise. *Int J Sports Med* 28:148-156, 2007.
49. GARRANDES, F., S.S. COLSON, M. PENSINI, O. SEYNNES, and P. LEGROS. Neuromuscular fatigue profile in endurance-trained and power-trained athletes. *Med Sci Sports Exerc* 39:149-158, 2007.
50. GILLAM, G.M. Effects of frequency of weight training on muscle strength enhancement. *J Sports Med* 21:432-436, 1981.
51. GOLLNICK, P.D., R.B. ARMSTRONG, B. SALTIN, C.W.T. SAUBERT, W.L. SEMBROWICH, and R.E. SHEPHERD. Effect of training on enzyme activity and fiber composition of human skeletal muscle. *J Appl Physiol* 34:107-111, 1973.

52. GOTO, K., M. HIGASHIYAMA, N. ISHII, and K. TAKAMATSU. Prior endurance exercise attenuates growth hormone response to subsequent resistance exercise. *Eur J Appl Physiol* 94:333-338, 2005.

53. GRANTIN, K. Contributions regarding the systematization of physical exercises. *Theory and Practice of Physical Culture* 9:27-37, 1940.

54. GUEZENNEC, Y., L. LEGER, F. LHOSTE, M. AYMONOD, and P.C. PESQUIES. Hormone and metabolite response to weight-lifting training sessions. *Int J Sports Med* 7:100-105, 1986.

55. HAFF, G.G., A.J. KOCH, J.A. POTTEIGER, K.E. KUPHAL, L.M. MAGEE, S.B. GREEN, and J.J. JAKICIC. Carbohydrate supplementation attenuates muscle glycogen loss during acute bouts of resistance exercise. *Int J Sport Nutr Exerc Metab* 10:326-339, 2000.

56. HAFF, G.G., M.J. LEHMKUHL, L.B. MCCOY, and M.H. STONE. Carbohydrate supplementation and resistance training. *J Strength Cond Res* 17:187-196, 2003.

57. HAFF, G.G., and A. WHITLEY. Low-carbohydrate diets and high-intensity anaerobic exercise. *Strength Cond* 24:42-53, 2002.

58. HALSON, S.L., M.W. BRIDGE, R. MEEUSEN, B. BUSSCHAERT, M. GLEESON, D.A. JONES, and A.E. JEUKENDRUP. Time course of performance changes and fatigue markers during intensified training in trained cyclists. *J Appl Physiol* 93:947-956, 2002.

59. HARRE, D. *Principles of sports training.* Berlin, Germany: Democratic Republic: Sportverlag, 1982.

60. HARRIS, R.C., R.H. EDWARDS, E. HULTMAN, L.O. NORDESJO, B. NYLIND, and K. SAHLIN. The time course of phosphorylcreatine resynthesis during recovery of the quadriceps muscle in man. *Pflugers Arch* 367:137-142, 1976.

61. HEIDT, R.S., JR., L.M. SWEETERMAN, R.L. CARLONAS, J.A. TRAUB, and F.X. TEKULVE. Avoidance of soccer injuries with preseason conditioning. *Am J Sports Med* 28:659-662, 2000.

62. HEPBURN, D., and R.J. MAUGHAN. Glycogen availability as a limiting factor in performance of isometric exercise. *J Physiol* 342:52P-53P, 1982.

63. HERMANSEN, L., and I. STENSVOLD. Production and removal of lactate during exercise in man. *Acta Physiol Scand* 86:191-201, 1972.

64. HIRVONEN, J., S. REHUNEN, H. RUSKO, and M. HARKONEN. Breakdown of high-energy phosphate compounds and lactate accumulation during short supramaximal exercise. *Eur J Appl Physiol* 56:253-259, 1987.

65. HULTMAN, E., J. BERGSTROM, and N.M. ANDERSON. Breakdown and resynthesis of phosphorylcreatine and adenosine triphosphate in connection with muscular work in man. *Scand J Clin Lab Invest* 19:56-66, 1967.

66. HULTMAN, E., and H. SJØHOLM. Biochemical causes of fatigue. In: *Human Muscle Power.* N.L. Jones, ed. Champaign, IL: Human Kinetics, 1986, pp. 343-363.

67. IMPELLIZZERI, F., A. SASSI, M. RODRIGUEZ-ALONSO, P. MOGNONI, and S. MARCORA. Exercise intensity during off-road cycling competitions. *Med Sci Sports Exerc* 34:1808-1813, 2002.

68. IVY, J.L., A.L. KATZ, C.L. CUTLER, W.M. SHERMAN, and E.F. COYLE. Muscle glycogen synthesis after exercise: effect of time of carbohydrate ingestion. *J Appl Physiol* 64:1480-1485, 1988.

69. IZQUIERDO, M., J. IBANEZ, J.J. GONZALEZ-BADILLO, K. HÄKKINEN, N.A. RATAMESS, W.J. KRAEMER, D.N. FRENCH, J. ESLAVA, A. ALTADILL, X. ASIAIN, and E.M. GOROSTIAGA. Differential effects of strength training leading to failure versus not to failure on hormonal responses, strength, and muscle power gains. *J Appl Physiol* 100:1647-1656, 2006.

70. JACOBS, I. Lactate, muscle glycogen and exercise performance in man. *Acta Physiol Scand Suppl* 495:1-35, 1981.

71. JAMURTAS, A.Z., Y. KOUTEDAKIS, V. PASCHALIS, T. TOFAS, C. YFANTI, A. TSIOKANOS, G. KOUKOULIS, D. KOURETAS, and D. LOUPOS. The effects of a single bout of exercise on resting energy expenditure and respiratory exchange ratio. *Eur J Appl Physiol* 92:393-398, 2004.

72. KARLSSON, J. Lactate in working muscles after prolonged exercise. *Acta Physiol Scand* 82:123-130, 1971.

73. KARLSSON, J., L.O. NORDESJÖ, L. JORFELDT, and B. SALTIN. Muscle lactate, ATP, and CP levels during exercise after physical training in man. *J Appl Physiol* 33:199-203, 1972.

74. KARLSSON, J., and B. OLLANDER. Muscle metabolites with exhaustive static exercise of different duration. *Acta Physiol Scand* 86:309-314, 1972.

75. KJAER, M., B. KIENS, M. HARGREAVES, and E.A. RICHTER. Influence of active muscle mass on glucose homeostasis during exercise in humans. *J Appl Physiol* 71:552-557, 1991.

76. KRAEMER, W.J., B.J. NOBLE, M.J. CLARK, and B.W. CULVER. Physiologic responses to heavy-resistance exercise with very short rest periods. *Int J Sports Med* 8:247-252, 1987.

77. LAFORGIA, J., R.T. WITHERS, and C.J. GORE. Effects of exercise intensity and duration on the excess post-exercise oxygen consumption. *J Sports Sci* 24:1247-1264, 2006.

78. LAURSEN, P.B., and D.G. JENKINS. The scientific basis for high-intensity interval training: optimising training programmes and maximising performance in highly trained endurance athletes. *Sports Med* 32:53-73, 2002.

79. LAURSEN, P.B., C.M. SHING, J.M. PEAKE, J.S. COOMBES, and D.G. JENKINS. Interval training

program optimization in highly trained endurance cyclists. *Med Sci Sports Exerc* 34:1801-1807, 2002.
80. LEBON, V., S. DUFOUR, K.F. PETERSEN, J. REN, B.M. JUCKER, L.A. SLEZAK, G.W. CLINE, D.L. ROTHMAN, and G.I. SHULMAN. Effect of triiodothyronine on mitochondrial energy coupling in human skeletal muscle. *J Clin Invest* 108:733-737, 2001.
81. MACDOUGALL, J.D., M.J. GIBALA, M.A. TARNOPOLSKY, J.R. MACDONALD, S.A. INTERISANO, and K.E. YARASHESKI. The time course for elevated muscle protein synthesis following heavy resistance exercise. *Can J Appl Physiol* 20:480-486, 1995.
82. MACDOUGALL, J.D., A.L. HICKS, J.R. MACDONALD, R.S. MCKELVIE, H.J. GREEN, and K.M. SMITH. Muscle performance and enzymatic adaptations to sprint interval training. *J Appl Physiol* 84:2138-2142, 1998.
83. MACDOUGALL, J.D., S. RAY, D.G. SALE, N. MCCARTNEY, P. LEE, and S. GARNER. Muscle substrate utilization and lactate production during weightlifting. *Can J Appl Physiol* 24:209-215, 1999.
84. MACINTOSH, B.R., and D.E. RASSIER. What is fatigue? *Can J Appl Physiol* 27:42-55, 2002.
85. MACINTYRE, D.L., S. SORICHTER, J. MAIR, A. BERG, and D.C. MCKENZIE. Markers of inflammation and myofibrillar proteins following eccentric exercise in humans. *Eur J Appl Physiol* 84:180-186, 2001.
86. MATHEWS, D., and E. FOX. *The Physiological Basis of Physical Education and Athletics*. Philadelphia: Saunders, 1976.
87. MAUGHAN, R., and M. GLEESON. *The Biochemical Basis of Sports Performance*. New York: Oxford University Press, 2004.
88. MCARDLE, W.D., F.I. KATCH, and V.L. KATCH. *Exercise Physiology: Energy, Nutrition, and Human Performance*. 6th ed. Baltimore: Lippincott, Williams & Wilkins, 2007.
89. MCCANN, D.J., P.A. MOLE, and J.R. CATON. Phosphocreatine kinetics in humans during exercise and recovery. *Med Sci Sports Exerc* 27:378-389, 1995.
90. MCMILLAN, J.L., M.H. STONE, J. SARTIN, R. KEITH, D. MARPLE, C. BROWN, and R.D. LEWIS. 20-hour physiological responses to a single weight-training session. *J Strength Cond Res* 7:9-21, 1993.
91. MELBY, C., C. SCHOLL, G. EDWARDS, and R. BULLOUGH. Effect of acute resistance exercise on postexercise energy expenditure and resting metabolic rate. *J Appl Physiol* 75:1847-1853, 1993.
92. MICHAUT, A., M. POUSSON, G. MILLET, J. BELLEVILLE, and J. VAN HOECKE. Maximal voluntary eccentric, isometric and concentric torque recovery following a concentric isokinetic exercise. *Int J Sports Med* 24:51-56, 2003.
92b. NEWSHOLME, E., A. LEECH, and G. DUESTER. *Keep on Running: The Science of Training and Performance*. West Sussex, UK: Wiley, 1994.
93. NICOL, C., J. AVELA, and P.V. KOMI. The stretch-shortening cycle: a model to study naturally occurring neuromuscular fatigue. *Sports Med* 36:977-999, 2006.
94. NIEMAN, D.C., and B.K. PEDERSEN. Exercise and immune function: recent developments. *Sports Med* 27:73-80, 1999.
95. PADILLA, S., I. MUJIKA, F. ANGULO, and J.J. GOIRIENA. Scientific approach to the 1-h cycling world record: a case study. *J Appl Physiol* 89:1522-1527, 2000.
96. PAROLIN, M.L., A. CHESLEY, M.P. MATSOS, L.L. SPRIET, N.L. JONES, and G.J. HEIGENHAUSER. Regulation of skeletal muscle glycogen phosphorylase and PDH during maximal intermittent exercise. *Am J Physiol* 277:E890-E900, 1999.
97. PETERSON, M.D., M.R. RHEA, and B.A. ALVAR. Applications of the dose-response for muscular strength development: a review of meta-analytic efficacy and reliability for designing training prescription. *J Strength Cond Res* 19:950-958, 2005.
98. PINCIVERO, D.M., and T.O. BOMPA. A physiological review of American football. *Sports Med* 23:247-260, 1997.
99. POWERS, S.K., and E.T. HOWLEY. *Exercise Physiology: Theory and Application to Fitness and Performance*. 5th ed. New York: McGraw-Hill, 2004.
100. PRATLEY, R., B. NICKLAS, M. RUBIN, J. MILLER, A. SMITH, M. SMITH, B. HURLEY, and A. GOLDBERG. Strength training increases resting metabolic rate and norepinephrine levels in healthy 50- to 65-yr-old men. *J Appl Physiol* 76:133-137, 1994.
101. RAHNAMA, N., T. REILLY, and A. LEES. Injury risk associated with playing actions during competitive soccer. *Br J Sports Med* 36:354-359, 2002.
102. SELYE, H. *The Stress of Life*. New York: McGraw-Hill, 1956.
103. SHERMAN, W.M. Carbohydrates, muscle glycogen, and muscle glycogen supercompensation. In: *Ergogenic Aids in Sport*. M.H. Williams, ed. Champaign IL: Human Kinetics, 1983, pp. 3-26.
104. SHERMAN, W.M., and G.S. WIMER. Insufficient dietary carbohydrate during training: does it impair athletic performance? *Int J Sport Nutr* 1:28-44, 1991.
105. SIFF, M.C., and Y.U. VERKHOSHANSKY. *Supertraining*. Denver, CO: Supertraining International, 1999.
106. STEPTO, N.K., D.T. MARTIN, K.E. FALLON, and J.A. HAWLEY. Metabolic demands of intense aer-

obic interval training in competitive cyclists. *Med Sci Sports Exerc* 33:303-310, 2001.

107. STONE, M.H., M.E. STONE, and W.A. SANDS. *Principles and Practice of Resistance Training.* Champaign, IL: Human Kinetics, 2007.

108. STONE, M.H., W.A. SANDS, and M.E. STONE. The downfall of sports science in the United States. *Strength and Cond J* 26:72-75, 2004.

109. SUH, S.H., I.Y. PAIK, and K. JACOBS. Regulation of blood glucose homeostasis during prolonged exercise. *Mol Cells* 23:272-279, 2007.

110. TESCH, P. Muscle fatigue in man: with special reference to lactate accumulation during short term intense exercise. *Acta Physiol Scand Suppl* 480:1-40, 1980.

111. TESCH, P.A., L.L. PLOUTZ-SNYDER, L. YSTRÖM, M. CASTRO, and G. DUDLEY. Skeletal muscle glycogen loss evoked by resistance exercise. *J Strength Cond Res* 12:67-73, 1998.

112. TOMLIN, D.L., and H.A. WENGER. The relationship between aerobic fitness and recovery from high intensity intermittent exercise. *Sports Med* 31:1-11, 2001.

113. K.A. VAN SOMEREN. The physiology of anaerobic endurance training. In: *The Physiology of Training.* G. Whyte, ed. Oxford, UK: Elsevier, 2006, pp. 88.

114. WADLEY, G., and P. LE ROSSIGNOL. The relationship between repeated sprint ability and the aerobic and anaerobic energy systems. *J Sci Med Sport* 1:100-110, 1998.

115. WESTERBLAD, H., D.G. ALLEN, and J. LANNERGREN. Muscle fatigue: lactic acid or inorganic phosphate the major cause? *News Physiol Sci* 17:17-21, 2002.

116. YAKOVLEV, N. *Sports Biochemistry.* Leipzig: Deutche Hochschule für, Körperkultur, 1967.

117. YASPELKIS, B.B.D., J.G. PATTERSON, P.A. ANDERLA, Z. DING, and J.L. IVY. Carbohydrate supplementation spares muscle glycogen during variable-intensity exercise. *J Appl Physiol* 75:1477-1485, 1993.

118. ZAINUDDIN, Z., P. SACCO, M. NEWTON, and K. NOSAKA. Light concentric exercise has a temporarily analgesic effect on delayed-onset muscle soreness, but no effect on recovery from eccentric exercise. *Appl Physiol Nutr Metab* 31:126-134, 2006.

119. ZATSIORSKY, V.M., and W.J. KRAEMER. *Science and Practice of Strength Training.* 2nd ed. Champaign, IL: Human Kinetics, 2006.

Chapter 2

1. ABERNETHY, P.J., J. JURIMAE, P.A. LOGAN, A.W. TAYLOR, and R.E. THAYER. Acute and chronic response of skeletal muscle to resistance exercise. *Sports Med* 17:22-38, 1994.

2. ABERNETHY, P.J., R. THAYER, and A.W. TAYLOR. Acute and chronic responses of skeletal muscle to endurance and sprint exercise: a review. *Sports Med* 10:365-389, 1990.

3. ARMSTRONG, N., B.J. KIRBY, A.M. MCMANUS, and J.R. WELSMAN. Aerobic fitness of prepubescent children. *Ann Hum Biol* 22:427-441, 1995.

4. ATHERTON, P.J., J. BABRAJ, K. SMITH, J. SINGH, M.J. RENNIE, and H. WACKERHAGE. Selective activation of AMPK-PGC-1alpha or PKB-TSC2-mTOR signaling can explain specific adaptive responses to endurance or resistance training-like electrical muscle stimulation. *FASEB J* 19:786-788, 2005.

5. AVALOS, M., P. HELLARD, and J.C. CHATARD. Modeling the training-performance relationship using a mixed model in elite swimmers. *Med Sci Sports Exerc* 35:838-846, 2003.

6. BAAR, K. Training for endurance and strength: lessons from cell signaling. *Med Sci Sports Exerc* 38:1939-1944, 2006.

7. BAAR, K., G. NADER, and S. BODINE. Resistance exercise, muscle loading/unloading and the control of muscle mass. *Essays Biochem* 42:61-74, 2006.

8. BAKER, D. Cycle-length variants in periodized strength/power training. *Strength Cond* 29:10-17, 2007.

9. BALYI, I., and A. HAMILTON. Long-term athlete development: trainability in childhood and adolescence. *Olympic Coach* 16:4-9, 1993.

10. BANISTER, E.W., T.W. CALVERT, M.V. SAVAGE, and A. BACK. A system model of training for athletic performance. *Aus J Sports Med* 7:170-176, 1975.

11. BILLAT, L.V., J.P. KORALSZTEIN, and R.H. MORTON. Time in human endurance models: from empirical models to physiological models. *Sports Med* 27:359-379, 1999.

11b. BOMPA, T.O. Antrenamentul in perioada pregatitoare [Training methodology during the preparatory phase]. *Caiet pentru sporturi nautice* 3:22-28, 1956.

11c. BOMPA, T.O. *Theory and Methodology of Training.* Dubuque, Iowa: Kendall/Hunt Publishing Company, 1983.

11d. BOMPA, T.O. *Periodization of Strength: The New Wave in Strength Training.* Toronto: Veritas, 1993.

12. BREWER, C. Athlete development: principles into practice. In: *SPEC: Coaches and Sports Sciences Symposium.* Johnson City, TN: East Tennessee State University, 2007, pp. 1-44.

13. BRUIN, G., H. KUIPERS, H.A. KEIZER, and G.J. VANDER VUSSE. Adaptation and overtraining in horses subjected to increasing training loads. *J Appl Physiol* 76:1908-1913, 1994.

14. BUSHMAN, B., G. MASTERSON, and J. NELSEN. Anaerobic power performance and the menstrual

cycle: eumenorrheic and oral contraceptive users. *J Sports Med Phys Fitness* 46:132-137, 2006.
15. CAINE, D.J., and J. BROEKHOFF. Maturity assessment: available preventive measure against physical and psychological insult to the young athlete? *Phys Sportsmed.* 15:70, 1987.
16. CALVERT, T.W., E.W. BANISTER, and M.V. SAVAGE. A systems model of the effects of training on physical performance. *SMS Systems, Man, and Cybernetics* 2:94-102, 1976.
17. CAO, W. Training differences between males and females. In: *Proceedings of the Weightlifting Symposium: Ancient Olympia, Greece*, A. Lukácsfalvi and F. Takács, eds. International Weightlifting Federation: Budapest, Hungary.1993, pp. 97-101.
18. CARLSON, R. The socialization of elite tennis players in Sweden: an analysis of the players' background and development. *Sociol Sport J* 5:241-256, 1988.
19. CHEUVRONT, S.N., R. CARTER, K.C. DERUISSEAU, and R.J. MOFFATT. Running performance differences between men and women: an update. *Sports Med* 35:1017-1024, 2005.
20. COAST, J.R., J.S. BLEVINS, and B.A. WILSON. Do gender differences in running performance disappear with distance? *Can J Appl Physiol* 29:139-145, 2004.
21. COFFEY, V.G., and J.A. HAWLEY. The molecular bases of training adaptation. *Sports Med* 37:737-763, 2007.
22. COLIBABA, E.D., and I. BOTA. *Jocurile Sportive: Teoria si Medodica.* Bucuresti: Editura Aldin, 1998.
23. COUTTS, A.J., L.K. WALLACE, and K.M. SLATTERY. Monitoring changes in performance, physiology, biochemistry, and psychology during overreaching and recovery in triathletes. *Int J Sports Med* 28:125-134, 2007.
24. DENCKER, M., O. THORSSON, M.K. KARLSSON, C. LINDEN, S. EIBERG, P. WOLLMER, and L.B. ANDERSEN. Gender differences and determinants of aerobic fitness in children aged 8-11 years. *Eur J Appl Physiol* 99:19-26, 2007.
25. DRABIK, J. *Children and Sports Training.* Island Pond, VT: Stadion, 1995.
26. FAIGENBAUM, A.D. Strength training for children and adolescents. *Clin Sports Med* 19:593-619, 2000.
27. FAIGENBAUM, A.D., and W.L. WESTCOTT. *Strength and Power for Young Athletes.* Champaign, IL: Human Kinetics, 2000.
28. FLECK, S., and W.J. KRAEMER. *Designing Resistance Training Programs.* 3rd ed. Champaign, IL: Human Kinetics, 2004.
29. FORD, L.E., A.J. DETTERLINE, K.K. HO, and W. CAO. Gender- and height-related limits of muscle strength in world weightlifting champions. *J Appl Physiol* 89:1061-1064, 2000.
30. FOSTER, C. Monitoring training in athletes with reference to overtraining syndrome. *Med Sci Sports Exerc* 30:1164-1168, 1998.
31. FRY, A.C. The role of training intensity in resistance exercise overtraining and overreaching. In: *Overtraining in Sport.* R.B. Kreider, A.C. Fry, and M.L. O'Toole, eds. Champaign, IL: Human Kinetics, 1998, pp. 107-127.
32. FRY, A.C., and W.J. KRAEMER. Resistance exercise overtraining and overreaching: neuroendocrine responses. *Sports Med* 23:106-129, 1997.
33. FRY, A.C., W.J. KRAEMER, M.H. STONE, L.P. KOZIRIS, J.T. THRUSH, and S.J. FLECK. Relationships between serum testosterone, cortisol, and weightlifting performance. *J Strength Cond Res.* 14:338-343, 2000.
34. FRY, A.C., W.J. KRAEMER, M.H. STONE, B.J. WARREN, S.J. FLECK, J.T. KEARNEY, and S.E. GORDON. Endocrine responses to overreaching before and after 1 year of weightlifting. *Can J Appl Physiol* 19:400-410, 1994.
35. FUSTER, V., A. JEREZ, and A. ORTEGA. Anthropometry and strength relationship: male-female differences. *Anthropol Anz* 56:49-56, 1998.
36. GARHAMMER, J. A comparison of maximal power outputs between elite male and female weightlifters in competition. *Int J Sport Biomech* 7:3-11, 1991.
37. GRGANTOV, Z., D. NEDOVIC, and R. KATIC. Integration of technical and situation efficacy into the morphological system in young female volleyball players. *Coll Antropol* 31:267-273, 2007.
38. GURD, B., and P. KLENTROU. Physical and pubertal development in young male gymnasts. *J Appl Physiol* 95:1011-1015, 2003.
39. HAFF, G.G., M. BURGENER, A.D. FAIGENBAUM, J.L. KILGORE, M.E. LAVALLE, M. NITKA, M. RIPPETOE, and C. PROULX. Roundtable discussion: youth resistance training. *Strength Cond J* 25:49-64, 2003.
40. HÄKKINEN, K. Neuromuscular and hormonal adaptations during strength and power training: a review. *J Sports Med Phys Fitness* 29:9-26, 1989.
41. HÄKKINEN, K., and M. KALLINEN. Distribution of strength training volume into one or two daily sessions and neuromuscular adaptations in female athletes. *Electromyogr Clin Neurophysiol* 34:117-124, 1994.
42. HÄKKINEN, K., K.L. KESKINEN, M. ALEN, P.V. KOMI, and H. KAUHANEN. Serum hormone concentrations during prolonged training in elite endurance-trained and strength-trained athletes. *Eur J Appl Physiol* 59:233-238, 1989.
43. HÄKKINEN, K., A. PAKARINEN, M. ALEN, H. KAUHANEN, and P.V. KOMI. Daily hormonal and neuromuscular responses to intensive strength training in 1 week. *Int J Sports Med* 9:422-428, 1988.

44. HÄKKINEN, K., A. PAKARINEN, M. ALEN, H. KAUHANEN, and P.V. KOMI. Neuromuscular and hormonal adaptations in athletes to strength training in two years. *J Appl Physiol* 65:2406-2412, 1988.

45. HALSON, S.L., M.W. BRIDGE, R. MEEUSEN, B. BUSSCHAERT, M. GLEESON, D.A. JONES, and A.E. JEUKENDRUP. Time course of performance changes and fatigue markers during intensified training in trained cyclists. *J Appl Physiol* 93:947-956, 2002.

46. HARRE, D. *Trainingslehre*. Berlin, Germany: Sportverlag, 1982.

47. HARRIS, G.R., M.H. STONE, H.S. O'BRYANT, C.M. PROULX, and R.L. JOHNSON. Short-term performance effects of high power, high force, or combined weight-training methods. *J Strength Cond Res* 14:14-20, 2000.

48. HAWLEY, J.A. Adaptations of skeletal muscle to prolonged, intense endurance training. *Clin Exp Pharmacol Physiol* 29:218-222, 2002.

49. HELLARD, P., M. AVALOS, L. LACOSTE, F. BARALE, J.C. CHATARD, and G.P. MILLET. Assessing the limitations of the Banister model in monitoring training. *J Sports Sci* 24:509-520, 2006.

50. HELLEBRANDT, F., and S. HOUTZ. Mechanisms of muscle training in man: experimental demonstration of the overload principle. *Phys Ther Rev* 36:371-383, 1956.

51. HODGES, N.J., S. HAYES, R.R. HORN, and A.M. WILLIAMS. Changes in coordination, control and outcome as a result of extended practice on a novel motor skill. *Ergonomics* 48:1672-1685, 2005.

52. HOFFMAN, J.R., M. WENDELL, J. COOPER, and J. KANG. Comparison between linear and non-linear in-season training programs in freshman football players. *J Strength Cond Res* 17:561-565, 2003.

53. JANSE DE JONGE, X.A. Effects of the menstrual cycle on exercise performance. *Sports Med* 33:833-851, 2003.

54. JANSSEN, I., S.B. HEYMSFIELD, Z.M. WANG, and R. ROSS. Skeletal muscle mass and distribution in 468 men and women aged 18-88 yr. *J Appl Physiol* 89:81-88, 2000.

55. KALLINEN, M., and A. MARKKU. Aging, physical activity and sports injuries: an overview of common sports injuries in the elderly. *Sports Med* 20:41-52, 1995.

56. KATIC, R., M. CAVALA, and V. SRHOJ. Biomotor structures in elite female handball players. *Coll Antropol* 31:795-801, 2007.

57. KRAEMER, W.J., S.A. MAZZETTI, B.C. NINDL, L.A. GOTSHALK, J.S. VOLEK, J.A. BUSH, J.O. MARX, K. DOHI, A.L. GOMEZ, M. MILES, S.J. FLECK, R.U. NEWTON, and K. HÄKKINEN. Effect of resistance training on women's strength/power and occupational performances. *Med Sci Sports Exerc* 33:1011-1025, 2001.

58. KURZ, T. *Science of Sports Training*. 2nd ed. Island Pond, VT: Stadion, 2001.

59. LANGE, L. *Uber Funktionelle Anpassung*. Berlin, Germany: Springer Verlag, 1919.

60. LAUGHLIN, N.T., and P.L. BUSK. Relationships between selected muscle endurance tasks and gender. *J Strength Cond Res* 21:400-404, 2007.

61. MACKINNON, L.T., and S.L. HOOPER. Overtraining and overreaching: causes effects and prevention. In: *Exercise and Sport Science*. W.E. Garrett and D.T. Kirkendall, eds. Philadelphia: Lippincott Williams & Wilkins, 2000, pp. 487-498.

62. MATVEYEV, L.P. *Fundamentals of Sports Training*. Moscow: Fizkultua i Sport, 1977.

63. MATVEYEV, L.P. *Periodisterung Des Sportlichen Trainings*. Moscow: Fizkultura i Sport, 1972.

64. MAUD, P.J., and B.B. SHULTZ. Gender comparisons in anaerobic power and anaerobic capacity tests. *Br J Sports Med* 20:51-54, 1986.

65. MERO, A., H. KAUHANEN, E. PELTOLA, T. VUORIMAA, and P.V. KOMI. Physiological performance capacity in different prepubescent athletic groups. *J Sports Med Phys Fitness* 30:57-66, 1990.

66. MILLER, A.E., J.D. MACDOUGALL, M.A. TARNOPOLSKY, and D.G. SALE. Gender differences in strength and muscle fiber characteristics. *Eur J Appl Physiol Occup Physiol* 66:254-262, 1993.

67. NADER, G.A. Concurrent strength and endurance training: from molecules to man. *Med Sci Sports Exerc* 38:1965-1970, 2006.

68. NADER, G.A., T.J. MCLOUGHLIN, and K.A. ESSER. mTOR function in skeletal muscle hypertrophy: increased ribosomal RNA via cell cycle regulators. *Am J Physiol Cell Physiol* 289:C1457-C1465, 2005.

69. O'TOOLE, M.L. Overreaching and overtraining in endurance athletes. In: *Overtraining in Sport*. R.B. Kreider, A.C. Fry, and M.L. O'Toole, eds. Champaign, IL: Human Kinetics, 1998, pp. 3-18.

70. PLISK, S.S., and V. GAMBETTA. Tactical metabolic training: part 1. *Strength Cond* 19:44-53, 1997.

71. PLISK, S.S., and M.H. STONE. Periodization strategies. *Strength Cond* 25:19-37, 2003.

72. POLIQUIN, C. Five steps to increasing the effectiveness of your strength training program. *NSCA J.* 10:34-39, 1988.

73. RATEL, S., N. LAZAAR, C.A. WILLIAMS, M. BEDU, and P. DUCHE. Age differences in human skeletal muscle fatigue during high-intensity intermittent exercise. *Acta Paediatr* 92:1248-1254, 2003.

74. RHEA, M.R., R.L. HUNTER, and T.J. HUNTER. Competition modeling of American football: observational data and implications for high school, collegiate, and professional player conditioning. *J Strength Cond Res* 20:58-61, 2006.
75. RILLING, J.K., C.M. WORTHMAN, B.C. CAMPBELL, J.F. STALLINGS, and M. MBIZVA. Ratios of plasma and salivary testosterone throughout puberty: production versus bioavailability. *Steroids* 61:374-378, 1996.
76. ROBAZZA, C., L. BORTOLI, and Y. HANIN. Perceived effects of emotion intensity on athletic performance: a contingency-based individualized approach. *Res Q Exerc Sport* 77:372-385, 2006.
77. SATORI, J., and P. TSCHIENE. The further development of training theory: new elements and tendencies. *Sci Period Res Technol Sport* 8:Physical Training 8(4):W-1. 1988.
78. SCHMOLINSKY, G. *Track and Field: The East German Textbook of Athletics*. Toronto, ON, Canada: Sports Book Publisher, 2004.
79. SEILER, K.S., and G.O. KJERLAND. Quantifying training intensity distribution in elite endurance athletes: is there evidence for an "optimal" distribution? *Scand J Med Sci Sports* 16:49-56, 2006.
80. SEILER, S., J.J. DE KONING, and C. FOSTER. The fall and rise of the gender difference in elite anaerobic performance 1952-2006. *Med Sci Sports Exerc* 39:534-540, 2007.
81. SHARP, M.A., J.F. PATTON, J.J. KNAPIK, K. HAURET, R.P. MELLO, M. ITO, and P.N. FRYKMAN. Comparison of the physical fitness of men and women entering the U.S. Army: 1978-1998. *Med Sci Sports Exerc* 34:356-363, 2002.
82. SIFF, M.C., and Y.U. VERKHOSHANSKY. *Supertraining*. Denver, CO: Supertraining International, 1999.
83. SMITH, D.J. A framework for understanding the training process leading to elite performance. *Sports Med* 33:1103-1126, 2003.
84. STEYERS, J. Liukin good at 18. www.nbcolympics.com/gymnastics/news/newsid=100218.html.
85. STONE, M.H., and A.C. FRY. Increased training volume in strength/power athletes. In: *Overtraining in Sport*. R.B. Kreider, A.C. Fry, and M.L. O'Toole, eds. Champaign, IL: Human Kinetics, 1998, pp. 87-106.
86. STONE, M.H., R. KEITH, J.T. KEARNEY, G.D. WILSON, and S. FLECK, J. Overtraining: a review of the signs and symptoms of overtraining. *J Appl Sport Sci Res* 5:35-50, 1991.
87. STONE, M.H., H. O'BRYANT, and J. GARHAMMER. A hypothetical model for strength training. *J. Sports Med* 21:342-351, 1981.
88. STONE, M.H., K. SANBORN, H.S. O'BRYANT, M. HARTMAN, M.E. STONE, C. PROULX, B. WARD, and J. HRUBY. Maximum strength-power-performance relationships in collegiate throwers. *J Strength Cond Res* 17:739-745, 2003.
89. STONE, M.H., M.E. STONE, and W.A. SANDS. *Principles and Practice of Resistance Training*. Champaign, IL: Human Kinetics, 2007.
90. SUZUKI, S., T. SATO, A. MAEDA, and Y. TAKAHASHI. Program design based on a mathematical model using rating of perceived exertion for an elite Japanese sprinter: a case study. *J Strength Cond Res* 20:36-42, 2006.
91. TANAKA, H., and D.R. SEALS. Endurance exercise performance in masters athletes: age-associated changes and underlying physiological mechanisms. *J Physiol* 586:55-63, 2008.
92. TSCHIENE, P. A necessary direction in training: the integration of biological adaptation in the training program. *Coach Sport Sci J* 1:2-14, 1995.
93. VANDERBURGH, P.M., M. KUSANO, M. SHARP, and B. NINDL. Gender differences in muscular strength: an allometric model approach. *Biomed Sci Instrum* 33:100-105, 1997.
94. VERKHOSHANSKY, Y.U. *Fundamentals of Special Strength Training in Sport*. Livonia, MI: Sportivy Press, 1986.
95. VERKHOSHANSKY, Y.U. *Programming and Organization of Training*. Moscow: Fizkultura i Sport, 1985.
96. VIRU, A. *Adaptations in Sports Training*. Boca Raton, FL: CRC Press, 1995.
97. VIRU, A., and M. VIRU. *Biochemical Monitoring of Sport Training*. Champaign, IL: Human Kinetics, 2001.
98. WERCHOSHANSKI, J. Specific training principles for power. *Mod Athlete Coach* 17:11-13, 1979.
99. WILMORE, J.H., D.L. COSTILL, and W.L. KENNEY. *Physiology of Sport and Exercise*. 4th ed. Champaign, IL: Human Kinetics, 2008.
100. ZANCHI, N.E., and A.H. LANCHA, JR. Mechanical stimuli of skeletal muscle: implications on mTOR/p70s6k and protein synthesis. *Eur J Appl Physiol* 102:253-263, 2008.
101. ZATSIORSKY, V.M. *Science and Practice of Strength Training*. Champaign, IL: Human Kinetics, 1995.
102. ZATSIORSKY, V.M., and W.J. KRAEMER. *Science and Practice of Strength Training*. 2nd ed. Champaign, IL: Human Kinetics, 2006.

Chapter 3

1. BAKER, D., and S. NANCE. The relation between running speed and measures of strength and power in professional rugby league players. *J Strength Cond Res* 13:230-235, 1999.
2. BOMPA, T.O. *Periodization: Theory and Methodology of Training*. 4th ed. Champaign, IL: Human Kinetics, 1999.

3. BOMPA, T.O. *Total training for coaching team sports*. Toronto: Sport Books Publisher, 2006, page 22.
4. BRAVO, D.F., F.M. IMPELLIZZERI, E. RAMPININI, C. CASTAGNA, D. BISHOP, and U. WISLOFF. Sprint vs. interval training in football. *Int J Sports Med* 29:668-674, 2008.
5. BRET, C., A. RAHMANI, A.B. DUFOUR, L. MESSONNIER, and J.R. LACOUR. Leg strength and stiffness as ability factors in 100 m sprint running. *J Sports Med Phys Fitness* 42:274-281, 2002.
6. BURGOMASTER, K.A., G.J. HEIGENHAUSER, and M.J. GIBALA. Effect of short-term sprint interval training on human skeletal muscle carbohydrate metabolism during exercise and time-trial performance. *J Appl Physiol* 100:2041-2047, 2006.
7. BURGOMASTER, K.A., S.C. HUGHES, G.J. HEIGENHAUSER, S.N. BRADWELL, and M.J. GIBALA. Six sessions of sprint interval training increases muscle oxidative potential and cycle endurance capacity in humans. *J Appl Physiol* 98:1985-1990, 2005.
8. CAVANAGH, P.R., and K.R. WILLIAMS. The effect of stride length variation on oxygen uptake during distance running. *Med Sci Sports Exerc* 14:30-35, 1982.
9. CHIU, L.Z., A.C. FRY, B.K. SCHILLING, E.J. JOHNSON, and L.W. WEISS. Neuromuscular fatigue and potentiation following two successive high intensity resistance exercise sessions. *Eur J Appl Physiol* 92:385-392, 2004.
10. CONLEY, D.L., and G. KRAHENBUHL. Running economy and distance running performance of highly trained athletes. *Med Sci Sports Exerc* 14:357-360, 1980.
11. CRONIN, J.B., and K.T. HANSEN. Strength and power predictors of sports speed. *J Strength Cond Res* 19:349-357, 2005.
12. CURY, F., S. BIDDLE, P. SARRAZIN, and J.P. FAMOSE. Achievement goals and perceived ability predict investment in learning a sport task. *Br J Educ Psychol* 67:293-309, 1997.
13. DALLEAU, G., A. BELLI, M. BOURDIN, and J.R. LACOUR. The spring-mass model and the energy cost of treadmill running. *Eur J Appl Physiol Occup Physiol* 77:257-263, 1998.
14. DANIELS, J.T. A physiologist's view of running economy. *Med Sci Sports Exerc* 17:332-338, 1985.
15. DUNLAVY, J.K., W.A. SANDS, J.R. MCNEAL, M.H. STONE, S.A. SMITH, M. JEMNI, and G.G. HAFF. Strength performance assessment in a simulated men's gymnastics still rings cross. *J Sports Sci Med* 6:93-97, 2007.
16. ENDEMANN, F. Teaching throwing events. In: *The Throws: Contemporary Theory, Technique, and Training*. J. Jarver, ed. Mountain View, CA: Tafnews Press, 2000, pp. 11-14.
17. FLORESCU, C., V. DUMITRESCU, and A. PREDESCU. *Metodologia Desvoltari Calitatilor Fizice* [The Methodology of Developing Physical Qualities]. Bucharest: National Sports Council, 1969.
18. GIBALA, M.J., J.P. LITTLE, M. VAN ESSEN, G.P. WILKIN, K.A. BURGOMASTER, A. SAFDAR, S. RAHA, and M.A. TARNOPOLSKY. Short-term sprint interval versus traditional endurance training: similar initial adaptations in human skeletal muscle and exercise performance. *J Physiol* 575:901-911, 2006.
19. GODFREY, R.J. Cross-training. *Sports Exercise & Injury* 4:50-56, 1998.
20. HEISE, G.D., and P.E. MARTIN. Are variations in running economy in humans associated with ground reaction force characteristics? *Eur J Appl Physiol* 84:438-442, 2001.
21. HODGES, N.J., S. HAYES, R.R. HORN, and A.M. WILLIAMS. Changes in coordination, control and outcome as a result of extended practice on a novel motor skill. *Ergonomics* 48:1672-1685, 2005.
22. HUGHES, M.D., and R.M. BARTLETT. The use of performance indicators in performance analysis. *J Sports Sci* 20:739-754, 2002.
23. KANEKO, M., A. ITO, T. FUCHIMOTO, Y. SHISHIKURA, and J. TOYOOKA. Influence of running speed on the mechanical efficiency of sprinters and distance runners. In: *Biomechanics IX-B*. D.A. Winter et al., eds. Champaign, IL: Human Kinetics, 1985, pp. 307-312.
24. LAURSEN, P.B., C.M. SHING, J.M. PEAKE, J.S. COOMBES, and D.G. JENKINS. Interval training program optimization in highly trained endurance cyclists. *Med Sci Sports Exerc* 34:1801-1807, 2002.
25. MALTSEVA, N. Instructing young throwers. In: *The Throws: Contemporary Theory, Technique, and Training*. J. Jarver, ed. Mountain View, CA: Tafnews Press, 2000, pp. 15-17.
26. MEDVEDEV, A.S. *Sistema Mnogoletnyei Trenirovki V Tyazheloi Atletikye*. Moscow: Fizkultura i Sport, 1986.
27. MORGAN, D.W., and M. CRAIB. Physiological aspects of running economy. *Med Sci Sports Exerc* 24:456-461, 1992.
28. NUMMELA, A., T. KERANEN, and L.O. MIKKELSSON. Factors related to top running speed and economy. *Int J Sports Med* 28:655-661, 2007.
29. PLISK, S.S., and V. GAMBETTA. Tactical metabolic training: part 1. *Strength Cond* 19:44-53, 1997.
30. PLISK, S.S., and M.H. STONE. Periodization strategies. *Strength Cond* 25:19-37, 2003.
31. RAGLIN, J.S. The psychology of the marathoner: of one mind and many. *Sports Med* 37:404-407, 2007.

32. ROBINSON, J.M., M.H. STONE, R.L. JOHNSON, C.M. PENLAND, B.J. WARREN, and R.D. LEWIS. Effects of different weight training exercise/rest intervals on strength, power, and high intensity exercise endurance. *J. Strength Cond Res* 9:216-221, 1995.
33. SCHMIDT, R.A., and C.A. WRISBERG. *Motor Learning and Performance*. 3rd ed. Champaign, IL: Human Kinetics, 2004.
34. SCHMOLINSKY, G. *Track and Field: The East German Textbook of Athletics*. Toronto, ON, Canada: Sports Book Publisher, 2004.
35. SIFF, M.C., and Y.U. VERKHOSHANSKY. *Supertraining*. Denver, CO: Supertraining International, 1999.
36. SINITSIN, A. A few hints for novice discus throwers. In: *The Throws: Contemporary Theory, Technique, and Training*. J. Jarver, ed. Mountain View, CA: Tafnews, 2000, pp. 95-97.
37. SMITH, D.J. A framework for understanding the training process leading to elite performance. *Sports Med* 33:1103-1126, 2003.
38. STONE, M.H., and H.O. O'BRYANT. *Weight Training: A Scientific Approach*. Edina, MN: Burgess, 1987.
39. STONE, M.H., R. KEITH, J.T. KEARNEY, G.D. WILSON, and S. FLECK, J. Overtraining: a review of the signs and symptoms of overtraining. *J Appl Sport Sci Res* 5:35-50, 1991.
40. STONE, M.H., W.A. SANDS, K.C. PIERCE, R.U. NEWTON, G.G. HAFF, and J. CARLOCK. Maximum strength and strength training: a relationship to endurance? *Strength Cond J* 28:44-53, 2006.
41. STONE, M.H., M.E. STONE, and W.A. SANDS. *Principles and Practice of Resistance Training*. Champaign, IL: Human Kinetics, 2007.
42. SUINN, R.M. Mental practice in sport psychology: where have we been, where do we go? *Clin Psychol Sci Pract* 4:189-207, 1997.
43. TAN, J.C., and M.R. YEADON. Why do high jumpers use a curved approach? *J Sport Sci* 23:775-780, 2005.
44. TEODORESCU, L., and C. FLORESCU. Some directions regarding the perfection and mastery of technique and strategy. In: *The Content and Methodology of Training*. E. Ghibu, ed. Bucharest, Hungary: Stadion, 1971, pp. 66-81.
45. VAN-YPEREN, N.W., and J.L. DUDA. Goal orientations, beliefs about success, and performance improvement among young elite Dutch soccer players. *Scand J Med Sci Sports* 9:358-364, 1999.
46. WILLIAMS, S.J., and L.R. KENDALL. A profile of sports science research (1983-2003). *J Sci Med Sport* 10:193-200, 2007.
47. ZATSIORSKY, V.M. *Science and Practice of Strength Training*. Champaign, IL: Human Kinetics, 1995.

Chapter 4

1. *2002 USA Cycling Club Coach Manual*. Colorado Springs, CO: USA Cycling, 2002.
2. ABADEJEV, I. Basic training principles for Bulgarian elite. *Int Olympic Lifter* 3:12-13, 1976.
3. ABADEJEV, I. Basic training principles for Bulgarian elite. *Canadian Weightlifting Federation Official Newsletter* 5:13-18, 1976.
4. ABADEJEV, I. Basic training principles for Bulgarian elite. *New Brunswick Weightlifting Association Newsletter* 4:19-24, 1977.
5. ABADEJEV, I. Preparation of the Bulgarian weightlifters for the Olympic Games 1984. *Australian Weightlifter* October:25-29, 1981.
6. ABADJIEV, I., and B. FARADJIEV. *Training of Weight Lifters*. Sofia, Bulgaria: Medicina i Fizkultura, 1986.
7. ACEVEDO, E.O., and A.H. GOLDFARB. Increased training intensity effects on plasma lactate, ventilatory threshold, and endurance. *Med Sci Sports Exerc* 21:563-568, 1989.
8. AJÁN, T., and L. BAROGA. *Weightlifting: Fitness for All Sports*. Budapest: International Weightlifting Federation, 1988.
9. ALLEN, H., and A.R. COGGAN. *Training and Racing with a Power Meter*. Boulder, CO: Velo Press, 2006.
10. BARNETT, A. Using recovery modalities between training sessions in elite athletes: does it help? *Sports Med* 36:781-796, 2006.
11. BEN ABDELKRIM, N., S. EL FAZAA, and J. EL ATI. Time-motion analysis and physiological data of elite under-19-year-old basketball players during competition. *Br J Sports Med* 41:69-75; discussion 75, 2007.
12. BILLAT, V.L., B. FLECHET, B. PETIT, G. MURIAUX, and J.P. KORALSZTEIN. Interval training at VO2max: effects on aerobic performance and overtraining markers. *Med Sci Sports Exerc* 31:156-163, 1999.
13. BOMPA, T.O. *Periodization: Theory and Methodology of Training*. 4th ed. Champaign, IL: Human Kinetics, 1999.
14. BOMPA, T.O., and M.C. CARRERA. *Periodization Training for Sports: Science-Based Strength and Conditioning Plans for 20 Sports*. 2nd ed. Champaign, IL: Human Kinetics, 2005.
15. BROOKS, G.A., T.D. FAHEY, T.P. WHITE, and K.M. BALDWIN. *Exercise Physiology: Human Bioenergetics and Its Application*. 3rd ed. Mountain View, CA: Mayfield, 2000.
16. BURKE, L., and V. DEAKIN. *Clincial Sports Nutrition*. Roseville, Australia: McGraw-Hill Australia, 2000.
17. COFFEY, V.G., and J.A. HAWLEY. The molecular bases of training adaptation. *Sports Med* 37:737-763, 2007.

18. CONLEY, M. Bioenergetics of exercise training. In: *Essentials of Strength Training and Conditioning.* T.R. Baechle and R.W. Earle, eds. Champaign, IL: Human Kinetics, 2000, pp. 73-90.
19. CONLEY, M.S., M.H. STONE, H.S. O'BRYANT, R.L. JOHNSON, D.R. HONEYCUTT, and T.P. HOKE. Peak power versus power at maximal oxygen uptake. In: *Proceedings of the National Strength and Conditioning Association Annual Convention,* Las Vegas, NV, 1993.
20. DEDRICK, M.E., and P.M. CLARKSON. The effects of eccentric exercise on motor performance in young and older women. *Eur J Appl Physiol Occup Physiol* 60:183-186, 1990.
21. ENISELER, N. Heart rate and blood lactate concentrations as predictors of physiological load on elite soccer players during various soccer training activities. *J Strength Cond Res* 19:799-804, 2005.
22. FARIA, E.W., D.L. PARKER, and I.E. FARIA. The science of cycling: physiology and training—part 1. *Sports Med* 35:285-312, 2005.
23. FARIA, E.W., D.L. PARKER, and I.E. FARIA. The science of cycling: factors affecting performance—part 2. *Sports Med* 35:313-337, 2005.
24. FISKERSTRAND, Å., and K.S. SEILER. Training and performance characteristics among Norwegian international rowers 1970-2001. *Scand J Med Sci Sports* 14:303-310, 2004.
25. FLECK, S., and W.J. KRAEMER. *Designing Resistance Training Programs.* 3rd ed. Champaign, IL: Human Kinetics, 2004.
26. FRÖBÖSE, I., A. VERDONCK, F. DUESBERG, and C. MUCHA. Effects of various load intensities in the framework of postoperative stationary endurance training on performance deficit of the quadriceps muscle of the thigh. *Z Orthop Ihre Grenzgeb* 131:164-167, 1993.
27. FRY, A.C., and W.J. KRAEMER. Resistance exercise overtraining and overreaching: neuroendocrine responses. *Sports Med* 23:106-129, 1997.
28. FRY, R.W., A.R. MORTON, and D. KEAST. Overtraining in athletes: an update. *Sports Med* 12:32-65, 1991.
29. GABBETT, T.J. Science of rugby league football: a review. *J Sports Sci* 23:961-976, 2005.
30. GARHAMMER, J., and B. TAKANO. Training for weightlifting. In: *Strength and Power in Sport.* P.V. Komi, ed. Oxford, UK: Blackwell Scientific, 2003, pp. 502-515.
31. GILLAM, G.M. Effects of frequency of weight training on muscle strength enhancement. *J Sports Med* 21:432-436, 1981.
32. HAFF, G.G., A. WHITLEY, and J.A. POTTEIGER. A brief review: explosive exercises and sports performance. *Natl Strength Cond Assoc* 23:13-20, 2001.
33. HÄKKINEN, K., and M. KALLINEN. Distribution of strength training volume into one or two daily sessions and neuromuscular adaptations in female athletes. *Electromyogr Clin Neurophysiol* 34:117-124, 1994.
34. HARRE, D. *Trainingslehre.* Berlin, Germany: Sportverlag, 1982.
35. HAUSSWIRTH, C., D. LEHENAFF, P. DREANO, and K. SAVONEN. Effects of cycling alone or in a sheltered position on subsequent running performance during a triathlon. *Med Sci Sports Exerc* 31:599-604, 1999.
36. HOWE, C., and A.R. COGGAN, *The Road Cyclist's Guide to Training by Power.* 2003, Training Smart Online. http://www.trainingsmartonline.com/images/Free_Triathlon_Articles/Power_Cycling_Training.pdf
37. ILIUTA, G., and C. DUMITRESCU. Medical and physiological criteria for the assessing and directing of athletes' training. *Sportul de Performanta Bucareti* 53:49-64, 1998.
38. JONES, L. Training programs: do Bulgarian methods lead the way for the USA? *Weightlifting USA* 9:10-11, 1991.
39. KOMI, P.V. *Strength and Power in Sport.* Oxford, UK: Blackwell Scientific, 1991.
40. KOMI, P.V. *Strength and Power in Sport.* 2nd ed. Malden, MA: Blackwell Scientific, 2003.
41. LANIER, A.B. Use of nonsteroidal anti-inflammatory drugs following exercise-induced muscle injury. *Sports Med* 33:177-186, 2003.
42. LAURSEN, P.B., and D.G. JENKINS. The scientific basis for high-intensity interval training: optimising training programmes and maximising performance in highly trained endurance athletes. *Sports Med* 32:53-73, 2002.
43. LAURSEN, P.B., C.M. SHING, J.M. PEAKE, J.S. COOMBES, and D.G. JENKINS. Interval training program optimization in highly trained endurance cyclists. *Med Sci Sports Exerc* 34:1801-1807, 2002.
44. LAURSEN, P.B., C.M. SHING, J.M. PEAKE, J.S. COOMBES, and D.G. JENKINS. Influence of high-intensity interval training on adaptations in well-trained cyclists. *J Strength Cond Res* 19:527-533, 2005.
45. LEUTSHENKO, A.V., and A.L. BERESTOVSKAYA. The main elements in the planning of training for elite discus throwers. In: *The Throws: Contemporary Theory, Technique, and Training.* J. Jarver, ed. Mountain View, CA: Tafnews Press, 2000, pp. 106-108.
46. LUEBBERS, P.E., J.A. POTTEIGER, M.W. HULVER, J.P. THYFAULT, M.J. CARPER, and R.H. LOCKWOOD. Effects of plyometric training and recovery on vertical jump performance and anaerobic power. *J Strength Cond Res* 17:704-709, 2003.

47. LYMAN, S., G.S. FLEISIG, J.W. WATERBOR, E.M. FUNKHOUSER, L. PULLEY, J.R. ANDREWS, E.D. OSINSKI, and J.M. ROSEMAN. Longitudinal study of elbow and shoulder pain in youth baseball pitchers. *Med Sci Sports Exerc* 33:1803-1810, 2001.

48. MATVEYEV, L.P. *Fundamentals of Sports Training*. Moscow: Fizkultua i Sport, 1977.

49. MAUGHAN, R., and M. GLEESON. *The Biochemical Basis of Sports Performance*. New York: Oxford University Press, 2004.

50. MCARDLE, W.D., F.I. KATCH, and V.L. KATCH. *Exercise Physiology: Energy, Nutrition, and Human Performance*. 6th ed. Baltimore: Lippincott, Williams & Wilkins, 2007.

51. MONEDERO, J., and B. DONNE. Effect of recovery interventions on lactate removal and subsequent performance. *Int J Sports Med* 21:593-597, 2000.

52. MORTON, R.H., J.R. FITZ-CLARKE, and E.W. BANISTER. Modeling human performance in running. *J Appl Physiol* 69:1171-1177, 1990.

53. MUJIKA, I., and S. PADILLA. Detraining: loss of training-induced physiological and performance adaptations: part I: short term insufficient training stimulus. *Sports Med* 30:79-87, 2000.

54. MUJIKA, I., and S. PADILLA. Detraining: loss of training-induced physiological and performance adaptations: part II: long term insufficient training stimulus. *Sports Med* 30:145-154, 2000.

55. NOAKES, T.D. *Lore of Running*. 4th ed. Champaign, IL: Human Kinetics, 2001.

56. OLBRECT, J. *The Science of Winning: Planning, Periodizing, and Optimizing Swim Training*. Luton, UK: Swimshop, 2000.

57. OSGNACH, C., S. POSER, R. BERNARDINI, R. RINALDO, and P.E. DI PRAMPERO. Energy cost and metabolic power in elite soccer: a new match analysis approach. *Med Sci Sports Exerc* 42:170-178, 2010.

58. PETERSON, M.D., M.R. RHEA, and B.A. ALVAR. Applications of the dose-response for muscular strength development: a review of meta-analytic efficacy and reliability for designing training prescription. *J Strength Cond Res* 19:950-958, 2005.

59. PLATONOV, V.N. *Teoria General del Entrenamiento Deportivo Olimpico*. Badalona, Spain: Paidotribo Editorial, 2002.

60. PLISK, S.S., and M.H. STONE. Periodization strategies. *Strength Cond* 25:19-37, 2003.

61. POTTEIGER, J.A. Aerobic endurance exercise training. In: *Essentials of Strength Training and Conditioning*. T.R. Baechle and R.W. Earle, eds. Champaign, IL: Human Kinetics, 2000, pp. 495-509.

62. RHEA, M.R., B.A. ALVAR, L.N. BURKETT, and S.D. BALL. A meta-analysis to determine the dose response for strength development. *Med Sci Sports Exerc* 35:456-464, 2003.

63. SCHMOLINSKY, G. *Track and Field: The East German Textbook of Athletics*. Toronto, ON, Canada: Sports Book Publisher, 2004.

64. SIFF, M.C., and Y.U. VERKHOSHANSKY. *Supertraining*. Denver, CO: Supertraining International, 1999.

65. SIMONEAU, J.A., G. LORTIE, M.R. BOULAY, M. MARCOTTE, M.C. THIBAULT, and C. BOUCHARD. Effects of two high-intensity intermittent training programs interspaced by detraining on human skeletal muscle and performance. *Eur J Appl Physiol Occup Physiol* 56:516-521, 1987.

66. SKURVYDAS, A., V. DUDONIENE, A. KALVENAS, and A. ZUOZA. Skeletal muscle fatigue in long-distance runners, sprinters and untrained men after repeated drop jumps performed at maximal intensity. *Scand J Med Sci Sports* 12:34-39, 2002.

67. SMITH, D.J. A framework for understanding the training process leading to elite performance. *Sports Med* 33:1103-1126, 2003.

68. SMITH, T.P., L.R. MCNAUGHTON, and K.J. MARSHALL. Effects of 4-wk training using Vmax/Tmax on VO_{2max} and performance in athletes. *Med Sci Sports Exerc* 31:892-896, 1999.

69. SPENCER, M., D. BISHOP, B. DAWSON, and C. GOODMAN. Physiological and metabolic responses of repeated-sprint activities: specific to field-based team sports. *Sports Med* 35:1025-1044, 2005.

70. STEPTO, N.K., D.T. MARTIN, K.E. FALLON, and J.A. HAWLEY. Metabolic demands of intense aerobic interval training in competitive cyclists. *Med Sci Sports Exerc* 33:303-310, 2001.

71. STOLEN, T., K. CHAMARI, C. CASTAGNA, and U. WISLOFF. Physiology of soccer: an update. *Sports Med* 35:501-536, 2005.

72. STONE, M.H., R. KEITH, J.T. KEARNEY, G.D. WILSON, and S. FLECK, J. Overtraining: a review of the signs and symptoms of overtraining. *J Appl Sport Sci Res* 5:35-50, 1991.

73. STONE, M.H., and H.O. O'BRYANT. *Weight Training: A Scientific Approach*. Edina, MN: Burgess, 1987.

74. STONE, M.H., M.E. STONE, and W.A. SANDS. *Principles and Practice of Resistance Training*. Champaign, IL: Human Kinetics, 2007.

75. WERNBOM, M., J. AUGUSTSSON, and R. THOMEE. The influence of frequency, intensity, volume and mode of strength training on whole muscle cross-sectional area in humans. *Sports Med* 37:225-264, 2007.

76. ZATSIORSKY, V.M. Intensity of strength training fact and theory: Russian and Eastern European approach. *NSCA J* 14:46-57, 1992.

77. ZATSIORSKY, V.M. *Science and Practice of Strength Training.* Champaign, IL: Human Kinetics, 1995.
78. ZATSIORSKY, V.M. and W.J. KRAEMER. *Science and Practice of Strength Training.* 2nd ed. Champaign, IL: Human Kinetics, 2006.

Chapter 5

1. BOMPA, T.O. *Periodization: Theory and Methodology of Training.* 4th ed. Champaign, IL: Human Kinetics, 1999.
2. BOMPA, T.O. *Theory and Methodology of Training: The Key to Athletic Performance.* Dubuque, IA: Kendall/Hunt, 1994.
3. BOMPA, T.O. *Total Training for Coaching Team Sports: A Self Help Guide.* Toronto, CA: Sports Books Publisher, 2006.
4. BOMPA, T.O., and M.C. CARRERA. *Periodization Training For Sports: Science-Based Strength and Conditioning Plans for 20 Sports.* 2nd ed. Champaign, IL: Human Kinetics, 2005.
5. BOMPA, T.O. Antrenamentul in perioada pregatitoare [Training methodology during the preparatory phase]. *Caiet pentru sporturi nautice* 3:22-28, 1956.
6. BOMPA, T. *Antrenamentul in Diferite Perioade de Pregatire* [Training Content in Different Stages of Preparation]. Timisoara, Romania: Cjefs, 1960.
7. BOMPA, T. *Periodization of Strength for Power Sports.* In: International Conference on Advancements in Sports Training. Moscow, 1965.
8. BOMPA, T. Periodization of strength. *Sports Review* 1:26–31, 1965b.
9. BOMPA, T.O. *Theory and Methodology of Training.* Dubuque, Iowa: Kendall/Hunt Publishing Company, 1983.
10. BOMPA, T.O. *Periodization of Strength: The new wave in Strength Training.* Toronto: Veritas, 1993.
11. DE LORME, T.L., and A.L. WATKINS. *Progression Resistance Exercises.* New York: Appleton-Century-Crofts, 1951.
12. FARROW, D., W. YOUNG, and L. BRUCE. The development of a test of reactive agility for netball: a new methodology. *J Sci Med Sport* 8:52-60, 2005.
13. FLECK, S.J., and W.J. KRAEMER. *Designing Resistance Training Programs.* 2nd ed. Champaign, IL: Human Kinetics, 1997.
14. FLECK, S., and W.J. KRAEMER. *Designing Resistance Training Programs.* 3rd ed. Champaign, IL: Human Kinetics, 2004.
15. FREEMAN, W.H. *Peak When It Counts Periodization for American Track & Field.* 4th ed. Mountain View, CA: Tafnews Press, 2001.
16. HOFF, J., U. WISLØFF, L.C. ENGEN, O.J. KEMI, and J. HELGERUD. Soccer specific aerobic endurance training. *Br J Sports Med* 36:218-221, 2002.
17. ISSURIN, V. Block periodization versus traditional training theory: a review. *J Sports Med Phys Fitness* 48:65-75, 2008.
18. KRAEMER, W.J., D.N. FRENCH, N.J. PAXTON, K. HÄKKINEN, J.S. VOLEK, W.J. SEBASTIANELLI, M. PUTUKIAN, R.U. NEWTON, M.R. RUBIN, A.L. GOMEZ, J.D. VESCOVI, N.A. RATAMESS, S.J. FLECK, J.M. LYNCH, and H.G. KNUTTGEN. Changes in exercise performance and hormonal concentrations over a big ten soccer season in starters and nonstarters. *J Strength Cond Res* 18:121-128, 2004.
19. KRAEMER, W.J., L.P. KOZIRIS, N.A. RATAMESS, K. HÄKKINEN, T.R.-M. NT, A.C. FRY, S.E. GORDON, J.S. VOLEK, D.N. FRENCH, M.R. RUBIN, A.L. GOMEZ, M.J. SHARMAN, J. MICHAEL LYNCH, M. IZQUIERDO, R.U. NEWTON, and S.J. FLECK. Detraining produces minimal changes in physical performance and hormonal variables in recreationally strength-trained men. *J Strength Cond Res* 16:373-382, 2002.
20. KRAEMER, W.J., J.S. VOLEK, J.A. BUSH, M. PUTUKIAN, and W.J. SEBASTIANELLI. Hormonal responses to consecutive days of heavy-resistance exercise with or without nutritional supplementation. *J Appl Physiol* 85:1544-1555, 1998.
21. LAURSEN, P.B., and D.G. JENKINS. The scientific basis for high-intensity interval training: optimising training programmes and maximising performance in highly trained endurance athletes. *Sports Med* 32:53-73, 2002.
22. MALLO, J., and E. NAVARRO. Physical load imposed on soccer players during small-sided training games. *J Sports Med Phys Fitness* 48:166-171, 2008.
23. MATVEYEV, L.P. *Fundamentals of Sports Training.* Moscow: Fizkultua i Sport, 1977.
24. MATVEYEV, L.P. *Periodisterung Des Sportlichen Trainings.* Moscow: Fizkultura i Sport, 1972.
25. MATVEYEV, L. *Periodization of Sports Training.* Moscow: Fizkultura i Sport, 1965.
26. MIKKOLA, J., H. RUSKO, A. NUMMELA, T. POLLARI, and K. HÄKKINEN. Concurrent endurance and explosive type strength training improves neuromuscular and anaerobic characteristics in young distance runners. *Int J Sports Med* 28:602-611, 2007.
27. NÁDORI, L. *Training and Competition.* Budapest: Sport, 1962.
28. NÁDORI, L., and I. GRANEK. *Theoretical and Methodological Basis of Training Planning With Special Considerations Within a Microcycle.* Lincoln, NE: NSCA, 1989.
29. OZOLIN, N. *Sovremennaia Systema Sportivnoi Trenirovky* [Athlete's Training System for Competition]. Moscow: Fizkultura i Sport, 1971.

30. PLATONOV, B.H. Theory of annual training: background, status, discussions, ways to modernize. In: *Theory and Practice of Physical Culture* 9:18-34, 2009.
31. SIEGLER, J., S. GASKILL, and B. RUBY. Changes evaluated in soccer-specific power endurance either with or without a 10-week, in-season, intermittent, high-intensity training protocol. *J Strength Cond Res* 17:379-387, 2003.
32. STONE, M.H., and C. KARATZEFERI. Connective tissue and bone response to strength training. In: *Encyclopaedia of Sports Medicine: Strength and Power in Sports*. P.V. Komi, ed. Oxford, UK: Blackwell, 2003. pp. 343-360.
33. STONE, M.H., R. KEITH, J.T. KEARNEY, G.D. WILSON, and S. FLECK, J. Overtraining: a review of the signs and symptoms of overtraining. *J Appl Sport Sci Res* 5:35-50, 1991.
34. STONE, M.H., and H.S. O'BRYANT. Letter to the editor. *J Strength Cond Res* 9:125-127, 1995.
35. STONE, M.H., and H.O. O'BRYANT. *Weight Training: A Scientific Approach*. Edina, MN: Burgess, 1987.
36. STONE, M.H., H. O'BRYANT, and J. GARHAMMER. A hypothetical model for strength training. *J. Sports Med.* 21:342-351, 1981.
37. STONE, M.H., H.S. O'BRYANT, and J. GARHAMMER. A theoretical model of strength training. *NSCA J.* 3:36-39, 1982.
38. STONE, M.H., H.S. O'BRYANT, L. MCCOY, R. COGLIANESE, M. LEHMKUHL, and B. SCHILLING. Power and maximum strength relationships during performance of dynamic and static weighted jumps. *J Strength Cond Res* 17:140-147, 2003.
39. STONE, M.H., K. SANBORN, H.S. O'BRYANT, M. HARTMAN, M.E. STONE, C. PROULX, B. WARD, and J. HRUBY. Maximum strength-power-performance relationships in collegiate throwers. *J Strength Cond Res* 17:739-745, 2003.
40. STONE, M.H., W.A. SANDS, J. CARLOCK, S. CALLAN, D. DICKIE, K. DAIGLE, J. COTTON, S.L. SMITH, and M. HARTMAN. The importance of isometric maximum strength and peak rate-of-force development in sprint cycling. *J Strength Cond Res* 18:878-884, 2004.
41. STONE, M.H., W.A. SANDS, K.C. PIERCE, J. CARLOCK, M. CARDINALE, and R.U. NEWTON. Relationship of maximum strength to weightlifting performance. *Med Sci Sports Exerc* 37:1037-1043, 2005.
42. STONE, M.H., W.A. SANDS, K.C. PIERCE, R.U. NEWTON, G.G. HAFF, and J. CARLOCK. Maximum strength and strength training: a relationship to endurance? *Strength Cond J* 28:44-53, 2006.
43. STONE, M.H., M.E. STONE, and W.A. SANDS. *Principles and Practice of Resistance Training*. Champaign, IL: Human Kinetics, 2007.
44. TANAKA, H., and T. SWENSEN. Impact of resistance training on endurance performance: a new form of cross-training? *Sports Med* 25:191-200, 1998.
45. TOMLIN, D.L., and H.A. WENGER. The relationship between aerobic fitness and recovery from high intensity intermittent exercise. *Sports Med* 31(1):1-11, 2001.
46. VERKHOSHANSKY, Y.U. *Fundamentals of Special Strength Training in Sport*. Livonia, MI: Sportivy Press, 1986.
47. VERKHOSHANSKY, Y.U. Perspectives in the development of speed-strength preparation in the development of jumpers. *Track and Field* 9:11-12, 1966.
48. VERKHOSHANSKY, Y.U. *Programming and Organization of Training*. Moscow: Fizkultura i Sport, 1985.
49. VERKHOSHANSKY, Y.U. *Special Strength Training: A Practical Manual for Coaches*. Muskegon, MI: Ultimate Athlete Concepts, 2006.
50. YOUNG, W.B., R. JAMES, and I. MONTGOMERY. Is muscle power related to running speed with changes of direction? *J Sports Med Phys Fitness* 42:282-288, 2002.

Chapter 6

1. ALLEN, D.G., J.A. LEE, and H. WESTERBLAD. Intracellular calcium and tension during fatigue in isolated single muscle fibres from Xenopus laevis. *J Physiol* 415:433-458, 1989.
2. BARCROFT, H., and O.G. EDHOLM. The effect of temperature on blood flow and deep temperature in the human forearm. *J Physiol* 102:5-20, 1943.
3. BARCROFT, J., and W.O. KING. The effect of temperature on the dissociation curve of blood. *J Physiol* 39:374-384, 1909.
4. BISHOP, D. Warm up I: potential mechanisms and the effects of passive warm up on exercise performance. *Sports Med* 33:439-454, 2003.
5. BISHOP, D. Warm up II: performance changes following active warm up and how to structure the warm up. *Sports Med* 33:483-498, 2003.
6. BISHOP, D., D. BONETTI, and M. SPENCER. The effect of an intermittent, high-intensity warm-up on supramaximal kayak ergometer performance. *J Sports Sci* 21:13-20, 2003.
7. BOGDANIS, G.C., M.E. NEVILL, H.K. LAKOMY, C.M. GRAHAM, and G. LOUIS. Effects of active recovery on power output during repeated maximal sprint cycling. *Eur J Appl Physiol Occup Physiol* 74:461-469, 1996.

8. BOMPA, T.O. *Total Training for Coaching Team Sports: A Self Help Guide*. Toronto, ON, Canada: Sports Books Publisher, 2006.
9. BOMPA, T.O., and M. CARRERA. *Conditioning Young Athletes*. Champaign, IL: Human Kinetics, 2015.
10. BURKE, L., and V. DEAKIN. *Clinical Sports Nutrition*. Roseville, Australia: McGraw-Hill Australia, 2000.
11. CHEUNG, K., P. HUME, and L. MAXWELL. Delayed onset muscle soreness: treatment strategies and performance factors. *Sports Med* 33:145-164, 2003.
12. CHIU, L.Z., A.C. FRY, L.W. WEISS, B.K. SCHILLING, L.E. BROWN, and S.L. SMITH. Postactivation potentiation response in athletic and recreationally trained individuals. *J Strength Cond Res* 17:671-677, 2003.
13. COGGAN, A.R., and E.F. COYLE. Carbohydrate ingestion during prolonged exercise: effects on metabolism and performance. *Exerc Sport Sci Rev* 19:1-40, 1991.
14. DAVIS, J.M. Central and peripheral factors in fatigue. *J Sports Sci* 13(spec no):S49-S53, 1995.
15. DAVIS, J.M., N.L. ALDERSON, and R.S. WELSH. Serotonin and central nervous system fatigue: nutritional considerations. *Am J Clin Nutr* 72:573S-578S, 2000.
16. DAVIS, J.M., and S.P. BAILEY. Possible mechanisms of central nervous system fatigue during exercise. *Med Sci Sports Exerc* 29:45-57, 1997.
17. ENOKA, R.M. Activation order of motor axons in electrically evoked contractions. *Muscle Nerve* 25:763-764, 2002.
18. ENOKA, R.M. *Neuromechanics of Human Movement*. Champaign, IL: Human Kinetics, 2015.
19. ENOKA, R.M., and D.G. STUART. Neurobiology of muscle fatigue. *J Appl Physiol* 72:1631-1648, 1992.
20. FRY, A.C., B.K. SCHILLING, L.W. WEISS, and L.Z. CHIU. Beta2-adrenergic receptor downregulation and performance decrements during high-intensity resistance exercise overtraining, *J Appl Physiol* 101(6):1664-72, 1985.
21. GANDELSMAN, A., and K. SMIRNOV. *Physiologicheskie Osnovi Metodiki Sportivnoi Trenirovki* [The Physiological Foundations of Training]. Moscow: Fizkultura i Sport, 1970.
22. GRANGE, R.W., C.R. CORY, R. VANDENBOOM, and M.E. HOUSTON. Myosin phosphorylation augments force-displacement and force-velocity relationships of mouse fast muscle. *Am J Physiol* 269:C713-C724, 1995.
23. GRANGE, R.W., R. VANDENBOOM, J. XENI, and M.E. HOUSTON. Potentiation of in vitro concentric work in mouse fast muscle. *J Appl Physiol* 84:236-243, 1998.
24. GRODJINOVSKY, A., and J.R. MAGEL. Effect of warming up on running performance. *Res Q Exerc Sport* 41:116-119.
25. HAFF, G.G., R.T. HOBBS, E.E. HAFF, W.A. SANDS, K.C. PIERCE, and M.H. STONE. Cluster training: a novel method for introducing training program variation. *Strength Cond* 30:67-76, 2008.
26. HAFF, G.G., M.J. LEHMKUHL, L.B. MCCOY, and M.H. STONE. Carbohydrate supplementation and resistance training. *J Strength Cond Res* 17:187-196, 2003.
27. HÄKKINEN, K., and M. KALLINEN. Distribution of strength training volume into one or two daily sessions and neuromuscular adaptations in female athletes. *Electromyogr Clin Neurophysiol* 34:117-124, 1994.
28. HODGSON, M., D. DOCHERTY, and D. ROBBINS. Post-activation potentiation: underlying physiology and implications for motor performance. *Sports Med* 35:585-595, 2005.
29. HOLCOMB, W.R. Stretching and warm-up. In: *Essentials of Strength and Conditioning*. T.R. Baechle and R.W. Earle, eds. Champaign, IL: Human Kinetics, 2000. pp. 321-342.
30. HORNERY, D.J., D. FARROW, I. MUJIKA, and W. YOUNG. Fatigue in tennis: mechanisms of fatigue and effect on performance. *Sports Med* 37:199-212, 2007.
31. IVY, J., and R. PORTMAN. *The Future of Sports Nutrition: Nutrient Timing*. North Bergan, NJ: Basic Health, 2004.
32. LAFORGIA, J., R.T. WITHERS, and C.J. GORE. Effects of exercise intensity and duration on the excess post-exercise oxygen consumption. *J Sports Sci* 24:1247-1264, 2006.
33. LITTLE, T., and A.G. WILLIAMS. Effects of differential stretching protocols during warm-ups on high-speed motor capacities in professional soccer players. *J Strength Cond Res* 20:203-207, 2006.
34. MALAREKI, I. Investigation of physiological justification of so-called "warming up." *Acta Physiol Pol* 5:543-546, 1954.
35. MASSEY, B.H., W.R. JOHNSON, and G.F. KRAMER. Effect of warm-up exercise upon muscular performance using hypnosis to control the psychological variable. *Re. Q Exerc Sport* 32:63-71, 1961.
36. MATVEYEV, L. About the construction of training. *Modern Athlete and Coach* 32:12-16, 1994.
37. MATVEYEV, L.P. *Fundamentals of Sports Training*. Moscow: Fizkultua i Sport, 1977.
38. MATVEYEV, L.P. *Periodisterung Des Sportlichen Trainings*. Moscow: Fizkultura i Sport, 1972.
39. MAUGHAN, R., and M. GLEESON. *The Biochemical Basis of Sports Performance*. New York: Oxford University Press, 2004.

40. MCBRIDE, J.M., S. NIMPHIUS, and T.M. ERICKSON. The acute effects of heavy-load squats and loaded countermovement jumps on sprint performance. *J Strength Cond Res* 19:893-897, 2005.
41. MCMILLAN, J.L., M.H. STONE, J. SARTIN, R. KEITH, D. MARPLE, C. BROWN, and R.D. LEWIS. 20-hour physiological responses to a single weight-training session. *J Strength Cond Res* 7:9-21, 1993.
42. MCGILL, S.M. *Low Back Disorders: Evidence-Based Prevention and Rehabilitation*. 2nd ed. Champaign, IL: Human Kinetics, 2007.
43. MEDVEDEV, A.S. *Sistema Mnogoletnyei Trenirovki V Tyazheloi Atletikye*. Moscow: Fizkultura i Sport, 1986.
44. MIKA, A., P. MIKA, B. FERNHALL, and V.B. UNNITHAN. Comparison of recovery strategies on muscle performance after fatiguing exercise. *Am J Phys Med Rehabil* 86:474-481, 2007.
45. MONEDERO, J., and B. DONNE. Effect of recovery interventions on lactate removal and subsequent performance. *Int J Sports Med* 21:593-597, 2000.
46. NAGANE, M. Relationship of subjective chronic fatigue to academic performance. *Psychol Rep* 95:48-52, 2004.
47. NOAKES, T.D. Physiological models to understand exercise fatigue and the adaptations that predict or enhance athletic performance. *Scand J Med Sci Sports* 10:123-145, 2000.
48. PETERSEN, J., K. THORBORG, M.B. NIELSEN, E. BUDTZ-JERGENSEN, and P. Hölmich. Preventive effect of eccentric training on acute hamstring injuries in men's soccer: a cluster-randomized controlled trial. *Am J Sports Med* 39(11):2296-2303, 2011.
49. RADCLIFFE, J.C., and J.L. RADCLIFFE. Effects of different warm-up protocols on peak power output during a single response jump task [abstract]. *Med Sci Sports Exerc* 28:S189, 1996.
50. REILLY, T., and B. EKBLOM. The use of recovery methods post-exercise. *J Sport Sci* 23:619-627, 2005.
51. SAEZ SAEZ DE VILLARREAL, E., J.J. GONZALEZ-BADILLO, and M. IZQUIERDO. Optimal warm-up stimuli of muscle activation to enhance short and long-term acute jumping performance. *Eur J Appl Physiol* 100:393-401, 2007.
52. SALTIN, B., A.P. GAGGE, and J.A. STOLWIJK. Muscle temperature during submaximal exercise in man. *J Appl Physiol* 25:679-688, 1968.
53. SHRIER, I. Does stretching improve performance? A systematic and critical review of the literature. *Clin J Sports Med* 14:267-273, 2004.
54. ST CLAIR GIBSON, A., D.A. BADEN, M.I. LAMBERT, E.V. LAMBERT, Y.X. HARLEY, D. HAMPSON, V.A. RUSSELL, and T.D. NOAKES. The conscious perception of the sensation of fatigue. *Sports Med* 33:167-176, 2003.
55. STONE, M.H., W.A. SANDS, K.C. PIERCE, M.W. RAMSEY, and G.G. HAFF. Power and power potentiation among strength power athletes: preliminary study. *Int J Sports Physiol Perf* 3:55-67, 2008.
56. STONE, M.H., M.E. STONE, and W.A. SANDS. *Principles and Practice of Resistance Training*. Champaign, IL: Human Kinetics, 2007.
57. THORBORG, K., C. COUPPÉ, J. PETERSEN, S.P. MAGNUSSON, and P. Hölmich. Eccentric hip adduction and abduction strength in elite soccer players and matched controls: a cross-sectional study. *Br J Sports Med* 45(1):10-13, 2011.
58. WINCHESTER, J.B., A.G. NELSON, D. LANDIN, M.A. YOUNG, and I.C. SCHEXNAYDER. Static stretching impairs sprint performance in collegiate track and field athletes. *J Strength Cond Res* 22:13-19, 2008.
59. WOODS, C., R.D. HAWKINS, S. MALTBY, M. HULSE, A. THOMAS, and A. HODSON. The Football Association Medical Research Programme: an audit of injuries in professional football—analysis of hamstring injuries. *Br J Sports Med* 38(1):36-41, 2004.
60. WOODS, K., P. BISHOP, and E. JONES. Warm-up and stretching in the prevention of muscular injury. *Sports Med* 37:1089-1099, 2007.
61. YETTER, M., and G.L. MOIR. The acute effects of heavy back and front squats on speed during forty-meter sprint trials. *J Strength Cond Res* 22:159-165, 2008.
62. YOUNG, W.B., and D.G. BEHM. Effects of running, static stretching and practice jumps on explosive force production and jumping performance. *J Sports Med Phys Fitness* 43:21-27, 2003.
63. ZATSIORSKY, V.M. *Science and Practice of Strength Training*. Champaign, IL: Human Kinetics, 1995.
64. ZATSIORSKY, V.M., and W.J. KRAEMER. Science and Practice of Strength Training. 2nd Champaign, IL: Human Kinetics, 2006.

Chapter 7

1. ARAZI, H. S.S. MOSAVI, S.S. BASIR, and M.G. KARAM. The effects of different recovery conditions on blood lactate concentration and physiological variables after high intensity exercise in handball players. *Sport Sci* 5:13-17, 2012.
2. BROOKS, G.A., T.D. FAHEY, T.P. WHITE, and K.M. BALDWIN. *Exercise Physiology: Human Bioenergetics and Its Application*. 3rd ed. Mountain View, CA: Mayfield, 2000.
3. BURKE, L., and V. DEAKIN. *Clinical Sports Nutrition*. Roseville, Australia: McGraw-Hill Australia, 2000.

4. HALSON, S.L., M.W. BRIDGE, R. MEEUSEN, B. BUSSCHAERT, M. GLEESON, D.A. JONES, and A.E. JEUKENDRUP. Time course of performance changes and fatigue markers during intensified training in trained cyclists. *J Appl Physiol* 93:947-956, 2002.

5. HELLARD, P., M. AVALOS, G. MILLET, L. LACOSTE, F. BARALE, and J.C. CHATARD. Modeling the residual effects and threshold saturation of training: a case study of Olympic swimmers. *J Strength Cond Res* 19:67-75, 2005.

6. HEYMAN, E., B. DE GEUS, I. MERTENS, and R. MEEUSEN. Effects of four recovery methods on repeated maximal rock climbing performance. *Med Sci Sports Exerc* 41:1303-1310, 2009.

7. IVY, J., and R. PORTMAN. *The Future of Sports Nutrition: Nutrient Timing*. North Bergan, NJ: Basic Health, 2004.

8. KRUSTRUP, P., M. MOHR, A. STEENSBERG, J. BENCKE, M. KJAER, and J. BANGSBO. Muscle and blood metabolites during a soccer game: implications for sprint performance. *Med Sci Sports Exerc* 38:1165-1174, 2006.

9. MARTIN, N.A., R.F. ZOELLER, R.J. ROBERTSON, and S.M. LEPHART. The comparative effects of sports massage, active recovery, and rest in promoting blood lactate clearance after supramaximal leg exercise. *J Athl Train* 33:30-35, 1998.

10. MCARDLE, W.D., F.I. KATCH, and V.L. KATCH. *Exercise Physiology: Energy, Nutrition, and Human Performance*. 6th ed. Baltimore: Lippincott Williams & Wilkins, 2007.

11. MENZIES, P., C. MENZIES, L. MCINTYRE, P. PATERSON, J. WILSON, and O.J. KEMI. Blood lactate clearance during active recovery after an intense running bout depends on the intensity of the active recovery. *J Sports Sci* 28:975-982, 2010.

12. MUJIKA, I., and S. PADILLA. Scientific bases for precompetition tapering strategies. *Med Sci Sports Exerc* 35:1182-1187, 2003.

13. REILLY, T., and B. EKBLOM. The use of recovery methods post-exercise. *J Sport Sci* 23:619-627, 2005.

14. REILLY, T., and M. RIGBY. Effect of an active warm-down following competitive soccer. In: *Science and Football IV*. W. Spinks, T. Reilly, and A. Murphy, eds. London: Routledge, 2002, pp. 226-229.

15. STONE, M.H., M.E. STONE, and W.A. SANDS. *Principles and Practice of Resistance Training*. Champaign, IL: Human Kinetics, 2007.

16. WHITE, G.E., and G.D. WELLS. The effect of on-hill active recovery performed between runs on blood lactate concentration and fatigue in alpine ski racers. *J Strength Cond Res* 29, 800-806, 2015.

Chapter 8

1. ANDERSEN, L.L., J.L. ANDERSEN, S.P. MAGNUSSON, C. SUETTA, J.L. MADSEN, L.R. CHRISTENSEN, and P. AAGAARD. Changes in the human muscle force-velocity relationship in response to resistance training and subsequent detraining. *J Appl Physiol* 99:87-94, 2005.

2. BOMPA, T.O. *Theory and Methodology of Training*. Dubuque, Iowa: Kendall/Hunt Publishing Company, 1983.

3. BOMPA, T.O. *Periodization: Theory and Methodology of Training*. 4th ed. Champaign, IL: Human Kinetics, 1999.

4. COYLE, E.F., W.H. MARTIN, III, D.R. SINACORE, M.J. JOYNER, J.M. HAGBERG, and J.O. HOLLOSZY. Time course of loss of adaptations after stopping prolonged intense endurance training. *J Appl Physiol* 57:1857-1864, 1984.

5. DUNLAVY, J.K., W.A. SANDS, J.R. MCNEAL, M.H. STONE, S.A. SMITH, M. JEMNI, and G.G. HAFF. Strength performance assessment in a simulated men's gymnastics still rings cross. *J Sports Sci Med* 6:93-97, 2007.

6. FRY, R.W., A.R. MORTON, and D. KEAST. Overtraining in athletes: an update. *Sports Med* 12:32-65, 1991.

7. FRY, A.C. The role of training intensity in resistance exercise overtraining and overreaching. In: *Overtraining in Sport*. R.B. Kreider, A.C. Fry, and M.L. O'Toole, eds. Champaign, IL: Human Kinetics, 1998. pp. 107-127.

8. HAFF, G.G., J.M. CARLOCK, M.J. HARTMAN, J.L. KILGORE, N. KAWAMORI, J.R. JACKSON, R.T. MORRIS, W.A. SANDS, and M.H. STONE. Force-time curve characteristics of dynamic and isometric muscle actions of elite women Olympic weightlifters. *J Strength Cond Res* 19:741-748, 2005.

9. HAFF, G.G., J.R. JACKSON, N. KAWAMORI, J.M. CARLOCK, M.J. HARTMAN, J.L. KILGORE, R.T. MORRIS, M.W. RAMSEY, W.A. SANDS, and M.H. STONE. Force-time curve characteristics and hormonal alterations during an eleven-week training period in elite women weightlifters. *J Strength Cond Res* 22:433-446, 2008.

10. HÄKKINEN, K., and P.V. KOMI. Electromyographic changes during strength training and detraining. *Med Sci Sports Exerc* 15:455-460, 1983.

11. HARMAN, E., and C. PANDORF. Principles of test selection and administration. In: *Essentials of Strength Training and Conditioning*. T.R. Baechle and R.W. Earle, eds. Champaign, IL: Human Kinetics, 2000, pp. 275-286.

12. HAWLEY, J.A. Interaction of exercise and diet to maximise training adaptation. *Asia Pac J Clin Nutr* 14:S35, 2005.

13. HORTOBAGYI, T., J.A. HOUMARD, J.R. STEVENSON, D.D. FRASER, R.A. JOHNS, and R.G. ISRAEL. The effects of detraining on power athletes. *Med Sci Sports Exerc* 25:929-935, 1993.
14. HOUMARD, J.A., T. HORTOBAGYI, R.A. JOHNS, N.J. BRUNO, C.C. NUTE, M.H. SHINEBARGER, and J.W. WELBORN. Effect of short-term training cessation on performance measures in distance runners. *Int J Sports Med* 13:572-576, 1992.
15. IZQUIERDO, M., J. IBANEZ, J.J. GONZALEZ-BADILLO, N.A. RATAMESS, W.J. KRAEMER, K. HÄKKINEN, H. BONNABAU, C. GRANADOS, D.N. FRENCH, and E.M. GOROSTIAGA. Detraining and tapering effects on hormonal responses and strength performance. *J Strength Cond Res* 21:768-775, 2007.
16. KRAEMER, W.J., L.P. KOZIRIS, N.A. RATAMESS, K. HÄKKINEN, T.R.-M. NT, A.C. FRY, S.E. GORDON, J.S. VOLEK, D.N. FRENCH, M.R. RUBIN, A.L. GOMEZ, M.J. SHARMAN, J. MICHAEL LYNCH, M. IZQUIERDO, R.U. NEWTON, and S.J. FLECK. Detraining produces minimal changes in physical performance and hormonal variables in recreationally strength-trained men. *J Strength Cond Res* 16:373-382, 2002.
17. KRAEMER, W.J., J.S. VOLEK, J.A. BUSH, M. PUTUKIAN, and W.J. SEBASTIANELLI. Hormonal responses to consecutive days of heavy-resistance exercise with or without nutritional supplementation. *J Appl Physiol* 85:1544-1555, 1998.
18. KUIPERS, H., and H.A. KEIZER. Overtraining in elite athletes: review and directions for the future. *Sports Med* 6:79-92, 1988.
19. MAUGHAN, R. Physiology of sport. *Br J Hosp Med (Lond)* 68:376-379, 2007.
20. MUJIKA, I., and S. PADILLA. Detraining: loss of training-induced physiological and performance adaptations: part I: short term insufficient training stimulus. *Sports Med* 30:79-87, 2000.
21. MUJIKA, I., and S. PADILLA. Detraining: loss of training-induced physiological and performance adaptations: part II: Long term insufficient training stimulus. *Sports Med* 30:145-154, 2000.
22. MUJIKA, I., and S. PADILLA. Muscular characteristics of detraining in humans. *Med Sci Sports Exerc* 33:1297-1303, 2001.
23. SMITH, D.J., S.R. NORRIS, and J.M. HOGG. Performance evaluation of swimmers: scientific tools. *Sports Med* 32:539-554, 2002.
24. STARON, R.S., M.J. LEONARDI, D.L. KARAPONDO, E.S. MALICKY, J.E. FALKEL, F.C. HAGERMAN, and R.S. HIKIDA. Strength and skeletal muscle adaptations in heavy-resistance-trained women after detraining and retraining. *J Appl Physiol* 70:631-640, 1991.
25. STONE, M.H., and H.O. O'BRYANT. *Weight Training: A Scientific Approach*. Edina, MN: Burgess, 1987.
26. STONE, M.H., K. SANBORN, H.S. O'BRYANT, M. HARTMAN, M.E. STONE, C. PROULX, B. WARD, and J. HRUBY. Maximum strength-power-performance relationships in collegiate throwers. *J Strength Cond Res* 17:739-745, 2003.
27. STONE, M.H., W.A. SANDS, K.C. PIERCE, J. CARLOCK, M. CARDINALE, and R.U. NEWTON. Relationship of maximum strength to weightlifting performance. *Med Sci Sports Exerc* 37:1037-1043, 2005.
28. VIRU, A. *Adaptations in Sports Training*. Boca Raton, FL: CRC Press, 1995.
29. ZATSIORSKY, V.M., and W.J. KRAEMER. *Science and Practice of Strength Training*. 2nd ed. Champaign, IL: Human Kinetics, 2006.

Chapter 9

1. AJÁN, T., and L. BAROGA. *Weightlifting: Fitness for All Sports*. Budapest: International Weightlifting Federation, 1988.
2. BANISTER, E.W., J.B. CARTER, and P.C. ZARKADAS. Training theory and taper: validation in triathlon athletes. *Eur J Appl Physiol Occup Physiol* 79:182-191, 1999.
3. BOMPA, T.O. *Theory and Methodology of Training: The Key to Athletic Performance*. Dubuque, IA: Kendall/Hunt, 1994.
4. BOSQUET, L., L. LEGER, and P. LEGROS. Methods to determine aerobic endurance. *Sports Med* 32:675-700, 2002.
5. BUSSO, T. Variable dose-response relationship between exercise training and performance. *Med Sci Sports Exerc* 35:1188-1195, 2003.
6. BUSSO, T., K. HÄKKINEN, A. PAKARINEN, H. KAUHANEN, P.V. KOMI, and J.R. LACOUR. Hormonal adaptations and modeled responses in elite weightlifters during 6 weeks of training. *Eur J Appl Physiol* 64:381-386, 1992.
6b. CHTOUROU, H., A. CHAOUACHI, T. DRISS, M. DOGUI, D.G. BEHM, K. CHAMARI, and N. SOUISSI. The effect of training at the same time of day and tapering period on the diurnal variation of short exercise performances. *J Strength Cond Res* 26(3):697-708, 2012.
7. COUTTS, A., P. REABURN, T.J. PIVA, and A. MURPHY. Changes in selected biochemical, muscular strength, power, and endurance measures during deliberate overreaching and tapering in rugby league players. *Int J Sports Med* 28:116-124, 2007.
8. DICK, F.W. *Sports Training Principles*. 4th ed. London: A & C Black, 2002.
9. DRABIK, J. *Children and Sports Training*. Island Pond, VT: Stadion, 1995.
10. FLYNN, M.G., F.X. PIZZA, J.B. BOONE, JR., F.F. ANDRES, T.A. MICHAUD, and J.R. RODRIGUEZ-ZAYAS. Indices of training stress during

competitive running and swimming seasons. *Int J Sports Med* 15:21-26, 1994.

11. GIBALA, M.J., J.D. MACDOUGALL, and D.G. SALE. The effects of tapering on strength performance in trained athletes. *Int J Sports Med* 15:492-497, 1994.

12. GJURKOW, D. Annual competition and training program for senior weightlifters. In: *Proceedings of the Weightlifting Symposium: Ancient Olympia/Greece 1993*. Á. Lukácsfalvi and F. Takács, eds. Budapest: International Weightlifting Federation, 1993, pp. 103-115.

13. GRAVES, J.E., M.L. POLLOCK, D. FOSTER, S.H. LEGGETT, D.M. CARPENTER, R. VUOSO, and A. JONES. Effect of training frequency and specificity on isometric lumbar extension strength. *Spine* 15:504-509, 1990.

14. GRAVES, J.E., M.L. POLLOCK, S.H. LEGGETT, R.W. BRAITH, D.M. CARPENTER, and L.E. BISHOP. Effect of reduced training frequency on muscular strength. *Int J Sports Med* 9:316-319, 1988.

15. HARRE, D. *Trainingslehre*. Berlin, Germany: Sportverlag, 1982.

16. HELLARD, P., M. AVALOS, G. MILLET, L. LACOSTE, F. BARALE, and J.C. CHATARD. Modeling the residual effects and threshold saturation of training: a case study of Olympic swimmers. *J Strength Cond Res* 19:67-75, 2005.

17. HICKSON, R.C., C. FOSTER, M.L. POLLOCK, T.M. GALASSI, and S. RICH. Reduced training intensities and loss of aerobic power, endurance, and cardiac growth. *J Appl Physiol* 58:492-499, 1985.

18. HICKSON, R.C., and M.A. ROSENKOETTER. Reduced training frequencies and maintenance of increased aerobic power. *Med Sci Sports Exerc* 13:13-16, 1981.

19. HOOPER, S.L., L.T. MACKINNON, and E.M. GINN. Effects of three tapering techniques on the performance, forces and psychometric measures of competitive swimmers. *Eur J Appl Physiol Occup Physiol* 78:258-263, 1998.

20. HOOPER, S.L., L.T. MACKINNON, and A. HOWARD. Physiological and psychometric variables for monitoring recovery during tapering for major competition. *Med Sci Sports Exerc* 31:1205-1210, 1999.

21. HOUMARD, J.A. Tapering for the competitive cyclist. *Performance Conditioning for Cyclists* 2:1-8, 1996.

22. HOUMARD, J.A., D.L. COSTILL, J.B. MITCHELL, S.H. PARK, W.J. FINK, and J.M. BURNS. Testosterone, cortisol, and creatine kinase levels in male distance runners during reduced training. *Int J Sports Med* 11:41-45, 1990.

23. HOUMARD, J.A., D.L. COSTILL, J.B. MITCHELL, S.H. PARK, R.C. HICKNER, and J.N. ROEMMICH. Reduced training maintains performance in distance runners. *Int J Sports Med* 11:46-52, 1990.

24. HOUMARD, J.A., and R.A. JOHNS. Effects of taper on swim performance: practical implications. *Sports Med* 17:224-232, 1994.

25. HOUMARD, J.A., J.P. KIRWAN, M.G. FLYNN, and J.B. MITCHELL. Effects of reduced training on submaximal and maximal running responses. *Int J Sports Med* 10:30-33, 1989.

26. HOUMARD, J.A., B.K. SCOTT, C.L. JUSTICE, and T.C. CHENIER. The effects of taper on performance in distance runners. *Med Sci Sports Exerc* 26:624-631, 1994.

27. IZQUIERDO, M., J. IBANEZ, J.J. GONZALEZ-BADILLO, N.A. RATAMESS, W.J. KRAEMER, K. HÄKKINEN, H. BONNABAU, C. GRANADOS, D.N. FRENCH, and E.M. GOROSTIAGA. Detraining and tapering effects on hormonal responses and strength performance. *J Strength Cond Res* 21:768-775, 2007.

28. JOHNS, R.A., J.A. HOUMARD, R.W. KOBE, T. HORTOBAGYI, N.J. BRUNO, J.M. WELLS, and M.H. SHINEBARGER. Effects of taper on swim power, stroke distance, and performance. *Med Sci Sports Exerc* 24:1141-1146, 1992.

29. KAUHANEN, H. Organization of the coaching system of young weightlifters in Finland. In: *Proceedings of International Conference on Weightlifting and Strength Training*. Lahti, Finland, 1998, p. 137-140.

30. KUBUKELI, Z.N., T.D. NOAKES, and S.C. DENNIS. Training techniques to improve endurance exercise performances. *Sports Med* 32:489-509, 2002.

31. KUKUSHKIN, G.I. *System of Physical Education in the USSR*. Moscow: Raduga, 1983.

31b. LACEY, J., M. BRUGHELLI, M. MCGUIGAN, K. HANSEN, P. SAMOZINO, and J.B. MORIN. The effects of tapering on power-force-velocity profiling and jump performance in professional rugby league players, *J Strength Cond Res* 28(12):3567-3570, 2014.

32. MARTIN, D.T., J.C. SCIFRES, S.D. ZIMMERMAN, and J.G. WILKINSON. Effects of interval training and a taper on cycling performance and isokinetic leg strength. *Int J Sports Med* 15:485-491, 1994.

32b. MATVEYEV, L.P. Teorii postroenija sportivnoj trenirovki [Sport Training Design Theories]. *Teorija i praktica fiziceskoj kul'turi* [Theory and Practice of Physical Kulture]12:11-20, 1991.

32c. MATVEYEV, L., V. KALININ, and N. OZOLIN. Characteristics of athletic shape and methods of rationalizing the structure of the competitive phase. In: *Scientific Research Collection*. Moscow, 1974, pp. 4-23.

33. MCCONELL, G.K., D.L. COSTILL, J.J. WIDRICK, M.S. HICKEY, H. TANAKA, and P.B. GASTIN. Reduced training volume and intensity maintain aerobic capacity but not performance in distance runners. *Int J Sports Med* 14:33-37, 1993.
34. MUJIKA, I. The influence of training characteristics and tapering on the adaptation in highly trained individuals: a review. *Int J Sports Med* 19:439-446, 1998.
35. MUJIKA, I., T. BUSSO, L. LACOSTE, F. BARALE, A. GEYSSANT, and J.C. CHATARD. Modeled responses to training and taper in competitive swimmers. *Med Sci Sports Exerc* 28:251-258, 1996.
36. MUJIKA, I., J.C. CHATARD, and A. GEYSSANT. Effects of training and taper on blood leucocyte populations in competitive swimmers: relationships with cortisol and performance. *Int J Sports Med* 17:213-217, 1996.
37. MUJIKA, I., J.C. CHATARD, S. PADILLA, C.Y. GUEZENNEC, and A. GEYSSANT. Hormonal responses to training and its tapering off in competitive swimmers: relationships with performance. *Eur J Appl Physiol Occup Physiol* 74:361-366, 1996.
38. MUJIKA, I., A. GOYA, S. PADILLA, A. GRIJALBA, E. GOROSTIAGA, and J. IBANEZ. Physiological responses to a 6-d taper in middle-distance runners: influence of training intensity and volume. *Med Sci Sports Exerc* 32:511-517, 2000.
39. MUJIKA, I., A. GOYA, E. RUIZ, A. GRIJALBA, J. SANTISTEBAN, and S. PADILLA. Physiological and performance responses to a 6-day taper in middle-distance runners: influence of training frequency. *Int J Sports Med* 23:367-373, 2002.
40. MUJIKA, I., and S. PADILLA. Detraining: loss of training-induced physiological and performance adaptations: part I: short term insufficient training stimulus. *Sports Med* 30:79-87, 2000.
41. MUJIKA, I., and S. PADILLA. Scientific bases for precompetition tapering strategies. *Med Sci Sports Exerc* 35:1182-1187, 2003.
42. MUJIKA, I., S. PADILLA, A. GEYSSANT, and J.C. CHATARD. Hematological responses to training and taper in competitive swimmers: relationships with performance. *Arch Physiol Biochem* 105:379-385, 1998.
43. MUJIKA, I., S. PADILLA, and D. PYNE. Swimming performance changes during the final 3 weeks of training leading to the Sydney 2000 Olympic Games. *Int J Sports Med* 23:582-587, 2002.
44. MUJIKA, I., S. PADILLA, D. PYNE, and T. BUSSO. Physiological changes associated with the pre-event taper in athletes. *Sports Med* 34:891-927, 2004.
45. NABATNIKOWAS, M.Y. *Osnovy upravlienya podgotovki yunyky sportsmenov*. Moscow: Fizkultura i Sport, 1982.
46. NÁDORI, L., and I. GRANEK. *Theoretical and Methodological Basis of Training Planning With Special Considerations Within a Microcycle*. Lincoln, NE: NSCA, 1989.
47. NEARY, J.P., Y.N. BHAMBHANI, and D.C. MCKENZIE. Effects of different stepwise reduction taper protocols on cycling performance. *Can J Appl Physiol* 28:576-587, 2003.
48. NEARY, J.P., T.P. MARTIN, and H.A. QUINNEY. Effects of taper on endurance cycling capacity and single muscle fiber properties. *Med Sci Sports Exerc* 35:1875-1881, 2003.
49. NEARY, J.P., T.P. MARTIN, D.C. REID, R. BURNHAM, and H.A. QUINNEY. The effects of a reduced exercise duration taper programme on performance and muscle enzymes of endurance cyclists. *Eur J Appl Physiol Occup Physiol* 65:30-36, 1992.
50. NEUFER, P.D. The effect of detraining and reduced training on the physiological adaptations to aerobic exercise training. *Sports Med* 8:302-320, 1989.
51. NEUFER, P.D., D.L. COSTILL, R.A. FIELDING, M.G. FLYNN, and J.P. KIRWAN. Effect of reduced training on muscular strength and endurance in competitive swimmers. *Med Sci Sports Exerc* 19:486-490, 1987.
52. OLBRECT, J. *The Science of Winning: Planning, Periodizing, and Optimizing Swim Training*. Luton, UK: Swimshop, 2000.
52b. OZOLIN, N. *Sovremennaia Systema Sportivnoi Trenirovky* [Athlete's Training System for Competition]. Moscow: Fizkultura i Sport, 1971.
53. PAPOTI, M., L.E. MARTINS, S.A. CUNHA, A.M. ZAGATTO, and C.A. GOBATTO. Effects of taper on swimming force and swimmer performance after an experimental ten-week training program. *J Strength Cond Res* 21:538-542, 2007.
53b. PLATONOV, V.N. *L'Organizzazione dell'Allenamento e dell'Attività di Gara* [General Training Theory of Olympic Sports].Perugia, Italy: Calzetti & Mariucci, 2004.
54. PLISK, S.S., and M.H. STONE. Periodization strategies. *Strength Cond* 25:19-37, 2003.
55. RACKZEK, J. *Szkolenie mlodziezy w systemie sportu wyczynowego* [Youth Training in the Competitive Sport System]. Katowice, Poland: AWF, 1989.
56. RAGLIN, J.S., D.M. KOCEJA, J.M. STAGER, and C.A. HARMS. Mood, neuromuscular function, and performance during training in female swimmers. *Med Sci Sports Exerc* 28:372-377, 1996.
57. RIETJENS, G.J., H.A. KEIZER, H. KUIPERS, and W.H. SARIS. A reduction in training volume and intensity for 21 days does not impair performance in cyclists. *Br J Sports Med* 35:431-434, 2001.
58. SHEPLEY, B., J.D. MACDOUGALL, N. CIPRIANO, J.R. SUTTON, M.A. TARNOPOLSKY, and

G. COATES. Physiological effects of tapering in highly trained athletes. *J Appl Physiol* 72:706-711, 1992.
59. SMITH, D.J. A framework for understanding the training process leading to elite performance. *Sports Med* 33:1103-1126, 2003.
60. STONE, M.H., M.E. STONE, and W.A. SANDS. *Principles and Practice of Resistance Training.* Champaign, IL: Human Kinetics, 2007.
61. THOMAS, L., and T. BUSSO. A theoretical study of taper characteristics to optimize performance. *Med Sci Sports Exerc* 37:1615-1621, 2005.
62. TRAPPE, S., D. COSTILL, and R. THOMAS. Effect of swim taper on whole muscle and single muscle fiber contractile properties. *Med Sci Sports Exerc* 32:48-56, 2000.
63. ZARKADAS, P.C., J.B. CARTER, and E.W. BANISTER. Modelling the effect of taper on performance, maximal oxygen uptake, and the anaerobic threshold in endurance triathletes. *Adv Exp Med Biol* 393:179-186, 1995.
64. ZATSIORSKY, V.M. *Science and Practice of Strength Training.* Champaign, IL: Human Kinetics, 1995.
65. ZATSIORSKY, V.M., and W.J. KRAEMER. *Science and Practice of Strength Training.* 2nd ed. Champaign, IL: Human Kinetics, 2006.

Chapter 10

1. AAGAARD, P., J.L. ANDERSEN, P. DYHRE-POULSEN, A.M. LEFFERS, A. WAGNER, S.P. MAGNUSSON, J. HALKJAER-KRISTENSEN, and E.B. SIMONSEN. A mechanism for increased contractile strength of human pennate muscle in response to strength training: changes in muscle architecture. *J Physiol* 534:613-623, 2001.
2. AAGAARD, P., E.B. SIMONSEN, J.L. ANDERSEN, P. MAGNUSSON, and P. DYHRE-POULSEN. Increased rate of force development and neural drive of human skeletal muscle following resistance training. *J Appl Physiol* 93:1318-1326, 2002.
3. AAGAARD, P., E.B. SIMONSEN, J.L. ANDERSEN, S.P. MAGNUSSON, J. HALKJAER-KRISTENSEN, and P. DYHRE-POULSEN. Neural inhibition during maximal eccentric and concentric quadriceps contraction: effects of resistance training *J Appl Physiol* 89:2249-2257, 2000.
4. ABDESSEMED, D., P. DUCHE, C. HAUTIER, G. POUMARAT, and M. BEDU. Effect of recovery duration on muscular power and blood lactate during the bench press exercise. *Int J Sports Med* 20:368-373, 1999.
5. ADAMS, G.R., B.M. HATHER, K.M. BALDWIN, and G.A. DUDLEY. Skeletal muscle myosin heavy chain composition and resistance training. *J Appl Physiol* 74:911-915, 1993.
6. AHTIAINEN, J.P., A. PAKARINEN, M. ALEN, W.J. KRAEMER, and K. HÄKKINEN. Muscle hypertrophy, hormonal adaptations and strength development during strength training in strength-trained and untrained men. *Eur J Appl Physiol* 89:555-563, 2003.
7. AJÁN, T., and L. BAROGA. *Weightlifting: Fitness for All Sports.* Budapest: International Weightlifting Federation, 1988.
8. American College of Sports Medicine position stand: progressive models in resistance training for healthy adults. *Med Sci Sports Exerc* 34:364-380, 2002.
9. ANDERSEN, L.L., and P. AAGAARD. Influence of maximal muscle strength and intrinsic muscle contractile properties on contractile rate of force development. *Eur J Appl Physiol* 96:46-52, 2006.
10. BABRAJ et al., Collagen synthesis in human musculoskeletal tissues and skin. *Am J Physiol Endocrinol Metab.* 289 (5): E864-E869, 2005. 10.1152/ajpendo.00243.2005
11. BAKER, D. Comparison of upper-body strength and power between professional and college-aged rugby league players. *J Strength Cond Res* 15:30-35, 2001.
12. BAKER, D. A series of studies on the training of high-intensity muscle power in rugby league football players. *J Strength Cond Res* 15:198-209, 2001.
13. BAKER, D., and S. NANCE. The relation between running speed and measures of strength and power in professional rugby league players. *J Strength Cond Res* 13:230-235, 1999.
14. BARKER, M., T.J. WYATT, R.L. JOHNSON, M.H. STONE, H.S. O'BRYANT, C. POE, and M. KENT. Performance factors, physiological assessment, physical characteristic, and football playing ability. *J Strength Cond Res* 7:224-233, 1993.
15. BASTIAANS, J.J., A.B. VAN DIEMEN, T. VENEBERG, and A.E. JEUKENDRUP. The effects of replacing a portion of endurance training by explosive strength training on performance in trained cyclists. *Eur J Appl Physiol* 86:79-84, 2001.
16. BEHM, D., and D.G. SALE. Intended rather than actual movement velocity determines velocity-specific training response. *J Appl Physiol* 74:359-368, 1993.
17. BERGH, U., A. THORSTENSSON, B. SJODIN, B. HULTEN, K. PIEHL, and J. KARLSSON. Maximal oxygen uptake and muscle fiber types in trained and untrained humans. *Med Sci Sports* 10:151-154, 1978.
18. BILCHECK, H.M., W.J. KRAEMER, C.M. MARESH, and Z. M.A. The effect of isokinetic fatigue on recovery of maximal isokinetic concentric and eccentric strength in women. *J Strength Cond Res* 7:43-50, 1993.
19. BOBBERT, M.F., and A.J. VAN SOEST. Why do people jump the way they do? *Exerc Sport Sci Rev* 29:95-102, 2001.

20. BOMPA, T.O., and M.C. CARRERA. *Periodization Training for Sports: Science-Based Strength and Conditioning Plans for 20 Sports*. 2nd ed. Champaign, IL: Human Kinetics, 2005.
21. BOMPA, T.O. *Total Training for Coaching Team Sports: A Self Help Guide*. Toronto, CA: Sports Books Publisher, 2006.
22. BOMPA, T.O., and C.A. BUZZICHELLI. *Periodization Training for Sports*. 3rd ed. Champaign, IL: Human Kinetics, 2015.
23. BOUCHARD, C., F.T. DIONNE, J.A. SIMONEAU, and M.R. BOULAY. Genetics of aerobic and anaerobic performances. *Exerc Sport Sci Rev* 20:27-58, 1992.
24. BRET, C., A. RAHMANI, A.B. DUFOUR, L. MESSONNIER, and J.R. LACOUR. Leg strength and stiffness as ability factors in 100 m sprint running. *J Sports Med Phys Fitness* 42:274-281, 2002.
25. BRYZYCHI, M. Assessing Strength. *Fitness Manage* June:34-37, 2000.
26. BRYZYCHI, M. Strength testing: predicting a one rep max from reps to fatigue. *JOPERD* 64:88-90, 1993.
27. CAMPOS, G.E., T.J. LUECKE, H.K. WENDELN, K. TOMA, F.C. HAGERMAN, T.F. MURRAY, K.E. RAGG, N.A. RATAMESS, W.J. KRAEMER, and R.S. STARON. Muscular adaptations in response to three different resistance-training regimens: specificity of repetition maximum training zones. *Eur J Appl Physiol* 88:50-60, 2002.
28. CAVAGNA, G.A., F.P. SAIBENE, and R. MARGARIA. Effect of negative work on the amount of positive work performed by an isolated muscle. *J Appl Physiol* 20:157-158, 1965.
29. CHILIBECK, P.D., A.W. CALDER, D.G. SALE, and C.E. WEBBER. A comparison of strength and muscle mass increases during resistance training in young women. *Eur J Appl Physiol* 77:170-175, 1998.
30. CHIU, L.Z., A.C. FRY, B.K. SCHILLING, E.J. JOHNSON, and L.W. WEISS. Neuromuscular fatigue and potentiation following two successive high intensity resistance exercise sessions. *Eur J Appl Physiol* 92:385-392, 2004.
31. CHIU, L.Z., A.C. FRY, L.W. WEISS, B.K. SCHILLING, L.E. BROWN, and S.L. SMITH. Postactivation potentiation response in athletic and recreationally trained individuals. *J Strength Cond Res* 17:671-677, 2003.
32. CHRISTOU, M., I. SMILIOS, K. SOTIROPOULOS, K. VOLAKLIS, T. PILIANIDIS, and S.P. TOKMAKIDIS. Effects of resistance training on the physical capacities of adolescent soccer players. *J Strength Cond Res* 20:783-791, 2006.
33. CLARKSON, P.M., J.M. DEVANEY, H. GORDISH-DRESSMAN, P.D. THOMPSON, M.J. HUBAL, M. URSO, T.B. PRICE, T.J. ANGELOPOULOS, P.M. GORDON, N.M. MOYNA, L.S. PESCATELLO, P.S. VISICH, R.F. ZOELLER, R.L. SEIP, and E.P. HOFFMAN. ACTN3 genotype is associated with increases in muscle strength in response to resistance training in women. *J Appl Physiol* 99:154-163, 2005.
34. COFFEY, V.G., and J.A. HAWLEY. The molecular bases of training adaptation. *Sports Med* 37:737-763, 2007.
35. CRAMERI, R.M., H. LANGBERG, B. TEISNER, P. MAGNUSSON, H.D. SCHRÿDER, J.L. OLESEN, C.H. JENSEN, S. KOSKINEN, C. SUETTA, and M. KJAER. Enhanced procollagen processing in skeletal muscle after a single bout of eccentric loading in humans. *Matrix Biol* 23 (4):259–64, 2004.
36. CRONIN, J.B., and K.T. HANSEN. Strength and power predictors of sports speed. *J Strength Cond Res* 19:349-357, 2005.
37. CRONIN, J.B., P.J. MCNAIR, and R.N. MARSHALL. The role of maximal strength and load on initial power production. *Med Sci Sports Exerc* 32:1763-1769, 2000.
38. D'ANTONA, G., F. LANFRANCONI, M.A. PELLEGRINO, L. BROCCA, R. ADAMI, R. ROSSI, G. MORO, D. MIOTTI, M. CANEPARI, and R. BOTTINELLI. Skeletal muscle hypertrophy and structure and function of skeletal muscle fibres in male body builders. *J Physiol* 570:611-627, 2006.
39. DESCHENES, M. Short review: rate coding and motor unit recruitment patterns. *J Appl Sports Sci Res* 3:33-39, 1989.
40. DOESSING, S. and M. KJAER. Growth hormone and connective tissue in exercise. *Scand J Med Sci Sports* 15(4):202–210, 2005.
41. DONS, B., K. BOLLERUP, F. BONDE-PETERSEN, and S. HANCKE. The effect of weight-lifting exercise related to muscle fiber composition and muscle cross-sectional area in humans. *Eur J Appl Physiol* 40:95-106, 1979.
42. DRINKWATER, E.J., T.W. LAWTON, M.J. MCKENNA, R.P. LINDSELL, P.H. HUNT, and D.B. PYNE. Increased number of forced repetitions does not enhance strength development with resistance training. *J Strength Cond Res* 21:841-847, 2007.
43. DUCHATEAU, J., and K. HAINAUT. Isometric or dynamic training: differential effects on mechanical properties of a human muscle. *J Appl Physiol* 56:296-301, 1984.
44. DUCHATEAU, J., J.G. SEMMLER, and R.M. ENOKA. Training adaptations in the behavior of human motor units. *J Appl Physiol* 101:1766-1775, 2006.
45. EL-HEWIE, M.F. *Essentials of Weightlifting & Strength Training*. Lodi, NJ: Shaymaa, 2003.
46. EPLEY, B. *The Path to Athletic Power*. Champaign, IL: Human Kinetics, 2004.

47. FERRIS, D.P., J.F. SIGNORILE, and J.F. CARUSO. The relationship between physical and physiological variables and volleyball spiking velocity. *J Strength Cond Res* 9:32-36, 1995.

48. FLECK, S.J., and W.J. KRAEMER. *Designing Resistance Training Programs*. 2 ed. Champaign, IL: Human Kinetics, 1997.

49. FLECK, S., and W.J. KRAEMER. *Designing Resistance Training Programs*. 3rd ed. Champaign, IL: Human Kinetics, 2004.

50. FLORESCU, C., V. DUMITRESCU, and A. PREDESCU. *Metodologia Desvoltari Calitatilor Fizice* [The Methodology of Developing Physical Qualities]. Bucharest: National Sports Council, 1969.

51. FOLLAND, J.P., and A.G. WILLIAMS. The adaptations to strength training: morphological and neurological contributions to increased strength. *Sports Med* 37:145-168, 2007.

52. FROBOSE, I., A. VERDONCK, F. DUESBERG, and C. MUCHA. Effects of various load intensities in the framework of postoperative stationary endurance training on performance deficit of the quadriceps muscle of the thigh. *Z Orthop Ihre Grenzgeb* 131:164-167, 1993.

53. FRY, A.C. The role of resistance exercise intensity on muscle fibre adaptations. *Sports Med* 34:663-679, 2004.

54. FRY, A.C. The role of training intensity in resistance exercise overtraining and overreaching. In: *Overtraining in Sport*. R.B. Kreider, A.C. Fry, and M.L. O'Toole, eds. Champaign, IL: Human Kinetics, 1998, pp. 107-127.

55. FRY, A.C., and W.J. KRAEMER. Physical performance characteristics of American collegiate football players. *J Appl Sport Sci Res* 5:126-138, 1991.

56. FRY, A.C., B.K. SCHILLING, R.S. STARON, F.C. HAGERMAN, R.S. HIKIDA, and J.T. THRUSH. Muscle fiber characteristics and performance correlates of male Olympic-style weightlifters. *J Strength Cond Res* 17:746-754, 2003.

57. FRY, A.C., J.M. WEBBER, L.W. WEISS, M.P. HARBER, M. VACZI, and N.A. PATTISON. Muscle fiber characteristics of competitive power lifters. *J Strength Cond Res* 17:402-410, 2003.

58. GABBETT, T.J. Science of rugby league football: a review. *J Sports Sci* 23:961-976, 2005.

59. GABRIEL, D.A., G. KAMEN, and G. FROST. Neural adaptations to resistive exercise: mechanisms and recommendations for training practices. *Sports Med* 36:133-149, 2006.

60. GALLAGHER, P., S. TRAPPE, M. HARBER, A. CREER, S. MAZZETTI, T. TRAPPE, B. ALKNER, and P. TESCH. Effects of 84-days of bedrest and resistance training on single muscle fibre myosin heavy chain distribution in human vastus lateralis and soleus muscles. *Acta Physiol Scand* 185:61-69, 2005.

61. GARCÍA-RAMOS, A., P. PADIAL, G.G. HAFF, J. ARQÜELLES-CIENFUEGOS, M. GARCÍA-RAMOS, J. CONDE-PIPÓ, and B. FERICHE. Effect of different interrepetition rest periods on barbell velocity loss during the ballistic bench press exercise. *J Strength Cond Res* 29(9):2288-2296, 2015.

62. GISSIS, I., C. PAPADOPOULOS, V.I. KALAPOTHARAKOS, A. SOTIROPOULOS, G. KOMSIS, and E. MANOLOPOULOS. Strength and speed characteristics of elite, subelite, and recreational young soccer players. *Res Sports Med* 14:205-214, 2006.

63. GONZALEZ-BADILLO, J.J., M. IZQUIERDO, and E.M. GOROSTIAGA. Moderate volume of high relative training intensity produces greater strength gains compared with low and high volumes in competitive weightlifters. *J Strength Cond Res* 20:73-81, 2006.

64. GOTO, K., M. NAGASAWA, O. YANAGISAWA, T. KIZUKA, N. ISHII, and K. TAKAMATSU. Muscular adaptations to combinations of high- and low-intensity resistance exercises. *J Strength Cond Res* 18:730-737, 2004.

65. GROSSER, M., and A. NEUMEIER. *Tecnicas de Entrenamiento* [Training Techniques]. Barcelona, Spain: Martinez Roca, 1986.

66. HAFF, G.G., J.M. CARLOCK, M.J. HARTMAN, J.L. KILGORE, N. KAWAMORI, J.R. JACKSON, R.T. MORRIS, W.A. SANDS, and M.H. STONE. Force-time curve characteristics of dynamic and isometric muscle actions of elite women Olympic weightlifters. *J Strength Cond Res* 19:741-748, 2005.

67. HAFF, G.G., M.H. STONE, H.S. O'BRYANT, E. HARMAN, C.N. DINAN, R. JOHNSON, and K.H. HAN. Force-time dependent characteristics of dynamic and isometric muscle actions. *J Strength Cond Res* 11:269-272, 1997.

68. HAFF, G.G., A. WHITLEY, L.B. MCCOY, H.S. O'BRYANT, J.L. KILGORE, E.E. HAFF, K. PIERCE, and M.H. STONE. Effects of different set configurations on barbell velocity and displacement during a clean pull. *J Strength Cond Res* 17:95-103, 2003.

69. HAFF, G.G., A. WHITLEY, and J.A. POTTEIGER. A brief review: explosive exercises and sports performance. *Natl Strength Cond Assoc* 23:13-20, 2001.

70. HÄKKINEN, K. Neuromuscular adaptations during strength training, aging, detraining, and immobilization. *Crit Rev Phys Rehabil Med* 6:161-198, 1994.

71. HÄKKINEN, K., M. ALEN, M. KALLINEN, M. IZQUIERDO, K. JOKELAINEN, H. LASSILA, E. MALKIA, W.J. KRAEMER, and R.U. NEWTON.

Muscle CSA, force production, and activation of leg extensors during isometric and dynamic muscle actions in middle-aged and elderly men and women. *J Aging Phys Act* 6:232-247, 1998.

72. HÄKKINEN, K., and M. KALLINEN. Distribution of strength training volume into one or two daily sessions and neuromuscular adaptations in female athletes. *Electromyogr Clin Neurophysiol* 34:117-124, 1994.

73. HÄKKINEN, K., H. KAUHANEN, and T. KUOPPA. Neural, muscular and hormonal adaptations, changes in muscle strength and weightlifting results with respect to variations in training during one year follow-up period in Finnish elite weightlifters. *World Weightlifting (IWF)* 87:2-10, 1987.

74. HÄKKINEN, K., and P.V. KOMI. Changes in electrical and mechanical behavior of leg extensor muscles during heavy resistance strength training. *Scand J Sports Sci* 7:55-64, 1985.

75. HÄKKINEN, K., and P.V. KOMI. Effect of explosive type strength training on electromyographic and force production characteristics of leg extensor muscles during concentric and various stretch-shortening cycle exercises. *Scand J Sports Sci* 7:65-76, 1985.

76. HÄKKINEN, K., and P.V. KOMI. Training-induced changes in neuromuscular performance under voluntary and reflex conditions. *Eur J Appl Physiol Occup Physiol* 55:147-155, 1986.

77. HÄKKINEN, K., P.V. KOMI, M. ALEN, and H. KAUHANEN. EMG, muscle fibre and force production characteristics during a 1 year training period in elite weight-lifters. *Eur J Appl Physiol* 56:419-427, 1987.

78. HÄKKINEN, K., P.V. KOMI, and P.A. TESCH. Effect of combined concentric and eccentric strength training and detraining on force-time, muscle fiber and metabolic characteristics of leg extensor muscles. *Scand J Sports Sci* 3:50-58, 1981.

79. HÄKKINEN, K., R.U. NEWTON, S.E. GORDON, M. MCCORMICK, J.S. VOLEK, B.C. NINDL, L.A. GOTSHALK, W.W. CAMPBELL, W.J. EVANS, A. HÄKKINEN, B.J. HUMPHRIES, and W.J. KRAEMER. Changes in muscle morphology, electromyographic activity, and force production characteristics during progressive strength training in young and older men. *J Gerontol A Biol Sci Med Sci* 53:B415-423, 1998.

80. HÄKKINEN, K., A. PAKARINEN, M. ALEN, H. KAUHANEN, and P.V. KOMI. Neuromuscular and hormonal adaptations in athletes to strength training in two years. *J Appl Physiol* 65:2406-2412, 1988.

81. HARDEE, J.P., M.M. LAWRENCE, K.A. ZWETSLOOT, N.T. TRIPLETT, A.C. UTTER, and J.M. MCBRIDE. Effect of cluster set configurations on power clean technique. *J Sports Sci* 31(5):488-496, 2013.

82. HARDEE, J.P., N.T. TRIPLETT, A.C. UTTER, K.A. ZWETSLOOT, and J.M. MCBRIDE. Effect of interrepetition rest on power output in the power clean. *J Strength Cond Res* 26(4):883-889, 2012.

83. HARMAN, E. Resistance training modes: a biomechanical perspective. *Strength Cond* 16:59-65, 1994.

84. HARRIS, G.R., M.H. STONE, H.S. O'BRYANT, C.M. PROULX, and R.L. JOHNSON. Short-term performance effects of high power, high force, or combined weight-training methods. *J Strength Cond Res* 14:14-20, 2000.

85. HARRIS, R.C., R.H. EDWARDS, E. HULTMAN, L.O. NORDESJO, B. NYLIND, and K. SAHLIN. The time course of phosphorylcreatine resynthesis during recovery of the quadriceps muscle in man. *Pflugers Arch* 367:137-142, 1976.

86. HENNEMAN, E., G. SOMJEN, and D.O. CARPENTER. Excitability and inhibitability of motoneurons of different sizes. *J Neurophysiol* 28:599-620, 1965.

87. HIGBIE, E.J., K.J. CURETON, G.L. WARREN, III, and B.M. PRIOR. Effects of concentric and eccentric training on muscle strength, cross-sectional area, and neural activation. *J Appl Physiol* 81:2173-2181, 1996.

88. HOEGER, W.W.K., D.R. HOPKINS, S.L. BARETTE, and D.F. HALE. Relationship between repetitions and selected percentages of one repetition maximum: a comparison between untrained and trained males and females. *J Appl Sport Sci Res* 4:47-54, 1990.

89. HOFF, J., A. GRAN, and J. HELGERUD. Maximal strength training improves aerobic endurance performance. *Scand J Med Sci Sports* 12:288-295, 2002.

90. HOFF, J., and J. HELGERUD. Endurance and strength training for soccer players: physiological considerations. *Sports Med* 34:165-180, 2004.

91. HOFF, J., J. HELGERUD, and U. WISLOFF. Maximal strength training improves work economy in trained female cross-country skiers. *Med Sci Sports Exerc* 31:870-877, 1999.

92. HOFF, J., O.J. KEMI, and J. HELGERUD. Strength and endurance differences between elite and junior elite ice hockey players: the importance of allometric scaling. *Int J Sports Med* 26:537-541, 2005.

93. HOFFMAN, J.R., W.J. KRAEMER, A.C. FRY, M. DESCHENES, and M. KEMP. The effects of self-selection for frequency of training in a winter conditioning program for football. *J Appl Sport Sci Res* 4:76-82, 1990.

94. HOLTERMANN, A., K. ROELEVELD, B. VEREIJKEN, and G. ETTEMA. The effect of rate of force

development on maximal force production: acute and training-related aspects. *Eur J Appl Physiol* 99:605-613, 2007.

95. HOUSTON, M.E., E.A. FROESE, S.P. VALERIOTE, H.J. GREEN, and D.A. RANNEY. Muscle performance, morphology and metabolic capacity during strength training and detraining: a one leg model. *Eur J Appl Physiol* 51:25-35, 1983.

96. HOWARD, J.D., M.R. RITCHIE, D.A. GATER, D.R. GATER, and R.M. ENOKA. Determining factors of strength: physiological foundations. *National Strength and Conditioning Journal* 7(6):16-21, 1985.

97. HULTMAN, E., J. BERGSTROM, and N.M. ANDERSON. Breakdown and resynthesis of phosphorylcreatine and adenosine triphosphate in connection with muscular work in man. *Scand J Clin Lab Invest* 19:56-66, 1967.

98. HULTMAN, E., and H. SJOHOLM. Biochemical causes of fatigue. In: *Human Muscle Power*. N.L. Jones, ed. Champaign, IL: Human Kinetics, 1986, pp. 343-363.

99. HUMPHRIES, B., E. DUGAN, and T.L. DOYLE. Muscular fitness. In: *ACSM's Resource Manual for Guidelines for Exercise Testing and Prescription*. L.A. Kaminsky, ed. Baltimore: Lippincott Williams & Wilkins, 2006, pp. 206-224.

100. HUYGENS, W., M.A. THOMIS, M.W. PEETERS, R.F. VLIETINCK, and G.P. BEUNEN. Determinants and upper-limit heritabilities of skeletal muscle mass and strength. *Can J Appl Physiol* 29:186-200, 2004.

101. IVEY, F.M., S.M. ROTH, R.E. FERRELL, B.L. TRACY, J.T. LEMMER, D.E. HURLBUT, G.F. MARTEL, E.L. SIEGEL, J.L. FOZARD, E. JEFFREY METTER, J.L. FLEG, and B.F. HURLEY. Effects of age, gender, and myostatin genotype on the hypertrophic response to heavy resistance strength training. *J Gerontol A Biol Sci Med Sci* 55:M641-M648, 2000.

102. IZQUIERDO, M., J. IBANEZ, J.J. GONZALEZ-BADILLO, K. HÄKKINEN, N.A. RATAMESS, W.J. KRAEMER, D.N. FRENCH, J. ESLAVA, A. ALTADILL, X. ASIAIN, and E.M. GOROSTIAGA. Differential effects of strength training leading to failure versus not to failure on hormonal responses, strength, and muscle power gains. *J Appl Physiol* 100:1647-1656, 2006.

103. JENSEN, B.R., M. PILEGAARD, and G. SJOGAARD. Motor unit recruitment and rate coding in response to fatiguing shoulder abductions and subsequent recovery. *Eur J Appl Physiol* 83:190-199, 2000.

104. JONES, K., P. BISHOP, G. HUNTER, and G. FLEISIG. The effects of varying resistance-training loads on intermediate- and high-velocity-specific adaptations. *J Strength Cond Res* 15:349-356, 2001.

105. JONES, L. Coaching platform: advanced training programs. *Weightlifting USA* volume x issue 4: 8-11, 1992.

106. JUNG, A.P. The impact of resistance training on distance running performance. *Sports Med* 33:539-552, 2003.

107. KAMEN, G. The acquisition of maximal isometric plantar flexor strength: a force-time curve analysis. *J Motor Behav* 15:63-73, 1983.

108. KAMEN, G., and A. ROY. Motor unit synchronization in young and elderly adults. *Eur J Appl Physiol* 81:403-410, 2000.

109. KANEKO, M., T. FUCHIMOTO, H. TOJI, and K. SUEI. Training effect of different loads on the force–velocity relationship and mechanical power output in human muscle. *Scand J Sports Sci* 5:50-55, 1983.

110. KAWAMORI, N., and G.G. HAFF. The optimal training load for the development of muscular power. *J Strength Cond Res* 18:675-684, 2004.

111. KEMMLER, W.K., D. LAUBER, A. WASSERMANN, and J.L. MAYHEW. Predicting maximal strength in trained postmenopausal woman. *J Strength Cond Res* 20:838-842, 2006.

112. KJAER, M., H. LANGBERG, B.F. MILLER, R. BOUSHEL, R. CRAMERI, S. KOSKINEN, K. HEINEMEIER, J.L. OLESEN, S. DÿSSING, M. HANSEN, S.G. PEDERSEN, M.J. RENNIE, and P. MAGNUSSON. Metabolic activity and collagen turnover in human tendon in response to physical activity. *J Musculoskelet Neuronal Interact* 5(1):41-52, 2005.

113. KJAER, M., P. MAGNUSSON, M. KROGSGAARD, J. BOYSEN MÿLLER, J. OLESEN, K. HEINEMEIER, M. HANSEN, B. HARALDSON, S. KOSKINEN, B. ESMARCK, and H. LANGBERG. Extracellular matrix adaptation of tendon and skeletal muscle to exercise. *J Anat* 208(4):445-450, 2006.

114. KOMI, P.V. *Strength and Power in Sport*. 2nd ed. Malden, MA: Blackwell Scientific, 2003.

115. KOMI, P.V. Stretch-shortening cycle: a powerful model to study normal and fatigued muscle. *J Biomech* 33:1197-1206, 2000.

116. KOMI, P.V. Training of muscle strength and power: interaction of neuromotoric, hypertrophic, and mechanical factors. *Int J Sports Med* 7:10-15, 1986.

117. KRAEMER, W.J., A.C. FRY, B.J. WARREN, M.H. STONE, S.J. FLECK, J.T. KEARNEY, B.P. CONROY, C.M. MARESH, C.A. WESEMAN, N.T. TRIPLETT, and S.E. GORDON. Acute hormonal responses in elite junior weightlifters. *Int J Sports Med* 13:103-109, 1992.

118. KRAEMER, W.J., L. MARCHITELLI, S.E. GORDON, E. HARMAN, J.E. DZIADOS, R. MELLO, P. FRYKMAN, D. MCCURRY, and S.J. FLECK. Hormonal and growth factor responses to heavy

resistance exercise protocols. *J Appl Physiol* 69:1442-1450, 1990.

119. KRAVITZ, L., C. AKALAN, K. NOWICKI, and S.J. KINZEY. Prediction of 1 repetition maximum in high-school power lifters. *J Strength Cond Res* 17:167-172, 2003.

120. LANGBERG et al. Eccentric rehabilitation exercise increases peritendinous type I collagen synthesis in humans with Achilles tendinosis, *Scand J Med Sci Sports* 17(1):61-6, 2007.

121. LAWTON, T., J. CRONIN, E. DRINKWATER, R. LINDSELL, and D. PYNE. The effect of continuous repetition training and intra-set rest training on bench press strength and power. *J Sports Med Phys Fitness* 44:361-367, 2004.

122. LAWTON, T.W., J.B. CRONIN, and R.P. LINDSELL. Effect of interrepetition rest intervals on weight training repetition power output. *J Strength Cond Res* 20:172-176, 2006.

123. MACDOUGALL, J.D., G.C. ELDER, D.G. SALE, J.R. MOROZ, and J.R. SUTTON. Effects of strength training and immobilization on human muscle fibres. *Eur J Appl Physiol* 43:25-34, 1980.

124. MALISOUX, L., M. FRANCAUX, and D. THEISEN. What do single-fiber studies tell us about exercise training? *Med Sci Sports Exerc* 39:1051-1060, 2007.

125. MAYHEW, J.L., J.L. PRINSTER, J.S. WARE, D.L. ZIMMER, J.R. ARABAS, and M.G. BEMBEN. Muscular endurance repetitions to predict bench press strength in men of different training levels. *J Sports Med Phys Fitness* 35:108-113, 1995.

126. MCBRIDE, J.M., S. NIMPHIUS, and T.M. ERICKSON. The acute effects of heavy-load squats and loaded countermovement jumps on sprint performance. *J Strength Cond Res* 19:893-897, 2005.

127. MCBRIDE, J.M., T. TRIPLETT-MCBRIDE, A. DAVIE, and R.U. NEWTON. A comparison of strength and power characteristics between power lifters, Olympic lifters, and sprinters. *J Strength Cond Res* 13:58-66, 1999.

128. MCBRIDE, J.M., T. TRIPLETT-MCBRIDE, A. DAVIE, and R.U. NEWTON. The effect of heavy- vs. light-load jump squats on the development of strength, power, and speed. *J Strength Cond Res* 16:75-82, 2002.

129. MCCALL, G.E., W.C. BYRNES, S.J. FLECK, A. DICKINSON, and W.J. KRAEMER. Acute and chronic hormonal responses to resistance training designed to promote muscle hypertrophy. *Can J Appl Physiol* 24:96-107, 1999.

130. MELROSE, D.R., F.J. SPANIOL, M.E. BOHLING, and R.A. BONNETTE. Physiological and performance characteristics of adolescent club volleyball players. *J Strength Cond Res* 21:481-486, 2007.

131. MILLER, B.F., J.L. OLESEN, M. HANSEN, S. DÿSSING, R.M. CRAMERI, R.J. WELLING, H. LANGBERG, A. FLYVBJERG, M. KJAER, J.A. BABRAJ, K. SMITH, and M.J. RENNIE. Coordinated collagen and muscle protein synthesis in human patella tendon and quadriceps muscle after exercise. *J Physiol* 567(3):1021-1033, 2005.

132. MILNER-BROWN, H.S., R.B. STEIN, and R.G. LEE. Synchronization of human motor units: possible roles of exercise and supraspinal reflexes. *Electroencephalogr Clin Neurophysiol* 38:245-254, 1975.

133. MIRKOV, D.M., A. NEDELJKOVIC, S. MILANOVIC, and S. JARIC. Muscle strength testing: evaluation of tests of explosive force production. *Eur J Appl Physiol* 91:147-154, 2004.

134. MORITANI, T., W.M. SHERMAN, M. SHIBATA, T. MATSUMOTO, and M. SHINOHARA. Oxygen availability and motor unit activity in humans. *Eur J Appl Physiol Occup Physiol* 64:552-556, 1992.

135. MOSS, B.M., P.E. REFSNES, A. ABILDGAARD, K. NICOLAYSEN, and J. JENSEN. Effects of maximal effort strength training with different loads on dynamic strength, cross-sectional area, load-power and load-velocity relationships. *Eur J Appl Physiol* 75:193-199, 1997.

136. NOAKES, T.D. Implications of exercise testing for prediction of athletic performance: a contemporary perspective. *Med Sci Sports Exerc* 20:319-330, 1988.

137. NOAKES, T.D., K.H. MYBURGH, and R. SCHALL. Peak treadmill running velocity during the VO2 max test predicts running performance. *J Sports Sci* 8:35-45, 1990.

138. NORRBRAND, L., J.D. FLUCKEY, M. POZZO, and P.A. TESCH. Resistance training using eccentric overload induces early adaptations in skeletal muscle size. *Eur J Appl Physiol* 102:271-281, 2008.

139. ØSTERÅS, H., J. HELGERUD, and J. HOFF. Maximal strength-training effects on force–velocity and force-power relationships explain increases in aerobic performance in humans. *Eur J Appl Physiol* 88:255-263, 2002.

140. PAAVOLAINEN, L., K. HÄKKINEN, I. HAMALAINEN, A. NUMMELA, and H. RUSKO. Explosive-strength training improves 5-km running time by improving running economy and muscle power. *J Appl Physiol* 86:1527-1533, 1999.

141. PAAVOLAINEN, L., K. HÄKKINEN, and H. RUSKO. Effects of explosive type strength training on physical performance characteristics in cross-country skiers. *Eur J Appl Physiol Occup Physiol* 62:251-255, 1991.

142. PAPADIMITRIOU, I.D., C. PAPADOPOULOS, A. KOUVATSI, and C. TRIANTAPHYLLIDIS. The ACTN3 gene in elite Greek track and field athletes. *Int J Sports Med* 29:352-355, 2008.

143. PETERSON, M.D., B.A. ALVAR, and M.R. RHEA. The contribution of maximal force production to explosive movement among young collegiate athletes. *J Strength Cond Res* 20:867-873, 2006.
144. PETERSON, M.D., M.R. RHEA, and B.A. ALVAR. Applications of the dose-response for muscular strength development: a review of meta-analytic efficacy and reliability for designing training prescription. *J Strength Cond Res* 19:950-958, 2005.
145. PINCIVERO, D.M., W.S. GEAR, N.M. MOYNA, and R.J. ROBERTSON. The effects of rest interval on quadriceps torque and perceived exertion in healthy males. *J Sports Med Phys Fitness* 39:294-299, 1999.
146. PLISK, S.S., and M.H. STONE. Periodization strategies. *Strength Cond* 25:19-37, 2003.
147. POLLOCK, M.L., J.E. GRAVES, M.M. BAMMAN, S.H. LEGGETT, D.M. CARPENTER, C. CARR, J. CIRULLI, J. MATKOZICH, and M. FULTON. Frequency and volume of resistance training: effect on cervical extension strength. *Arch Phys Med Rehabil* 74:1080-1086, 1993.
148. PRINCE, F.P., R.S. HIKIDA, and F.C. HAGERMAN. Human muscle fiber types in power lifters, distance runners and untrained subjects. *Pflugers Arch* 363:19-26, 1976.
149. PRINCE, F.P., R.S. HIKIDA, F.C. HAGERMAN, R.S. STARON, and W.H. ALLEN. A morphometric analysis of human muscle fibers with relation to fiber types and adaptations to exercise. *J Neurol Sci* 49:165-179, 1981.
150. REYNOLDS, J.M., T.J. GORDON, and R.A. ROBERGS. Prediction of one repetition maximum strength from multiple repetition maximum testing and anthropometry. *J Strength Cond Res* 20:584-592, 2006.
151. RHEA, M.R., B.A. ALVAR, L.N. BURKETT, and S.D. BALL. A meta-analysis to determine the dose response for strength development. *Med Sci Sports Exerc* 35:456-464, 2003.
152. ROONEY, K.J., R.D. HERBERT, and R.J. BALNAVE. Fatigue contributes to the strength training stimulus. *Med Sci Sports Exerc* 26:1160-1164, 1994.
153. RUTHERFORD, O.M. and D.A. JONES. The role of learning and coordination in strength training. *Eur J Appl Physiol Occup Physiol* 55:100-105, 1986.
154. RYDWIK, E., C. KARLSSON, K. FRANDIN, and G. AKNER. Muscle strength testing with one repetition maximum in the arm/shoulder for people aged 75 +: test-retest reliability. *Clin Rehabil* 21:258-265, 2007.
155. SAHLIN, K., and J.M. REN. Relationship of contraction capacity to metabolic changes during recovery from a fatiguing contraction. *J Appl Physiol* 67:648-654, 1989.
156. SALE, D.G. Neural adaptation to resistance training. *Med Sci Sports Exerc* 20:S135-S145, 1988.
157. SCHMIDTBLEICHER, D. Strength training, part 2: structural analysis of motor strength qualities and its application to training. *Science Periodical on Research and Technology* 5:1-10, 1985.
158. SCHMIDTBLEICHER, D. 1984. *Sportliches Krafttraining*. Berlin: Jung, Haltong, und Bewegung bei Menchen.
159. SCHMIDTBLEICHER, D. Training for power events. In: *Strength and Power in Sport*. P.V. Komi, ed. Oxford, UK: Blackwell, 1992, pp. 381-385.
160. SEMMLER, J.G. Motor unit synchronization and neuromuscular performance. *Exerc Sport Sci Rev* 30:8-14, 2002.
161. SEMMLER, J.G., K.W. KORNATZ, D.V. DINENNO, S. ZHOU, and R.M. ENOKA. Motor unit synchronisation is enhanced during slow lengthening contractions of a hand muscle. *J Physiol* 545:681-695, 2002.
162. SEMMLER, J.G., and M.A. NORDSTROM. Motor unit discharge and force tremor in skill- and strength-trained individuals. *Exp Brain Res* 119:27-38, 1998.
163. SEMMLER, J.G., M.V. SALE, F.G. MEYER, and M.A. NORDSTROM. Motor-unit coherence and its relation with synchrony are influenced by training. *J Neurophysiol* 92:3320-3331, 2004.
164. SEYNNES, O.R., M. DE BOER, and M.V. NARICI. Early skeletal muscle hypertrophy and architectural changes in response to high-intensity resistance training. *J Appl Physiol* 102:368-373, 2007.
165. SFORZO, G.A., and P.R. TOUEY. Manipulating exercise order affects muscular performance during a resistance exercise training session. *J Strength Cond Res* 10:20-24, 1996.
166. SHAW, C.E., K.K. MCCULLY, and J.D. POSNER. Injuries during the one repetition maximum assessment in the elderly. *J Cardiopulm Rehabil* 15:283-287, 1995.
167. SHIMANO, T., W.J. KRAEMER, B.A. SPIERING, J.S. VOLEK, D.L. HATFIELD, R. SILVESTRE, J.L. VINGREN, M.S. FRAGALA, C.M. MARESH, S.J. FLECK, R.U. NEWTON, L.P. SPREUWENBERG, and K. HÄKKINEN. Relationship between the number of repetitions and selected percentages of one repetition maximum in free weight exercises in trained and untrained men. *J Strength Cond Res* 20:819-823, 2006.
168. SHOEPE, T.C., J.E. STELZER, D.P. GARNER, and J.J. WIDRICK. Functional adaptability of muscle fibers to long-term resistance exercise. *Med Sci Sports Exerc* 35:944-951, 2003.
169. SIFF, M.C., and Y.U. VERKHOSHANSKY. *Supertraining*. Denver, CO: Supertraining International, 1999.

170. SILVESTRE, R., W.J. KRAEMER, C. WEST, D.A. JUDELSON, B.A. SPIERING, J.L. VINGREN, D.L. HATFIELD, J.M. ANDERSON, and C.M. MARESH. Body composition and physical performance during a National Collegiate Athletic Association Division I men's soccer season. *J Strength Cond Res* 20:962-970, 2006.

171. SMITH, J.C., A.C. FRY, L.W. WEISS, Y. LI, and S.J. KINZEY. The effects of high-intensity exercise on a 10-second sprint cycle test. *J Strength Cond Res* 15:344-348, 2001.

172. STARON, R.S., E.S. MALICKY, M.J. LEONARDI, J.E. FALKEL, F.C. HAGERMAN, and G.A. DUDLEY. Muscle hypertrophy and fast fiber type conversions in heavy resistance-trained women. *Eur J Appl Physiol* 60:71-79, 1990.

173. STONE, M.H., T.J. CHANDLER, M.S. CONLEY, J.B. KRAMER, and M.E. STONE. Training to muscular failure: is it necessary? *Strength Cond* 18:44-51, 1996.

174. STONE, M.H., and H.O. O'BRYANT. *Weight Training: A Scientific Approach.* Edina, MN: Burgess, 1987.

175. STONE, M.H., H.S. O'BRYANT, B.K. SCHILLING, R.L. JOHNSON, K.C. PIERCE, G.G. HAFF, A.J. KOCH, and M. STONE. Periodization: effects of manipulating volume and intensity, part 1. *Strength Cond* 21:56-62, 1999.

176. STONE, M.H., H.S. O'BRYANT, B.K. SCHILLING, R.L. JOHNSON, K.C. PIERCE, G.G. HAFF, A.J. KOCH, and M. STONE. Periodization: effects of manipulating volume and intensity, part 2. *Strength Cond J* 21:54-60, 1999.

177. STONE, M.H., K. PIERCE, W.A. SANDS, and M. STONE. Weightlifting: program design. *Strength Cond* 28:10-17, 2006.

178. STONE, M.H., W.A. SANDS, K.C. PIERCE, J. CARLOCK, M. CARDINALE, and R.U. NEWTON. Relationship of maximum strength to weightlifting performance. *Med Sci Sports Exerc* 37:1037-1043, 2005.

179. STONE, M.H., W.A. SANDS, K.C. PIERCE, M.W. RAMSEY, and G.G. HAFF. Power and power potentiation among strength power athletes: preliminary study. *Int J Sports Physiol Perf* in press.

180. STONE, M.H., M.E. STONE, and W.A. SANDS. *Principles and Practice of Resistance Training.* Champaign, IL: Human Kinetics, 2007.

181. STULL, G.A., and D.H. CLARKE. Patterns of recovery following isometric and isotonic strength decrement. *Med Sci Sports* 3:135-139, 1971.

182. TAN, B. Manipulating resistance training program variables to optimize maximum strength in men: a review. *J Strength Cond Res* 13:289-304, 1999.

183. TANAKA, H., and T. SWENSEN. Impact of resistance training on endurance performance: a new form of cross-training? *Sports Med* 25:191-200, 1998.

184. TERZIS, G., G. GEORGIADIS, E. VASSILIADOU, and P. MANTA. Relationship between shot put performance and triceps brachia fiber type composition and power production. *Eur J Appl Physiol* 90:10-15, 2003.

185. TESCH, P.A., and J. KARLSSON. Muscle fiber types and size in trained and untrained muscles of elite athletes. *J Appl Physiol* 59:1716-1720, 1985.

186. TESCH, P.A., A. THORSSON, and P. KAISER. Muscle capillary supply and fiber type characteristics in weight and power lifters. *J Appl Physiol Respir Environ Exerc Physiol* 56(1):35-38, 1984.

187. TESCH, P.A., and L. LARSSON. Muscle hypertrophy in bodybuilders. *Eur J Appl Physiol Occup Physiol* 49(3):301-306, 1982.

188. THOMAS, M., M.A. FIATARONE, and R.A. FIELDING. Leg power in young women: relationship to body composition, strength, and function. *Med Sci Sports Exerc* 28:1321-1326, 1996.

189. THOMPSON, P.D., N. MOYNA, R. SEIP, T. PRICE, P. CLARKSON, T. ANGELOPOULOS, P. GORDON, L. PESCATELLO, P. VISICH, R. ZOELLER, J.M. DEVANEY, H. GORDISH, S. BILBIE, and E.P. HOFFMAN. Functional polymorphisms associated with human muscle size and strength. *Med Sci Sports Exerc* 36:1132-1139, 2004.

190. THORSTENSSON, A., B. HULTEN, W. VON DOBELN, and J. KARLSSON. Effect of strength training on enzyme activities and fibre characteristics in human skeletal muscle. *Acta Physiol Scand* 96:392-398, 1976.

191. TRAPPE, S., M. HARBER, A. CREER, P. GALLAGHER, D. SLIVKA, K. MINCHEV, and D. WHITSETT. Single muscle fiber adaptations with marathon training. *J Appl Physiol* 101:721-727, 2006.

192. VAN CUTSEM, M., J. DUCHATEAU, and K. HAINAUT. Changes in single motor unit behaviour contribute to the increase in contraction speed after dynamic training in humans. *J Physiol* 513(1):295-305, 1998.

193. VIITASALO, J.T. Rate of force development, muscle structure and fatigue. In: *Biomechanics VII-A: Proceedings of the 7th International Congress of Biomechanics.* A. Morecki, et al. eds. Warsaw, Poland: PWN, 1981, pp. 136-141.

194. VIITASALO, J.T., and P.V. KOMI. Interrelationships between electromyographic, mechanical, muscle structure and reflex time measurements in man. *Acta Physiol Scand* 111:97-103, 1981.

195. VOROBYEV, A.N. *A Textbook on Weightlifting.* Budapest: International Weightlifting Federation, 1978.

196. WERNBOM, M., J. AUGUSTSSON, and R. THOMEE. The influence of frequency, intensity,

volume and mode of strength training on whole muscle cross-sectional area in humans. *Sports Med* 37:225-264, 2007.

197. WESTCOTT, W.L. *Strength Fitness*. Boston: Allyn & Bacon, 1982.

198. WIDRICK, J.J., J.E. STELZER, T.C. SHOEPE, and D.P. GARNER. Functional properties of human muscle fibers after short-term resistance exercise training. *Am J Physiol Regul Integr Comp Physiol* 283:R408-R416, 2002.

199. WILLARDSON, J.M. A brief review: factors affecting the length of the rest interval between resistance exercise sets. *J Strength Cond Res* 20:978-984, 2006.

200. WILLIAMSON, D.L., P.M. GALLAGHER, C.C. CARROLL, U. RAUE, and S.W. TRAPPE. Reduction in hybrid single muscle fiber proportions with resistance training in humans. *J Appl Physiol* 91:1955-1961, 2001.

201. Wilmore and Costill, *Training for Sport and Activity: The Physiological Basis of the Conditioning Process*. Champaign, IL: Human Kinetics, 1993.

202. WILSON, G.J., R.U. NEWTON, A.J. MURPHY, and B.J. HUMPHRIES. The optimal training load for the development of dynamic athletic performance. *Med Sci Sports Exerc* 25:1279-1286, 1993.

203. YAMAMOTO, L.M., R.M. LOPEZ, J.F. KLAU, D.J. CASA, W.J. KRAEMER, and C.M. MARESH. The effects of resistance training on endurance distance running performance among highly trained runners: a systematic review. *J Strength Cond Res* 22:2036-2044. 2008.

204. YAO, W., R.J. FUGLEVAND, and R.M. ENOKA. Motor-unit synchronization increases EMG amplitude and decreases force steadiness of simulated contractions. *J Neurophysiol* 83:441-452, 2000.

205. YETTER, M. and G.L. MOIR. The acute effects of heavy back and front squats on speed during forty-meter sprint trials. *J Strength Cond Res* 22:159-165. 2008.

206. YOUNG, W.B., A. JENNER, and K. GRIFFITHS. Acute enhancement of power performance from heavy load squats. *J. Strength Cond Res* 12:82-84, 1998.

207. ZATSIORSKY, V.M. *Science and Practice of Strength Training*. Champaign, IL: Human Kinetics, 1995.

208. ZATSIORSKY, V.M., and W.J. KRAEMER. *Science and Practice of Strength Training*. 2nd ed. Champaign, IL: Human Kinetics, 2006.

Chapter 11

1. *2002 USA Cycling Club Coach Manual*. Colorado Springs, CO: USA Cycling, 2002.

2. AAGAARD, P., E.B. SIMONSEN, J.L. ANDERSEN, P. MAGNUSSON, and P. DYHRE-POULSEN. Increased rate of force development and neural drive of human skeletal muscle following resistance training. *J Appl Physiol* 93:1318-1326, 2002.

3. ABERNETHY, P.J., R. THAYER, and A.W. TAYLOR. Acute and chronic responses of skeletal muscle to endurance and sprint exercise. A review. *Sports Med* 10:365-389, 1990.

4. ACEVEDO, E.O., and A.H. GOLDFARB. Increased training intensity effects on plasma lactate, ventilatory threshold, and endurance. *Med Sci Sports Exerc* 21:563-568, 1989.

4b. AKENHEAD, R., P.R. HAYES, K.G. THOMPSON, and D. FRENCH. Diminutions of acceleration and deceleration output during professional football match play. *J Sci Med Sport* 16(6):556-561, 2013.

5. BAILEY, S.P., and R.R. PATE. Feasibility of improving running economy. *Sports Med* 12:228-236, 1991.

6. BAKER, D., and S. NANCE. The relation between running speed and measures of strength and power in professional rugby league players. *J Strength Cond Res* 13:230-235, 1999.

7. BALSOM, P.D., J.Y. SEGER, B. SJÖDIN, and B. EKBLOM. Maximal-intensity intermittent exercise: effect of recovery duration. *Int J Sports Med* 13:528-533, 1992.

8. BALSOM, P.D., J.Y. SEGER, B. SJÖDIN, and B. EKBLOM. Physiological responses to maximal intensity intermittent exercise. *Eur J Appl Physiol* 65:144-149, 1992.

8b. BANGSBO, J., F.M. IAIA, and P. KRUSTRUP. The Yo-Yo intermittent recovery test: a useful tool for evaluation of physical performance in intermittent sports. *Sports Med* 38(1):37-51, 2008.

9. BASSETT, D.R., Jr., and E.T. HOWLEY. Limiting factors for maximum oxygen uptake and determinants of endurance performance. *Med Sci Sports Exerc* 32:70-84, 2000.

10. BASSETT, D.R., Jr., and E.T. HOWLEY. Maximal oxygen uptake: "classical" versus "contemporary: viewpoints. *Med Sci Sports Exerc* 29:591-603, 1997.

11. BASTIAANS, J.J., A.B. VAN DIEMEN, T. VENEBERG, and A.E. JEUKENDRUP. The effects of replacing a portion of endurance training by explosive strength training on performance in trained cyclists. *Eur J Appl Physiol* 86:79-84, 2001.

12. BEHM, D.G., and D.G. SALE. Intended rather than actual movement velocity determines velocity-specific training response. *J Appl Physiol* 74:359-368, 1993.

13. BEHM, D.G., and D.G. SALE. Velocity specificity of resistance training. *Sports Med* 15:374-388, 1993.

14. BENTLEY, D.J., J. NEWELL, and D. BISHOP. Incremental exercise test design and analysis: implications for performance diagnostics in endurance athletes. *Sports Med* 37:575-586, 2007.

15. BERGLUND, B., B. EKBLOM, E. EKBLOM, L. BERGLUND, A. KALLNER, P. REINEBO, and S. LINDEBERG. The Swedish Blood Pass project. *Scand J Med Sci Sports* 17:292-297, 2007.

16. BILLAT, L.V. Interval training for performance: a scientific and empirical practice. Special recommendations for middle- and long-distance running. Part I: aerobic interval training. *Sports Med* 31(1):13-31, 2001.

17. BILLAT, L.V. Interval training for performance: a scientific and empirical practice. Special recommendations for middle- and long-distance running. Part II: anaerobic interval training. *Sports Med* 31:75-90, 2001.

17b. BILLAT, V., J.C. RENOUX, J. PINOTEAU, B. PETIT, and J.P. KORALSZTEIN. Times to exhaustion at 90, 100 and 105% of velocity at VO2 max (maximal aerobic speed) and critical speed in elite long-distance runners, *Arch Physiol Biochem*.103(2):129-35, 1995.

17c. BILLAT, V., B. FLECHET, B. PETIT, G. MURIAUX, and J.P. KORALSZTEIN. Interval training at VO2max: effects on aerobic performance and overtraining markers. *Med Sci Sports Exerc* 31(1):156-163, 1999.

17d. BILLAT, V., J.C. RENOUX, J. PINOTEAU, B. PETIT, and J.P. KORALSZTEIN. Times to exhaustion at 100% of velocity at VO2max and modelling of the time-limit/velocity relationship in elite long-distance runners. *Eur J Appl Physiol* 69:271-273, 1994.

17e. BILLAT, V., and J.P. KORALSZTEIN. Significance of the velocity at VO2max and time to exhaustion at this velocity. *Sports Med.* 22(2):90-108, 1996.

17f. BISCIOTTI, G.N. Utilizziamo bene l'intermittente. *Il Nuovo Calcio* 114:110-114, 2002.

17g. BONEN, A. The expression of lactate transporters (MCT1 and MCT4) in heart and muscle. *Eur J Appl Physiol* 86(1):6-11, 2001.

18. BOSQUET, L., L. LEGER, and P. LEGROS. Methods to determine aerobic endurance. *Sports Med* 32:675-700, 2002.

19. BRANSFORD, D.R., and E.T. HOWLEY. Oxygen cost of running in trained and untrained men and women. *Med Sci Sports* 9:41-44, 1977.

20. BURGOMASTER, K.A., G.J. HEIGENHAUSER, and M.J. GIBALA. Effect of short-term sprint interval training on human skeletal muscle carbohydrate metabolism during exercise and time-trial performance. *J Appl Physiol* 100:2041-2047, 2006.

21. BURGOMASTER, K.A., S.C. HUGHES, G.J. HEIGENHAUSER, S.N. BRADWELL, and M.J. GIBALA. Six sessions of sprint interval training increases muscle oxidative potential and cycle endurance capacity in humans. *J Appl Physiol* 98:1985-1990, 2005.

22. BURLESON, M.A., JR., H.S. O'BRYANT, M.H. STONE, M.A. COLLINS, and T. TRIPLETT-MCBRIDE. Effect of weight training exercise and treadmill exercise on post-exercise oxygen consumption. *Med Sci Sports Exerc* 30:518-522, 1998.

23. BURTSCHER, M., M. FAULHABER, M. FLATZ, R. LIKAR, and W. NACHBAUER. Effects of short-term acclimatization to altitude (3200 m) on aerobic and anaerobic exercise performance. *Int J Sports Med* 27:629-635, 2006.

24. CARTER, H., A.M. JONES, and J.H. DOUST. Effect of 6 weeks of endurance training on the lactate minimum speed. *J Sports Sci* 17:957-967, 1999.

25. CERRETELLI, P., G. AMBROSOLI, and M. FUMAGALLI. Anaerobic recovery in man. *Eur J Appl Physiol Occup Physiol* 34:141-148, 1975.

26. COGGAN, A.R., R.J. SPINA, M.A. ROGERS, D.S. KING, M. BROWN, P.M. NEMETH, and J.O. HOLLOSZY. Histochemical and enzymatic characteristics of skeletal muscle in master athletes. *J Appl Physiol* 68:1896-1901, 1990.

27. CONLEY, D.L., and G.S. KRAHENBUHL. Running economy and distance running performance of highly trained athletes. *Med Sci Sports Exerc* 12:357-360, 1980.

28. CONLEY, M. Bioenergetics of exercise training. In: *Essentials of Strength Training and Conditioning*. T.R. Baechle and R.W. Earle, eds. Champaign, IL: Human Kinetics, 2000, pp. 73-90.

29. CONLEY, M.S., M.H. STONE, H.S. O'BRYANT, R.L. JOHNSON, D.R. HONEYCUTT, and T.P. HOKE. Peak power versus power at maximal oxygen uptake. In: *Proceedings of National Strength and Conditioning Association Annual Convention*. Las Vegas, NV, 1993.

30. COSTILL, D.L., W.J. FINK, and M.L. POLLOCK. Muscle fiber composition and enzyme activities of elite distance runners. *Med Sci Sports* 8:96-100, 1976.

31. COSTILL, D.L., M.G. FLYNN, J.P. KIRWAN, J.A. HOUMARD, J.B. MITCHELL, R. THOMAS, and S.H. PARK. Effects of repeated days of intensified training on muscle glycogen and swimming performance. *Med Sci Sports Exerc* 20:249-254, 1988.

32. COSTILL, D.L., R. THOMAS, R.A. ROBERGS, D. PASCOE, C. LAMBERT, S. BARR, and W.J. FINK. Adaptations to swimming training: influence of training volume. *Med Sci Sports Exerc* 23:371-377, 1991.

33. COSTILL, D.L., H. THOMASON, and E. ROBERTS. Fractional utilization of the aerobic capacity during distance running. *Med Sci Sports* 5:248-252, 1973.

34. COYLE, E.F. Improved muscular efficiency displayed as Tour de France champion matures. *J Appl Physiol* 98:2191-2196, 2005.

35. COYLE, E.F. Integration of the physiological factors determining endurance performance ability. *Exerc Sport Sci Rev* 23:25-63, 1995.
36. COYLE, E.F., A.R. COGGAN, M.K. HOPPER, and T.J. WALTERS. Determinants of endurance in well-trained cyclists. *J Appl Physiol* 64:2622-2630, 1988.
37. CRONIN, J.B. and K.T. HANSEN. Strength and power predictors of sports speed. *J Strength Cond Res* 19:349-357, 2005.
37b. DAUSSIN, F.N., E. PONSOT, S.P. DUFOUR, E. LONSDORFER-WOLF, S. DOUTRELEAU, B. GENY, F. PIQUARD, and R. RICHARD. Improvement of VO2max by cardiac output and oxygen extraction adaptation during intermittent versus continuous endurance training. *Eur J Appl Physiol* 101: 377-383, 2007.
37b. WUNDERSITZ, D.W., C. JOSMAN, R. GUPTA, K.J. NETTO, P.B. GASTIN, and S. ROBERTSON. Classification of team sport activities using a single wearable tracking device, *J Biomech* 48(15):3975-3981, 2015.
38. DAWSON, B., M. FITZSIMONS, S. GREEN, C. GOODMAN, M. CAREY, and K. COLE. Changes in performance, muscle metabolites, enzymes and fibre types after short sprint training. *Eur J Appl Physiol* 78:163-169, 1998.
39. DEMPSEY, J.A., P.G. HANSON, and K.S. HENDERSON. Exercise-induced arterial hypoxaemia in healthy human subjects at sea level. *J Physiol* 355:161-175, 1984.
40. DENADAI, B.S., M.J. ORTIZ, C.C. GRECO, and M.T. DE MELLO. Interval training at 95% and 100% of the velocity at VO2 max: effects on aerobic physiological indexes and running performance. *Appl Physiol Nutr Metab* 31:737-743, 2006.
40b. DI PRAMPERO, P.E., and C. OSGNACH. Impegno metabolico del calciatore: teorie e realtà. [Metabolic effort of the soccer player: theories and reality], Milan, 2013, Slideshare. https://www.slideshare.net/exelio/impegno-metabolico-del-calciatore.
40c. DI PRAMPERO, P.E., A. BOTTER, and C. OSGNACH. The energy cost of sprint running and the role of metabolic power in setting top performances, *Eur J Appl Physiol* 115(3):451-469, 2015.
41. DUDLEY, G.A., W.M. ABRAHAM, and R.L. TERJUNG. Influence of exercise intensity and duration on biochemical adaptations in skeletal muscle. *J Appl Physiol* 53:844-850, 1982.
42. DUDLEY, G.A., and R. DJAMIL. Incompatibility of endurance- and strength-training modes of exercise. *J Appl Physiol* 59:1446-1451, 1985.
43. DUMKE, C.L., D.W. BROCK, B.H. HELMS, and G.G. HAFF. Heart rate at lactate threshold and cycling time trials. *J Strength Cond Res* 20:601-607, 2006.
44. EKBLOM, B., G. WILSON, and P.O. ASTRAND. Central circulation during exercise after venesection and reinfusion of red blood cells. *J Appl Physiol* 40:379-383, 1976.
45. ELLIOTT, M.C., P.P. WAGNER, and L. CHIU. Power athletes and distance training: physiological and biomechanical rationale for change. *Sports Med* 37:47-57, 2007.
46. ESTEVE-LANAO, J., C. FOSTER, S. SEILER, and A. LUCIA. Impact of training intensity distribution on performance in endurance athletes. *J Strength Cond Res* 21:943-949, 2007.
46b. ESTEVE-LANAO, J., A.F. SAN JUAN, C.P. EARNEST, C. FOSTER, and A. LUCIA. How do endurance runners actually train? Relationship with competition performance. *Med Sci Sports Exerc* 37(3):496-504, 2005.
47. FARRELL, P.A., J.H. WILMORE, E.F. COYLE, J.E. BILLING, and D.L. COSTILL. Plasma lactate accumulation and distance running performance. *Med Sci Sports* 11:338-344, 1979.
48. FARRELL, P.A., J.H. WILMORE, E.F. COYLE, J.E. BILLING, and D.L. COSTILL. Plasma lactate accumulation and distance running performance. 1979.*Med Sci Sports Exerc* 25:1091-1097; discussion 1089-1090, 1993.
49. FAULKNER, J.A., J. KOLLIAS, C.B. FAVOUR, E.R. BUSKIRK, and B. BALKE. Maximum aerobic capacity and running performance at altitude. *J Appl Physiol* 24:685-691, 1968.
49b. FAVERO, T.G., and K.J. STOLL. Seasonal improvements in VO2Max among women's college soccer players with one-day per week aerobic interval training. *Kinesiologia Slovenica* 22(2):14-21, 2016.
50. FLECK, S. Bridging the gap: interval training: physiological basis. *NSCA J* 5:40-63, 1983.
51. FLECK, S., and W.J. KRAEMER. *Designing Resistance Training Programs*. 3rd ed. Champaign, IL: Human Kinetics, 2004.
52. FOSTER, C., L.L. HECTOR, R. WELSH, M. SCHRAGER, M.A. GREEN, and A.C. SNYDER. Effects of specific versus cross-training on running performance. *Eur J Appl Physiol Occup Physiol* 70:367-372, 1995.
53. FRANCH, J., K. MADSEN, M.S. DJURHUUS, and P.K. PEDERSEN. Improved running economy following intensified training correlates with reduced ventilatory demands. *Med Sci Sports Exerc* 30:1250-1256, 1998.
54. FRIEL, J. *Total Heart Rate Training*. Berkley, CA: Ulysses Press, 2006.
55. FRY, A.C., C.A. ALLEMEIER, and R.S. STARON. Correlation between percentage fiber type area and myosin heavy chain content in human skeletal muscle. *Eur J Appl Physiol Occup Physiol* 68:246-251, 1994.

56. GABBETT, T., T. KING, and D. JENKINS. Applied physiology of rugby league. *Sports Med* 38:119-138, 2008.
56b. GABBETT, T.J. GPS analysis of elite women's field hockey training and competition. *J Strength Cond Res* 24(5):1321-1324, 2010.
56c. GABBETT, T.J. Skill-based conditioning games as an alternative to traditional conditioning for rugby league players. *J Strength Cond Res* 20:309-314, 2006.
57. GIBALA, M.J. High-intensity interval training: a time-efficient strategy for health promotion? *Curr Sports Med Rep* 6:211-213, 2007.
58. GIBALA, M.J., J.P. LITTLE, M. VAN ESSEN, G.P. WILKIN, K.A. BURGOMASTER, A. SAFDAR, S. RAHA, and M.A. TARNOPOLSKY. Short-term sprint interval versus traditional endurance training: similar initial adaptations in human skeletal muscle and exercise performance. *J Physiol* 575:901-911, 2006.
59. GLEDHILL, N., D. COX, and R. JAMNIK. Endurance athletes' stroke volume does not plateau: major advantage is diastolic function. *Med Sci Sports Exerc* 26:1116-1121, 1994.
60. HÄKKINEN, K., A. MERO, and H. KAUHANEN. Specificity of endurance, sprint and strength training on physical performance capacity in young athletes. *J Sports Med Phys Fitness* 29:27-35, 1989.
61. HÄKKINEN, K. and E. MYLLYLA. Acute effects of muscle fatigue and recovery on force production and relaxation in endurance, power and strength athletes. *J Sports Med Phys Fitness* 30:5-12, 1990.
61b. HALSON, S.L., and A.E. JEUKENDRUP. Does overtraining exist? an analysis of overreaching and overtraining research. *Sports Med* 34:967-981, 2004.
62. HELGERUD, J., L.C. ENGEN, U. WISLOFF, and J. HOFF. Aerobic endurance training improves soccer performance. *Med Sci Sports Exerc* 33:1925-1931, 2001.
63. HENNESSY, L.C. and A.W.S. WATSON. The interference effects of training for strength and endurance simultaneously. *J Strength Cond Res* 8:12-19, 1994.
64. HENRIKSSON, J. Effects of physical training on the metabolism of skeletal muscle. *Diabetes Care* 15:1701-1711, 1992.
65. HENRITZE, J., A. WELTMAN, R.L. SCHURRER, and K. BARLOW. Effects of training at and above the lactate threshold on the lactate threshold and maximal oxygen uptake. *Eur J Appl Physiol Occup Physiol* 54:84-88, 1985.
66. HICKSON, R.C., B.A. DVORAK, E.M. GOROSTIAGA, T.T. KUROWSKI, and C. FOSTER. Potential for strength and endurance training to amplify endurance performance. *J Appl Physiol* 65:2285-2290, 1988.
66b. HICKSON, R.C., J.M. HAGBERG, R.K. CONLEE, D.A. JONES, A.A. EHSANI, and W.W. WINDER. Effect of training on hormonal responses to exercise in competitive swimmers. *Eur J Appl Physiol Occup Physiol* 41(3):211-219, 1979.
67. HILL-HAAS, S., D. BISHOP, B. DAWSON, C. GOODMAN, and J. EDGE. Effects of rest interval during high-repetition resistance training on strength, aerobic fitness, and repeated-sprint ability. *J Sports Sci* 25:619-628, 2007.
68. HOFF, J., A. GRAN, and J. HELGERUD. Maximal strength training improves aerobic endurance performance. *Scand J Med Sci Sports* 12:288-295. 2002.
69. HOLLOSZY, J.O. and E.F. COYLE. Adaptations of skeletal muscle to endurance exercise and their metabolic consequences. *J Appl Physiol* 56:831-838, 1984.
70. HOWALD, H., H. HOPPELER, H. CLAASSEN, O. MATHIEU, and R. STRAUB. Influences of endurance training on the ultrastructural composition of the different muscle fiber types in humans. *Pflugers Arch* 403:369-376, 1985.
71. INGJER, F. Capillary supply and mitochondrial content of different skeletal muscle fiber types in untrained and endurance-trained men. A histochemical and ultrastructural study. *Eur J Appl Physiol Occup Physiol* 40:197-209, 1979.
72. JACKSON, N.P., M.S. HICKEY, and R.F. REISER, II. High resistance/low repetition vs. low resistance/high repetition training: effects on performance of trained cyclists. *J Strength Cond Res* 21:289-295, 2007.
72b. JEZOVi, D., M. VIGAS, P. TATiR, R. KVETNANSK›, K. NAZAR, H. KACIUBA-UŚCILKO, and S. KOZLOWSKI. Plasma testosterone and catecholamine responses to physical exercise of different intensities in men. *Eur J Appl Physiol Occup Physiol* 54(1):62–66, 1985.
73. JOHNSTON, R.E., T.J. QUINN, R. KERTZER, and N.B. VROMAN. Strength training in female distance runners: impact on running economy. *J Strength Cond Res* 11:224-229, 1997.
74. JONES, A.M. A five year physiological case study of an Olympic runner. *Br J Sports Med* 32:39-43, 1998.
75. JONES, A.M., and H. CARTER. The effect of endurance training on parameters of aerobic fitness. *Sports Med* 29:373-386, 2000.
76. JOYNER, M.J., and E.F. COYLE. Endurance exercise performance: the physiology of champions. *J Physiol* 586:35-44, 2008.
77. JUNG, A.P. The impact of resistance training on distance running performance. *Sports Med* 33:539-552, 2003.
78. KEITH, S.P., I. JACOBS, and T.M. MCLELLAN. Adaptations to training at the individual anaerobic

threshold. *Eur J Appl Physiol Occup Physiol* 65:316-323, 1992.

79. KINDERMANN, W., G. SIMON, and J. KEUL. The significance of the aerobic-anaerobic transition for the determination of work load intensities during endurance training. *Eur J Appl Physiol Occup Physiol* 42:25-34, 1979.

80. KLAUSEN, K., L.B. ANDERSEN, and I. PELLE. Adaptive changes in work capacity, skeletal muscle capillarization and enzyme levels during training and detraining. *Acta Physiol Scand* 113:9-16, 1981.

81. KORHONEN, M.T., A. CRISTEA, M. ALEN, K. HAKKINEN, S. SIPILA, A. MERO, J.T. VIITASALO, L. LARSSON, and H. SUOMINEN. Aging, muscle fiber type, and contractile function in sprint-trained athletes. *J Appl Physiol* 101:906-917, 2006.

82. KRAEMER, W.J., D.N. FRENCH, N.J. PAXTON, K. HÄKKINEN, J.S. VOLEK, W.J. SEBASTIANELLI, M. PUTUKIAN, R.U. NEWTON, M.R. RUBIN, A.L. GOMEZ, J.D. VESCOVI, N.A. RATAMESS, S.J. FLECK, J.M. LYNCH, and H.G. KNUTTGEN. Changes in exercise performance and hormonal concentrations over a big ten soccer season in starters and nonstarters. *J Strength Cond Res* 18:121-128, 2004.

83. KRAEMER, W.J., J.F. PATTON, S.E. GORDON, E.A. HARMAN, M.R. DESCHENES, K. REYNOLDS, R.U. NEWTON, N.T. TRIPLETT, and J.E. DZIADOS. Compatibility of high-intensity strength and endurance training on hormonal and skeletal muscle adaptations. *J Appl Physiol* 78:976-989, 1995.

83b. KRUSTRUP, P., M. MOHR, T. ARMSTRUP, T. RYSGAARD, J. JOHANSEN, A. STEENSBERG, P.K. PEDERSEN, and J. BANGSBO. The Yo-Yo intermittent recovery test: physiological response, reliability, and validity. *Med Sci Sports Exerc* 35(4):697-705, 2003.

84. KUBUKELI, Z.N., T.D. NOAKES, and S.C. DENNIS. Training techniques to improve endurance exercise performances. *Sports Med* 32:489-509, 2002.

85. KYROLAINEN, H., J. AVELA, J.M. MCBRIDE, S. KOSKINEN, J.L. ANDERSEN, S. SIPILA, T.E. TAKALA, and P.V. KOMI. Effects of power training on muscle structure and neuromuscular performance. *Scand J Med Sci Sports* 15:58-64, 2005.

86. LAURSEN, P.B., M.A. BLANCHARD, and D.G. JENKINS. Acute high-intensity interval training improves Tvent and peak power output in highly trained males. *Can J Appl Physiol* 27:336-348, 2002.

87. LAURSEN, P.B., and D.G. JENKINS. The scientific basis for high-intensity interval training: optimising training programmes and maximising performance in highly trained endurance athletes. *Sports Med* 32:53-73, 2002.

88. LAURSEN, P.B., E.C. RHODES, R.H. LANGILL, D.C. MCKENZIE, and J.E. TAUNTON. Relationship of exercise test variables to cycling performance in an Ironman triathlon. *Eur J Appl Physiol* 87:433-440, 2002.

89. LAURSEN, P.B., E.C. RHODES, R.H. LANGILL, J.E. TAUNTON, and D.C. MCKENZIE. Exercise-induced arterial hypoxemia is not different during cycling and running in triathletes. *Scand J Med Sci Sports* 15:113-117, 2005.

90. LAURSEN, P.B., C.M. SHING, J.M. PEAKE, J.S. COOMBES, and D.G. JENKINS. Influence of high-intensity interval training on adaptations in well-trained cyclists. *J Strength Cond Res* 19:527-533, 2005.

91. LAURSEN, P.B., C.M. SHING, J.M. PEAKE, J.S. COOMBES, and D.G. JENKINS. Interval training program optimization in highly trained endurance cyclists. *Med Sci Sports Exerc* 34:1801-1807, 2002.

92. LEVINE, B.D. V/od/O2max: what do we know, and what do we still need to know? *J Physiol* 586:25-34, 2008.

93. LINOSSIER, M.T., D. DORMOIS, C. PERIER, J. FREY, A. GEYSSANT, and C. DENIS. Enzyme adaptations of human skeletal muscle during bicycle short-sprint training and detraining. *Acta Physiol Scand* 161:439-445, 1997.

94. LITTLE, T., and A.G. WILLIAMS. Effects of sprint duration and exercise: rest ratio on repeated sprint performance and physiological responses in professional soccer players. *J Strength Cond Res* 21:646-648, 2007.

95. MACDOUGALL, J.D., A.L. HICKS, J.R. MACDONALD, R.S. MCKELVIE, H.J. GREEN, and K.M. SMITH. Muscle performance and enzymatic adaptations to sprint interval training. *J Appl Physiol* 84:2138-2142, 1998.

96. MARCINIK, E.J., J. POTTS, G. SCHLABACH, S. WILL, P. DAWSON, and B.F. HURLEY. Effects of strength training on lactate threshold and endurance performance. *Med Sci Sports Exerc* 23:739-743, 1991.

97. MAYHEW, J.L. Oxygen cost and energy expenditure of running in trained runners. *Br J Sports Med* 11:116-121, 1977.

98. MCARDLE, W.D., F.I. KATCH, and V.L. KATCH. *Exercise Physiology: Energy, Nutrition, and Human Performance*. 6th ed. Baltimore: Lippincott Williams & Wilkins, 2007.

99. MCGEE, D., T.C. JESSEE, M.H. STONE, and D. BLESSING. Leg and hip endurance adaptations to three weight-training programs. *J Appl Sport Sci Res* 6:92-85, 1992.

100. MCGUIRE, B.J., and T.W. SECOMB. Estimation of capillary density in human skeletal muscle based on maximal oxygen consumption rates. *Am J Physiol Heart Circ Physiol* 285:H2382-2391, 2003.

101. MCKENNA, M.J., A.R. HARMER, S.F. FRASER, and J.L. LI. Effects of training on potassium, calcium and hydrogen ion regulation in skeletal muscle and blood during exercise. *Acta Physiol Scand* 156:335-346, 1996.

102. MEDBO, J.I., and S. BURGERS. Effect of training on the anaerobic capacity. *Med Sci Sports Exerc* 22:501-507, 1990.

102b. MICHELI, M.L., E.CASTELLINI, and M. MARELLA. Il condizionamento aerobico. *L'Allenatore*, 2008.

103. MIDGLEY, A.W., L.R. MCNAUGHTON, and A.M. JONES. Training to enhance the physiological determinants of long-distance running performance: can valid recommendations be given to runners and coaches based on current scientific knowledge? *Sports Med* 37:857-880, 2007.

104. MIKKOLA, J., H. RUSKO, A. NUMMELA, T. POLLARI, and K. HÄKKINEN. Concurrent endurance and explosive type strength training improves neuromuscular and anaerobic characteristics in young distance runners. *Int J Sports Med* 28:602-611, 2007.

105. MILLER, T.A., R. THIERRY-AGUILERA, J.J. CONGLETON, A.A. AMENDOLA, M.J. CLARK, S.F. CROUSE, S.M. MARTIN, and O.C. JENKINS. Seasonal changes in VO2max among Division 1A collegiate women soccer players. *J Strength Cond Res* 21:48-51, 2007.

105b. MOHR, M., P. KRUSTRUP, and J. BANGSBO. Match performance of high-standard soccer players with special reference to development of fatigue. *J Sports Sci* 21(7):519-528, 2003.

106. MONTGOMERY, D.L. Physiology of ice hockey. *Sports Med* 5:99-126, 1988.

107. MORGAN, D.W., D.R. BRANSFORD, D.L. COSTILL, J.T. DANIELS, E.T. HOWLEY, and G.S. KRAHENBUHL. Variation in the aerobic demand of running among trained and untrained subjects. *Med Sci Sports Exerc* 27:404-409, 1995.

108. NADER, G.A. Concurrent strength and endurance training: from molecules to man. *Med Sci Sports Exerc* 38:1965-1970, 2006.

109. NIELSEN, H.B. Arterial desaturation during exercise in man: implication for O2 uptake and work capacity. *Scand J Med Sci Sports* 13:339-358, 2003.

109b. OSGNACH, C., S. POSER, R. BERNARDINI, R. RINALDO, and P.E. DI PRAMPERO. Energy cost and metabolic power in elite soccer: a new match analysis approach. *Med Sci Sports Exerc* 42:170-178, 2010.

110. PAAVOLAINEN, L., K. HÄKKINEN, I. HAMALAINEN, A. NUMMELA, and H. RUSKO. Explosive-strength training improves 5-km running time by improving running economy and muscle power. *J Appl Physiol* 86:1527-1533, 1999.

111. PAAVOLAINEN, L., K. HÄKKINEN, and H. RUSKO. Effects of explosive type strength training on physical performance characteristics in cross-country skiers. *Eur J Appl Physiol Occup Physiol* 62:251-255, 1991.

112. PINCIVERO, D.M., and T.O. BOMPA. A physiological review of American football. *Sports Med* 23:247-260, 1997.

113. PLISK, S.S. Anaerobic metabolic conditioning: a brief review of theory, strategy and practical application. *J Appl Sport Sci Res* 5:22-34, 1991.

114. PLISK, S.S. Speed, agility, and speed-endurance development. In: *Essentials of Strength Training and Conditioning*. T.R. Baechle and R.W. Earle, eds. Champaign, IL: Human Kinetics, 2008.

115. PLISK, S.S., and V. GAMBETTA. Tactical metabolic training: part 1. *Strength Cond* 19:44-53, 1997.

116. PLISK, S.S., and M.H. STONE. Periodization strategies. *Strength Cond* 25:19-37, 2003.

117. POLLOCK, M.L. The quantification of endurance training programs. *Exerc Sport Sci Rev* 1:155-188, 1973.

118. POTTEIGER, J.A. Aerobic endurance exercise training. In: *Essentials of Strength Training and Conditioning*. T.R. Baechle and R.W. Earle, eds. Champaign, IL: Human Kinetics, 2000, pp. 495-509.

119. POWERS, S.K., and E.T. HOWLEY. *Exercise Physiology: Theory and Application to Fitness and Performance*. 5th ed. New York: McGraw-Hill, 2004.

120. POWERS, S.K., J. LAWLER, J.A. DEMPSEY, S. DODD, and G. LANDRY. Effects of incomplete pulmonary gas exchange on VO2 max. *J Appl Physiol* 66:2491-2495, 1989.

120b. PROIETTI, R. *La Corsa*. Città di Castello, Italy: Edizioni Nuova Prhomos, 1999.

121. RAMPININI, E., F.M. IMPELLIZZERI, C. CASTAGNA, G. ABT, K. CHAMARI, A. SASSI, and S.M. MARCORA. Factors influencing physiological responses to small-sided soccer games. *J Sports Sci* 25:659-666, 2007.

122. REILLY, T., C.N. DOWZER, and N.T. CABLE. The physiology of deep-water running. *J Sports Sci* 21:959-972, 2003.

123. REILLY, T., and B. EKBLOM. The use of recovery methods post-exercise. *J Sports Sci* 23:619-627, 2005.

124. REINDELL, H., and H. ROSKAMM. Ein Beitrag zu den physiologischen Grundlagen des Intervall training unter besonderer Berücksichtigug des Kreilaufes. *Schweiz Z Sportmed* 7:1-8, 1959.

125. ROBINSON, J.M., M.H. STONE, R.L. JOHNSON, C.M. PENLAND, B.J. WARREN, and R.D. LEWIS. Effects of different weight training exercise/rest intervals on strength, power, and high intensity exercise endurance. *J Strength Cond Res* 9:216-221, 1995.
126. RODAS, G., J.L. VENTURA, J.A. CADEFAU, R. CUSSO, and J. PARRA. A short training programme for the rapid improvement of both aerobic and anaerobic metabolism. *Eur J Appl Physiol* 82:480-486, 2000.
127. RODRIGUEZ, L.P., J. LOPEZ-REGO, J.A. CALBET, R. VALERO, E. VARELA, and J. PONCE. Effects of training status on fibers of the musculus vastus lateralis in professional road cyclists. *Am J Phys Med Rehabil* 81:651-660, 2002.
128. RUBAL, B.J., J.M. MOODY, S. DAMORE, S.R. BUNKER, and N.M. DIAZ. Left ventricular performance of the athletic heart during upright exercise: a heart rate-controlled study. *Med Sci Sports Exerc* 18:134-140, 1986.
129. RUBIO, J. Devising an efficient training plan. In: *Run Strong*. K. Beck, ed. Champaign, IL: Human Kinetics, 2005, pp. 41-58.
130. SALTIN, B. Hemodynamic adaptations to exercise. *Am J Cardiol* 55:42D-47D, 1985.
131. SALTIN, B., and P.O. ASTRAND. Maximal oxygen uptake in athletes. *J Appl Physiol* 23:353-358, 1967.
132. SALTIN, B., J. HENRIKSSON, E. NYGAARD, P. ANDERSEN, and E. JANSSON. Fiber types and metabolic potentials of skeletal muscles in sedentary man and endurance runners. *Ann N Y Acad Sci* 301:3-29, 1977.
133. SCHMIDT, W., N. MAASSEN, U. TEGTBUR, and K.M. BRAUMANN. Changes in plasma volume and red cell formation after a marathon competition. *Eur J Appl Physiol Occup Physiol* 58:453-458, 1989.
134. SCHUMACHER, Y.O., D. GRATHWOHL, J.M. BARTUREN, M. WOLLENWEBER, L. HEINRICH, A. SCHMID, G. HUBER, and J. KEUL. Haemoglobin, haematocrit and red blood cell indices in elite cyclists. Are the control values for blood testing valid? *Int J Sports Med* 21:380-385, 2000.
135. SCHUMACHER, Y.O., A. SCHMID, D. GRATHWOHL, D. BULTERMANN, and A. BERG. Hematological indices and iron status in athletes of various sports and performances. *Med Sci Sports Exerc* 34:869-875, 2002.
135b. SEILER, K.S., and G.O. KJERLAND. Quantifying training intensity distribution in elite endurance athletes: is there evidence for an "optimal" distribution? *Scand J Med Sci Sports* 16(1):49-56, 2006.
136. SHONO, N., H. URATA, B. SALTIN, M. MIZUNO, T. HARADA, M. SHINDO, and H. TANAKA. Effects of low intensity aerobic training on skeletal muscle capillary and blood lipoprotein profiles. *J Atheroscler Thromb* 9:78-85, 2002.
137. SILVESTRE, R., W.J. KRAEMER, C. WEST, D.A. JUDELSON, B.A. SPIERING, J.L. VINGREN, D.L. HATFIELD, J.M. ANDERSON, and C.M. MARESH. Body composition and physical performance during a National Collegiate Athletic Association Division I men's soccer season. *J Strength Cond Res* 20:962-970, 2006.
138. SJÖDIN, B., and I. JACOBS. Onset of blood lactate accumulation and marathon running performance. *Int J Sports Med* 2:23-26, 1981.
139. SJÖDIN, B., I. JACOBS, and J. SVEDENHAG. Changes in onset of blood lactate accumulation (OBLA) and muscle enzymes after training at OBLA. *Eur J Appl Physiol Occup Physiol* 49:45-57, 1982.
140. SJÖDIN, B, and J. SVEDENHAG. Applied physiology of marathon running. *Sports Med* 2:83-99, 1985.
141. SLEAMAKER, R., and R. BROWNING. *Serious Training for Endurance Athletes*. 2nd ed. Champaign, IL: Human Kinetics, 1996.
141b. SLETTALÿKKEN, G., and B.R. RÿNNESTAD. High-intensity interval training every second week maintains VO2max in soccer players during off-season, *J Strength Cond Res.*; 28(7):1946-1951, 2014.
142. SMITH, T.P., L.R. MCNAUGHTON, and K.J. MARSHALL. Effects of 4-wk training using Vmax/Tmax on V/od/O2max and performance in athletes. *Med Sci Sports Exerc* 31:892-896, 1999.
143. SPRIET, L.L., M.I. LINDINGER, R.S. MCKELVIE, G.J. HEIGENHAUSER, and N.L. JONES. Muscle glycogenolysis and H+ concentration during maximal intermittent cycling. *J Appl Physiol* 66:8-13, 1989.
144. STEPTO, N.K., J.A. HAWLEY, S.C. DENNIS, and W.G. HOPKINS. Effects of different interval-training programs on cycling time-trial performance. *Med Sci Sports Exerc* 31:736-741, 1999.
145. STEPTO, N.K., D.T. MARTIN, K.E. FALLON, and J.A. HAWLEY. Metabolic demands of intense aerobic interval training in competitive cyclists. *Med Sci Sports Exerc* 33:303-310, 2001.
146. STONE, M.H., and H.O. O'BRYANT. *Weight Training: A Scientific Approach*. Edina, MN: Burgess, 1987.
147. STONE, M.H., W.A. SANDS, K.C. PIERCE, R.U. NEWTON, G.G. HAFF, and J. CARLOCK. Maximum strength and strength training: a relationship to endurance? *Strength Cond J* 28:44-53, 2006.

148. STONE, M.H., M.E. STONE, and W.A. SANDS. *Principles and Practice of Resistance Training.* Champaign, IL: Human Kinetics, 2007.
149. SUTER, E., W. HERZOG, J. SOKOLOSKY, J.P. WILEY, and B.R. MACINTOSH. Muscle fiber type distribution as estimated by Cybex testing and by muscle biopsy. *Med Sci Sports Exerc* 25:363-370, 1993.
150. SVEDAHL, K., and B.R. MACINTOSH. Anaerobic threshold: the concept and methods of measurement. *Can J Appl Physiol* 28:299-323, 2003.
151. SVEDENHAG, J., J. HENRIKSSON, and A. JUHLIN-DANNFELT. Beta-adrenergic blockade and training in human subjects: effects on muscle metabolic capacity. *Am J Physiol* 247:E305-311, 1984.
152. TABATA, I., K. IRISAWA, M. KOUZAKI, K. NISHIMURA, F. OGITA, and M. MIYACHI. Metabolic profile of high intensity intermittent exercises. *Med Sci Sports Exerc* 29:390-395, 1997.
153. TANAKA, H., and T. SWENSEN. Impact of resistance training on endurance performance. A new form of cross-training? *Sports Med* 25:191-200, 1998.
153b. TOMLIN, D.L., and H.A. WENGER. The relationship between aerobic fitness and recovery from high intensity intermittent exercise. *Sports Med* 31(1):1-11, 2001.
154. TRAPPE, S., M. HARBER, A. CREER, P. GALLAGHER, D. SLIVKA, K. MINCHEV, and D. WHITSETT. Single muscle fiber adaptations with marathon training. *J Appl Physiol* 101:721-727, 2006.
155. TURNER, A.M., M. OWINGS, and J.A. SCHWANE. Improvement in running economy after 6 weeks of plyometric training. *J Strength Cond Res* 17:60-67, 2003.
155b. VITTORI, C. Velocista resisti. *Universo Atletica* 17:19-20, 1991.
156. WANG, N., R.S. HIKIDA, R.S. STARON, and J.A. SIMONEAU. Muscle fiber types of women after resistance training–quantitative ultrastructure and enzyme activity. *Pflugers Arch* 424:494-502, 1993.
157. WELTMAN, A., R.L. SEIP, D. SNEAD, J.Y. WELTMAN, E.M. HASKVITZ, W.S. EVANS, J.D. VELDHUIS, and A.D. ROGOL. Exercise training at and above the lactate threshold in previously untrained women. *Int J Sports Med* 13:257-263, 1992.
158. WESTGARTH-TAYLOR, C., J.A. HAWLEY, S. RICKARD, K.H. MYBURGH, T.D. NOAKES, and S.C. DENNIS. Metabolic and performance adaptations to interval training in endurance-trained cyclists. *Eur J Appl Physiol* 75:298-304, 1997.
159. WESTON, A.R., K.H. MYBURGH, F.H. LINDSAY, S.C. DENNIS, T.D. NOAKES, and J.A. HAWLEY. Skeletal muscle buffering capacity and endurance performance after high-intensity interval training by well-trained cyclists. *Eur J Appl Physiol Occup Physiol* 75:7-13, 1997.
159b. WIGERNAES, I., A.T. HOSTMARK, S.B. STROMME, P. KIERULF, and K. BIRKELAND. Active recovery and post-exercise white blood cell count, free fatty acids, and hormones in endurance athletes. *Eur J Appl Physiol* 84(4):358-66, 2001.
160. WILMORE, J.H., D.L. COSTILL, and W.L. KENNEY. *Physiology of Sport and Exercise.* 4th ed. Champaign, IL: Human Kinetics, 2008.
161. WRIGHT, D.C., D.H. HAN, P.M. GARCIA-ROVES, P.C. GEIGER, T.E. JONES, and J.O. HOLLOSZY. Exercise-induced mitochondrial biogenesis begins before the increase in muscle PGC-1 alpha expression. *J Biol Chem* 282:194-199, 2007.
162. YOSHIDA, T., M. CHIDA, M. ICHIOKA, and Y. SUDA. Blood lactate parameters related to aerobic capacity and endurance performance. *Eur J Appl Physiol Occup Physiol* 56:7-11, 1987.
162b. ZAPICO, A.G., F.J. CALDERON, P.J. BENITO, C.B. GONZALEZ, A. PARISI, F. PIGOZZI, and V. DI SALVO. Evolution of physiological and haematological parameters with training load in elite male road cyclists: a longitudinal study. *J Sports Med Phys Fitness* 47:191-196, 2007.
163. ZAWADOWSKA, B., J. MAJERCZAK, D. SEMIK, J. KARASINSKI, L. KOLODZIEJSKI, W.M. KILARSKI, K. DUDA, and J.A. ZOLADZ. Characteristics of myosin profile in human vastus lateralis muscle in relation to training background. *Folia Histochem Cytobiol* 42:181-190, 2004.
164. ZHOU, B., R.K. CONLEE, R. JENSEN, G.W. FELLINGHAM, J.D. GEORGE, and A.G. FISHER. Stroke volume does not plateau during graded exercise in elite male distance runners. *Med Sci Sports Exerc* 33:1849-1854, 2001.
165. ZOLADZ, J.A., D. SEMIK, B. ZAWADOWSKA, J. MAJERCZAK, J. KARASINSKI, L. KOLODZIEJSKI, K. DUDA, and W.M. KILARSKI. Capillary density and capillary-to-fibre ratio in vastus lateralis muscle of untrained and trained men. *Folia Histochem Cytobiol* 43:11-17, 2005.

Chapter 12

1. ADRIAN, M.J., and J.M. COOPER. *Biomechanics of Human Movement.* 2nd ed. New York: WCB McGraw-Hill, 1995.
2. AE, M., A. ITO, and M. SUZUKI. The men's 100 metres. *New Studies in Athletics* 7:47-52, 1992.
3. ALLEMEIER, C.A., A.C. FRY, P. JOHNSON, R.S. HIKIDA, F.C. HAGERMAN, and R.S. STARON.

Effects of sprint cycle training on human skeletal muscle. *J Appl Physiol* 77:2385-2390, 1994.
4. ANDERSEN, J.L., H. KLITGAARD, and B. SALTIN. Myosin heavy chain isoforms in single fibres from m. vastus lateralis of sprinters: influence of training. *Acta Physiol Scand* 151:135-142, 1994.
5. ANDERSEN, J.L., and S. SCHIAFFINO. Mismatch between myosin heavy chain mRNA and protein distribution in human skeletal muscle fibers. *Am J Physiol* 272:C1881-1889, 1997.
6. BAKER, D., and S. NANCE. The relation between running speed and measures of strength and power in professional rugby league players. *J. Strength Cond. Res* 13:230-235, 1999.
7. BALSOM, P.D., J.Y. SEGER, B. SJODIN, and B. EKBLOM. Maximal-intensity intermittent exercise: effect of recovery duration. *Int J Sports Med* 13:528-533, 1992.
8. BALSOM, P.D., J.Y. SEGER, B. SJODIN, and B. EKBLOM. Physiological responses to maximal intensity intermittent exercise. *Eur J Appl Physiol* 65:144-149, 1992.
9. BANGSBO, J. The physiology of soccer–with special reference to intense intermittent exercise. *Acta Physiol Scand Suppl* 619:1-155, 1994.
10. BOGDANIS, G.C., M.E. NEVILL, L.H. BOOBIS, and H.K. LAKOMY. Contribution of phosphocreatine and aerobic metabolism to energy supply during repeated sprint exercise. *J Appl Physiol* 80:876-884, 1996.
11. BOGDANIS, G.C., M.E. NEVILL, H.K. LAKOMY, and L.H. BOOBIS. Power output and muscle metabolism during and following recovery from 10 and 20 s of maximal sprint exercise in humans. *Acta Physiol Scand* 163:261-272, 1998.
12. BOMPA, T.O. *Total Training for Coaching Team Sports: A Self Help Guide*. Toronto, CA: Sports Books Publisher, 2006.
13. BOMPA, T., and C. BUZZICHELLI. *Periodization Training for Sports*. 3rd ed. Champaign, IL: Human Kinetics, 2015.
14. BONDARCHUK, A.P. The role and sequence of using different training-load intensities. *Fit Sports Rev Int* 29:202-204, 1994.
15. BONDARCHUK, A.P. *Track and Field Training*. Kiev: Zdotovye, 1986.
16. BOTTINELLI, R., M.A. PELLEGRINO, M. CANEPARI, R. ROSSI, and C. REGGIANI. Specific contributions of various muscle fibre types to human muscle performance: an in vitro study. *J Electromyogr Kinesiol* 9:87-95, 1999.
17. BOTTINELLI, R., S. SCHIAFFINO, and C. REGGIANI. Force-velocity relations and myosin heavy chain isoform compositions of skinned fibres from rat skeletal muscle. *J Physiol* 437:655-672, 1991.

18. BRUGHELLI, M., J. CRONIN, and A. CHAOUACHI. Effects of running velocity on running kinetics and kinematics. *J Strength Cond Res* 25(4):933-939, 2011.
18b. BUCHHEIT, M., P. SAMOZINO, J.A. GLYNN, B.S. MICHAEL, H. AL HADDAD, A. MENDEZ-VILLANUEVA, and J.B. MORIN. Mechanical determinants of acceleration and maximal sprinting speed in highly trained young soccer players. *J Sports Sci* 32(20):1905-1913, 2014.
19. CADEFAU, J., J. CASADEMONT, J.M. GRAU, J. FERNANDEZ, A. BALAGUER, M. VERNET, R. CUSSO, and A. URBANO-MARQUEZ. Biochemical and histochemical adaptation to sprint training in young athletes. *Acta Physiol Scand* 140:341-351, 1990.
20. CARPENTIER, A., J. DUCHATEAU, and K. HAINAUT. Velocity dependent muscle strategy during plantarflexion in humans. *J Electromyogr Kinesiol* 6:225-233, 1996.
21. CHELLY, S.M., and C. DENIS. Leg power and hopping stiffness: relationship with sprint running performance. *Med Sci Sports Exerc* 33:326-333, 2001.
22. CONTRERAS, B., A.D. VIGOTSKY, B.J. SCHOENFELD, C. BEARDSLEY, D.T. MCMASTER, J.H. REYNEKE, and J.B. CRONIN. Effects of a six-week hip thrust vs. front squat resistance training program on performance in adolescent males: a randomized controlled trial. *J Strength Cond Res* 31(4):999-1008, 2017.
23. COSTILL, D.L., J. DANIELS, W. EVANS, W. FINK, G. KRAHENBUHL, and B. SALTIN. Skeletal muscle enzymes and fiber composition in male and female track athletes. *J Appl Physiol* 40:149-154, 1976.
24. CRONIN, J.B., and K.T. HANSEN. Strength and power predictors of sports speed. *J Strength Cond Res* 19:349-357, 2005.
25. DAWSON, B., M. FITZSIMONS, S. GREEN, C. GOODMAN, M. CAREY, and K. COLE. Changes in performance, muscle metabolites, enzymes and fibre types after short sprint training. *Eur J Appl Physiol* 78:163-169, 1998.
26. DELECLUSE, C. Influence of strength training on sprint running performance. Current findings and implications for training. *Sports Med* 24:147-156, 1997.
27. DELECLUSE, C.H., H. VAN COPPENOLLE, E. WILLEMS, R. DIELS, M. GORIS, M. VAN LEEMPUTTE, and M. VUYLSTEKE. Analysis of 100 m sprint performance as a multi-dimensional skill. *Journal of Human Movement Studies* 28:87-101, 1995.
28. DICK, F.W. Planning the programme. In: *Sports Training Principles*. London: A&C Black, 1997, pp. 253-304.

29. DIETZ, V., D. SCHMIDTBLEICHER, and J. NOTH. Neuronal mechanisms of human locomotion. *J Neurophysiol* 42:1212-1222, 1979.
30. DUTHIE, G., D. PYNE, and S. HOOPER. Applied physiology and game analysis of rugby union. *Sports Med* 33:973-991, 2003.
31. ESBJORNSSON, M., Y. HELLSTEN-WESTING, P.D. BALSOM, B. SJODIN, and E. JANSSON. Muscle fibre type changes with sprint training: effect of training pattern. *Acta Physiol Scand* 149:245-246, 1993.
32. ESBJORNSSON, M., C. SYLVEN, I. HOLM, and E. JANSSON. Fast twitch fibres may predict anaerobic performance in both females and males. *Int J Sports Med* 14:257-263, 1993.
33. FREEMAN, W.H. *Peak When it Counts: Periodization for American Track & Field*. 4th ed. Mountain View, CA: Tafnews Press, 2001.
34. GABBETT, T.J., J.N. KELLY, and J.M. SHEPPARD. Speed, change of direction speed, and reactive agility of rugby league players. *J Strength Cond Res* 22:174-181, 2008.
35. GOLLHOFER, A., A. SCHOPP, W. RAPP, and V. STROINIK. Changes in reflex excitability following isometric contraction in humans. *Eur J Appl Physiol Occup Physiol* 77:89-97, 1998.
36. GOTTLIEB, G.L., G.C. AGARWAL, and R.J. JAEGER. Response to sudden torques about ankle in man. IV. A functional role of alpha-gamma linkage. *J Neurophysiol* 46:179-190, 1981.
37. GRAY, H., and M.H. STONE. *Players Guide to ETSU Men's Soccer: Athlete Development*. Johnson City, TN: East Tennessee State University, 2008, p. 40.
38. HAFF, G.G., A. WHITLEY, and J.A. POTTEIGER. A brief review: explosive exercises and sports performance. *Natl Strength Cond Assoc* 23:13-20, 2001.
39. HÄKKINEN, K. and E. MYLLYLA. Acute effects of muscle fatigue and recovery on force production and relaxation in endurance, power and strength athletes. *J Sports Med Phys Fitness* 30:5-12, 1990.
40. HAMADA, T., D.G. SALE, and J.D. MACDOUGALL. Postactivation potentiation in endurance-trained male athletes. *Med Sci Sports Exerc* 32:403-411, 2000.
41. HARGREAVES, M., M.J. MCKENNA, D.G. JENKINS, S.A. WARMINGTON, J.L. LI, R.J. SNOW, and M.A. FEBBRAIO. Muscle metabolites and performance during high-intensity, intermittent exercise. *J Appl Physiol* 84:1687-1691, 1998.
42. HARRIDGE, S.D., R. BOTTINELLI, M. CANEPARI, M. PELLEGRINO, C. REGGIANI, M. ESBJORNSSON, P.D. BALSOM, and B. SALTIN. Sprint training, in vitro and in vivo muscle function, and myosin heavy chain expression. *J Appl Physiol* 84:442-449, 1998.
43. HELGERUD, J., L.C. ENGEN, U. WISLØFF, and J. HOFF. Aerobic endurance training improves soccer performance. *Med Sci Sports Exerc* 33:1925-1931, 2001.
44. HELGERUD, J., K. HOYDAL, E. WANG, T. KARLSEN, P. BERG, M. BJERKAAS, T. SIMONSEN, C. HELGESEN, N. HJORTH, R. BACH, and J. HOFF. Aerobic high-intensity intervals improve VO2max more than moderate training. *Med Sci Sports Exerc* 39:665-671, 2007.
45. HIRVONEN, J., S. REHUNEN, H. RUSKO, and M. HARKONEN. Breakdown of high-energy phosphate compounds and lactate accumulation during short supramaximal exercise. *Eur J Appl Physiol* 56:253-259, 1987.
46. HOFF, J., U. WISLØFF, L.C. ENGEN, O.J. KEMI, and J. HELGERUD. Soccer specific aerobic endurance training. *Br J Sports Med* 36:218-221, 2002.
47. JACOBS, I., M. ESBJORNSSON, C. SYLVEN, I. HOLM, and E. JANSSON. Sprint training effects on muscle myoglobin, enzymes, fiber types, and blood lactate. *Med Sci Sports Exerc* 19:368-374, 1987.
48. JANSSON, E., M. ESBJORNSSON, I. HOLM, and I. JACOBS. Increase in the proportion of fast-twitch muscle fibres by sprint training in males. *Acta Physiol Scand* 140:359-363, 1990.
49. JEFFREYS, I. *Total Soccer Fitness*. Monterey, CA: Coaches Choice, 2007.
50. JEFFREYS, I. Warm-up and stretching. In: *Essentials of Strength Training and Conditioning*. T.R. Baechle and R.W. Earle, eds. Champaign, IL: Human Kinetics, 2008, pp. 296-276.
51. JENKINS, D.G., S. BROOKS, and C. WILLIAMS. Improvements in multiple sprint ability with three weeks of training. *NZ J Sports Med* 22:2-5, 1994.
52. JONHAGEN, S., M.O. ERICSON, G. NEMETH, and E. ERIKSSON. Amplitude and timing of electromyographic activity during sprinting. *Scand J Med Sci Sports* 6:15-21, 1996.
53. KAWAMORI, N., K. NOSAKA, and R.U. NEWTON. Relationships between ground reaction impulse and sprint acceleration performance in team sport athletes. *J Strength Cond Res* 27(3):568-573, 2013.
54. KELLER, T.S., A.M. WEISBERGER, J.L. RAY, S.S. HASAN, R.G. SHIAVI, and D.M. SPENGLER. Relationship between vertical ground reaction force and speed during walking, slow jogging, and running. *Clin Biomech (Bristol, Avon)* 11:253-259, 1996.
55. KOMI, P.V. Stretch-shortening cycle. In: *Strength and Power in Sport*. P.V. Komi, ed. Oxford, UK: Blackwell Science, 2003, pp. 184-202.
56. KOMI, P.V. Training of muscle strength and power: interaction of neuromotoric, hypertrophic,

and mechanical factors. *Int J Sports Med* 7(suppl 1):10-15, 1986.
57. LAURSEN, P.B., and D.G. JENKINS. The scientific basis for high-intensity interval training: optimising training programmes and maximising performance in highly trained endurance athletes. *Sports Med* 32:53-73, 2002.
58. LILJEDAHL, M.E., I. HOLM, C. SYLVEN, and E. JANSSON. Different responses of skeletal muscle following sprint training in men and women. *Eur J Appl Physiol* 74:375-383, 1996.
59. LINNAMO, V., K. HAKKINEN, and P.V. KOMI. Neuromuscular fatigue and recovery in maximal compared to explosive strength loading. *Eur J Appl Physiol Occup Physiol* 77:176-181. 1998.
60. LINOSSIER, M.T., C. DENIS, D. DORMOIS, A. GEYSSANT, and J.R. LACOUR. Ergometric and metabolic adaptation to a 5-s sprint training programme. *Eur J Appl Physiol* 67:408-414, 1993.
61. LINOSSIER, M.T., D. DORMOIS, A. GEYSSANT, and C. DENIS. Performance and fibre characteristics of human skeletal muscle during short sprint training and detraining on a cycle ergometer. *Eur J Appl Physiol* 75:491-498, 1997.
62. LINOSSIER, M.T., D. DORMOIS, C. PERIER, J. FREY, A. GEYSSANT, and C. DENIS. Enzyme adaptations of human skeletal muscle during bicycle short-sprint training and detraining. *Acta Physiol Scand* 161:439-445, 1997.
63. LITTLE, T., and A.G. WILLIAMS. Specificity of acceleration, maximum speed, and agility in professional soccer players. *J Strength Cond Res* 19:76-78, 2005.
64. LOCATELLI, E. The importance of anaerobic glycolysis and stiffness in the sprints (60, 100, 200 metres) *N. Stud Athletics* 11:121-125, 1996.
65. MACKALA, K. Optimisation of performance through kinematic analysis of the different phases of the 100 metres, *N. Stud Athletics* 22(2):7-16, 2007.
66. MACDOUGALL, J.D., A.L. HICKS, J.R. MACDONALD, R.S. MCKELVIE, H.J. GREEN, and K.M. SMITH. Muscle performance and enzymatic adaptations to sprint interval training. *J Appl Physiol* 84:2138-2142, 1998.
67. MAUGHAN, R., and M. GLEESON. *The Biochemical Basis of Sports Performance*. New York: Oxford University Press, 2004.
68. MCBRIDE, J.M., T. TRIPLETT-MCBRIDE, A. DAVIE, and R.U. NEWTON. A comparison of strength and power characteristics between power lifters, Olympic lifters, and sprinters. *J Strength Cond Res* 13:58-66, 1999.
69. MCBRIDE, J.M., T. TRIPLETT-MCBRIDE, A. DAVIE, and R.U. NEWTON. The effect of heavy- vs. light-load jump squats on the development of strength, power, and speed. *J Strength Cond Res* 16:75-82, 2002.
70. MCKENNA, M.J., A.R. HARMER, S.F. FRASER, and J.L. LI. Effects of training on potassium, calcium and hydrogen ion regulation in skeletal muscle and blood during exercise. *Acta Physiol Scand* 156:335-346, 1996.
71. MCKENNA, M., and P.E. RICHES. A comparison of sprinting kinematics on two types of treadmill and over-ground. *Scand J Med Sci Sports* 17:649-655, 2007.
72. MERO, A., and P.V. KOMI. Effects of supramaximal velocity on biomechanical variables in sprinting. *Int J Sport Biomech* 1:240-252, 1985.
73. MERO, A., P. LUHTANEN, J.T. VIITASALO, and P.V. KOMI. Relationships between maximal running velocity, muscle fiber characteristics, force production and force relaxation of sprinters. *Scand J Sports Sci* 3:16-22, 1981.
74. MILLER, R.G., R.S. MOUSSAVI, A.T. GREEN, P.J. CARSON, and M.W. WEINER. The fatigue of rapid repetitive movements. *Neurology* 43:755-761, 1993.
75. MOIR, G., R. SANDERS, C. BUTTON, and M. GLAISTER. The effect of periodized resistance training on accelerative sprint performance. *Sports Biomech* 6:285-300, 2007.
76. MORENO, E. Developing quickness, part II. *Strength Cond J* 17:38-39, 1995.
77. MORIN, J.B., P. EDOUARD, and P. SAMOZINO. New insights into sprint biomechanics and determinants of elite 100m performance. *N. Stud Athletics* 28(3/4):87-104, 2013.
78. MURPHY, A.J., R.G. LOCKIE, and A.J. COUTTS. Kinematic determinants of early acceleration in field sport athletes. *J Sports Sci Med* 2:144-150, 2003.
79. NEGRETE, R., and J. BROPHY. The relationship between isokinetic open and closed chain lower extremity strength and functional performance. *J Sport Rehabil* 9:46-61, 2000.
80. NEVILL, M.E., L.H. BOOBIS, S. BROOKS, and C. WILLIAMS. Effect of training on muscle metabolism during treadmill sprinting. *J Appl Physiol* 67:2376-2382, 1989.
81. NUMMELA, A., H. RUSKO, and A. MERO. EMG activities and ground reaction forces during fatigued and nonfatigued sprinting. *Med Sci Sports Exerc* 26:605-609, 1994.
82. NUMMELA, A., T. KERÄNEN, and L.O. MIKKELSSON. Factors related to top running speed and economy. *Int J Sports Med* 28(8):655-661, 2007.
83. PARRA, J., J.A. CADEFAU, G. RODAS, N. AMIGO, and R. CUSSO. The distribution of rest periods affects performance and adaptations of energy metabolism induced by high-intensity training

in human muscle. *Acta Physiol Scand* 169:157-165, 2000.
84. PETTE, D. The adaptive potential of skeletal muscle fibers. *Can J Appl Physiol* 27:423-448, 2002.
85. PETTE, D., and R.S. STARON. Myosin isoforms, muscle fiber types, and transitions. *Microsc Res Tech* 50:500-509, 2000.
86. PLISK, S.S. The angle on agility. *Training and Conditioning* 10:37-43, 2000.
87. PLISK, S.S. Speed, agility, and speed-endurance development. In: *Essentials of Strength Training and Conditioning*. T.R. Baechle and R.W. Earle, eds. Champaign, IL: Human Kinetics, 2008.
88. PLISK, S.S., and V. GAMBETTA. Tactical metabolic training: part 1. *Strength Cond* 19:44-53, 1997.
89. PLISK, S.S., and M.H. STONE. Periodization strategies. *Strength Cond* 25:19-37, 2003.
90. RACINAIS, S., D. BISHOP, R. DENIS, G. LATTIER, A. MENDEZ-VILLANEUVA, and S. PERREY. Muscle deoxygenation and neural drive to the muscle during repeated sprint cycling. *Med Sci Sports Exerc* 39:268-274, 2007.
91. ROSS, A., and M. LEVERITT. Long-term metabolic and skeletal muscle adaptations to short-sprint training: implications for sprint training and tapering. *Sports Med* 31:1063-1082, 2001.
92. ROSS, A., M. LEVERITT, and S. RIEK. Neural influences on sprint running: training adaptations and acute responses. *Sports Med* 31:409-425, 2001.
93. SAYERS, M. Running technique for field sport players. *Sports Coach* Autumn: 26-27, 2000.
94. SHEPPARD, J.M., and W.B. YOUNG. Agility literature review: classifications, training and testing. *J Sports Sci* 24:919-932, 2006.
95. SIFF, M.C. *Supertraining*. 6th ed. Denver, CO: Supertraining Institute, 2003.
96. SIMONEAU, J.A., G. LORTIE, M.R. BOULAY, M. MARCOTTE, M.C. THIBAULT, and C. BOUCHARD. Human skeletal muscle fiber type alteration with high-intensity intermittent training. *Eur J Appl Physiol Occup Physiol* 54:250-253, 1985.
97. SPENCER, M., D. BISHOP, B. DAWSON, and C. GOODMAN. Physiological and metabolic responses of repeated-sprint activities : specific to field-based team sports. *Sports Med* 35:1025-1044, 2005.
98. SPRIET, L.L., M.I. LINDINGER, R.S. MCKELVIE, G.J. HEIGENHAUSER, and N.L. JONES. Muscle glycogenolysis and H+ concentration during maximal intermittent cycling. *J Appl Physiol* 66:8-13, 1989.
99. STACKHOUSE, S.K., D.S. REISMAN, and S.A. BINDER-MACLEOD. Challenging the role of pH in skeletal muscle fatigue. *Phys Ther* 81:1897-1903, 2001.
100. STONE, M.H., M.E. STONE, and W.A. SANDS. *Principles and Practice of Resistance Training*. Champaign, IL: Human Kinetics, 2007.
101. TESCH, P.A., J.E. WRIGHT, J.A. VOGEL, W.L. DANIELS, D.S. SHARP, and B. SJODIN. The influence of muscle metabolic characteristics on physical performance. *Eur J Appl Physiol Occup Physiol* 54:237-243, 1985.
102. THORSTENSSON, A., B. SJÖDIN, and J. KARLSSON. Enzyme activities and muscle strength after "sprint training" in man. *Acta Physiol Scand* 94:313-318, 1975.
103. TRAPPE, S., M. GODARD, P. GALLAGHER, C. CARROLL, G. ROWDEN, and D. PORTER. Resistance training improves single muscle fiber contractile function in older women. *Am J Physiol Cell Physiol* 281:C398-406, 2001.
104. TRAPPE, S., M. HARBER, A. CREER, P. GALLAGHER, D. SLIVKA, K. MINCHEV, and D. WHITSETT. Single muscle fiber adaptations with marathon training. *J Appl Physiol* 101:721-727, 2006.
105. TRAPPE, S., D. WILLIAMSON, M. GODARD, D. PORTER, G. ROWDEN, and D. COSTILL. Effect of resistance training on single muscle fiber contractile function in older men. *J Appl Physiol* 89:143-152, 2000.
106. VOLEK, J.S., and W.J. KRAEMER. Creatine supplementation: its effect on human muscular performance and body composition. *J Strength Cond Res* 10:200-210, 1996.
107. WESTON, A.R., K.H. MYBURGH, F.H. LINDSAY, S.C. DENNIS, T.D. NOAKES, and J.A. HAWLEY. Skeletal muscle buffering capacity and endurance performance after high-intensity interval training by well-trained cyclists. *Eur J Appl Physiol Occup Physiol* 75:7-13, 1997.
108. WILLIAMSON, D.L., P.M. GALLAGHER, C.C. CARROLL, U. RAUE, and S.W. TRAPPE. Reduction in hybrid single muscle fiber proportions with resistance training in humans. *J Appl Physiol* 91:1955-1961, 2001.
109. WILLIAMSON, D.L., M.P. GODARD, D.A. PORTER, D.L. COSTILL, and S.W. TRAPPE. Progressive resistance training reduces myosin heavy chain coexpression in single muscle fibers from older men. *J Appl Physiol* 88:627-633, 2000.
110. YOUNG, W., D. BENTON, G. DUTHIE, and J. PRYOR. Resistance training for short sprints and maximum-speed sprints. *Strength Cond* 23:7-13, 2001.
111. YOUNG, W.B., R. JAMES, and I. MONTGOMERY. Is muscle power related to running speed with changes of direction? *J Sports Med Phys Fitness* 42:282-288, 2002.
112. YOUNG, W.B., M.H. MCDOWELL, and B.J. SCARLETT. Specificity of sprint and agility training methods. *J Strength Cond Res* 15:315-319, 2001.

Index

Note: The italicized *f* and *t* following page numbers refer to figures and tables, respectively.

A

absolute density 85
absolute intensity 78
absolute strength 238
absolute volume 85
acceleration phase 107-108, 301, 308-309
accelerometers 247-248, 292-293
accessory (compensation) exercises 194
Accumulation-Transmutation-Realization (A.T.R.) 97
active rest or recovery
   for aerobic training 277
   in competitive microcycle 149-150
   in transition phase 176-177
acyclic combined skills 6
acyclic skills 6
adaptation
   in endurance training 109-110
   fatigue and 151
   maladaptation 8, 83
   performance gains and 10, 11*f*
   specialization and 33
   in strength training 235-237
   supercompensation and 12-19, 14*f*
   training load and 8-9, 9*f*
   training phases and 10-11
   training planning and 116
   types of 10
   volume and 83-84
adenosine diphosphate (ADP) 20
adenosine triphosphate (ATP)
   described 19
   in metabolic adaptation 10
   in sprint training 303
Aeneid, The (Virgil) 115
aerobic compensation training (CoT) 299
aerobic endurance
   versus anaerobic 53, 265
   anaerobic training for 266-267
   exercise economy in 273-274
   lactate threshold in 271-272, 272*f*, 273*f*
   muscles in 270-271
   performance factors overview 267*f*
   $\dot{V}O_2$max in 268-271, 272*f*
aerobic endurance training
   active rest in 277
   in competitive phase 169-170, 171
   in general subphase 167
   interval training in 266-267, 275, 278-283, 280*t*, 281*t*, 283*t*
   long slow distance training in 277-278, 279*t*
   methods overview 276-277, 277*t*
   microcycles for 158, 159*f*
   periodization of 109-110, 294-300, 296*f*
   strength training in 283-284, 284*f*
   tapers in 171-172, 172*f*
aerobic energy system. See oxidative system
aerobic interval training 279-280, 280*t*, 281*t*
aerobic power. See $\dot{V}O_2$max
aerobic threshold training (ATT) 299
age
   for specialization by sport 34, 34*t*-35*t*
   training capacity and 36
agility
   defined 106
   factors affecting 311*f*, 312-313
   strength and 229
   terms confused with 311
agility training
   in daily training sessions 126
   in microcycles 138
   periodization of 106-107, 106*f*, 319-322, 320*f*, 321*f*, 323*f*
   principles of 313-314
   in speed training 108-109
   training variables in 315-318, 317*t*
alactic system training (AST) 295-297
altitude exposure 269
American football
   competitive phase planning in 218-219
   energy sources in 27
   microcycle model for 323*f*
   rest intervals in 286-288
anaerobic endurance
   vs. aerobic 53, 265
   aerobic training and 284-285
anaerobic endurance phase 108
anaerobic endurance training
   for aerobic endurance 266-267
   competitive trial methods 290, 290*t*
   factors affecting 275-276
   interval training in 285-292, 285*t*, 286*t*, 288*t*
   periodization of 294-300, 296*f*
   strength training in 293-294
anaerobic energy systems. See glycolytic system; phosphagen (ATP-PC) system
anaerobic interval training 281, 283*t*
anaerobic threshold 271
anaerobic threshold training (AnTT) 298
anatomical adaptation phase 103, 260
annual plans. See also specific phases
   athlete readiness and 98, 181-182
   bi-cycle 178-179, 179*f*, 186, 187*f*
   competition calendar and 192-193, 199
   competitive phase 169-173, 172*f*, 173*f*
   compiling 192-193, 203*f*
   described 165-166
   elements overview 193
   individualization of 98, 184
   monocycle 177-178, 177*f*, 178*f*, 184-186, 185*f*
   multiple-peak 181, 181*f*, 191-192, 191*f*

371

annual plans. *See also specific phases (continued)*
   objectives in 197-198, 198t
   performance model analysis in 193-195, 194f
   performance prediction in 196-197, 197t
   periodization model in 202
   phase duration by plan type 182, 182t
   phases and cycles overview 93, 93f
   preparation model in 202-203, 204t, 205t
   preparatory phase 166-169, 167t
   retrospective analysis in 195-196, 195t
   for speed and agility training 319, 320f, 321f
   term usage 119
   test results and standards in 199-201, 202t
   transition phase 174-177
   tri-cycle 179-181, 180f, 186-189, 188f
   types overview 98, 98t
   when to create 192
AnTT (anaerobic threshold training) 298
arteriovenous oxygen difference 271
ascending pyramid loading 250-251, 251t
assessment sessions 120
AST (alactic system training) 295-297
asynchronous motor unit firing 234
athletic drills, in warm-ups 125
athletic formation phase 118
athletic shape 208
athletic testing and monitoring
   in annual plan 199-201, 202t
   in long-term plan 118-119
   in strength training 254-255, 259
   training models and 40-41
   using technology 292-293, 293f, 294f
   Yo-Yo Intermittent Recovery Test 287, 287t
ATP (adenosine triphosphate). *See* adenosine triphosphate
ATP-PC system. *See* phosphagen (ATP-PC) system
A.T.R. (Accumulation-Transmutation-Realization) 97
ATT (aerobic threshold training) 299

B
barbell velocity 247-248, 247t
baseball monocycle 101f
basic training zone 77
basketball monocycle chart 184-186, 185f
bi-cycle plans
   athlete readiness and 98, 182
   chart of 186, 187f
   in history of periodization 92
   model plans 101f, 178-179, 179f
bioenergetics. *See also energy systems*
   in anaerobic endurance 275
   defined 3
   intensity zones based on 74-76, 74t
   in interval training 285t
bioenergetic specificity 22, 23f, 25, 25t-27t
biological age 36
biomotor abilities. *See also specific abilities*
   defined 5
   dominance by sport 230f
   integration of 101-103, 102f
   periodization of 93, 99-101, 99f
   relationship between 229-231, 230f, 231f
   retrospective analysis of 196
   sport-specific training for 54-55
   in technical or tactical errors 67
   in training goal 3
block (term) 94
block periodization 97
body temperature, and warm-ups 123, 124
body weight exercises 239
Bompa, Tudor 92
Bondarchuk, A.P. 6-7
buffer, in strength training 245, 245f, 246f
buffering, of lactic acid 275, 304

C
calisthenics 54
capillary density 271
carbohydrates 21-22, 76
cardiac output 269-270, 269f
cardiorespiratory adaptation 10, 109
cardiovascular system 275-276
central fatigue 129
cessation phase 105, 262-263
change-of-direction speed 311f, 312-313
chronological age 36
cluster sets 252, 253t

compensation (accessory) exercises 194
compensation phase
   of adaptation 10-11
   in strength training 105-106, 263
   of supercompensation 16-17
competition calendar
   as aspect of annual plan 192-193, 199
   competition frequency 219-222, 220t, 221t
   in competition phase planning 216-217, 217f
competition classification 215-216
competition readiness
   as adaptation 11
   annual plan selection and 98, 182
   term usage 94
   volume and intensity in 72, 73f, 79
competitive training phase
   adaptation and 11
   in bi-cycle plans 179
   competition frequency and 219-222, 220t, 221t
   interval training during 291-292, 291t
   macrocycles for 162-163, 162f
   main competitive subphase 171-173
   microcycle dynamics 146f, 147-151, 148f
   in monocycle plans 178
   objectives of 94, 94f, 169, 222t
   planning methods 217-219, 218f, 219f, 220f
   precompetitive subphase 170-171
   rest and recovery in 149, 150
   special preparation period 173
   stress curve in 183, 183f
   structure of 170
   tapering subphase 171-173, 172f, 173f, 222, 223t
   in tri-cycle plans 180
competitive trial methods 290, 290t
complexity 85-86
concentrated loading 44-45, 45f
conjugated sequence loading 45-46, 46t
conversion phase 104-105, 261-262
cool-downs 127-128
Cooper, H.K. 11, 12, 12t
CoT (aerobic compensation training) 299

coupled successive system 45-46, 46*t*
creatine phosphokinase (CPK) 303
cross-country skiers competitive phase 219*f*
cross-over concept 22
cross-training 54
cumulative effect 11-12
cutting (term) 311
cyclic method of planning 218-219, 218*f*, 219*f*, 220*f*
cyclic skills 5-6
cycling
   drafting in 81-82
   heart rate-based training zones 77*t*
   power-based training zones 78, 78*t*

D
daily training sessions
   classification of 120-121
   cool-down in 127-128
   duration of 121, 128, 128*t*
   goals of 126
   introductions in 122
   main body of 125-126
   multiple daily sessions 132-133
   regeneration sessions 152*t*
   structure of 121-122
   supplementary 130, 130*t*
   warm-ups in 122-125, 123*t*
decision making, in agility 311*f*, 312
degree of training 207-208
delayed-onset muscle soreness (DOMS) 16
delayed training effect 11
density. See frequency
detraining load 42
detraining syndrome 174-176, 175*t*, 263
developmental macrocycles 161-162, 161*f*
developmental microcycles 146, 147*f*
differentiation 63-64
DOMS (delayed-onset muscle soreness) 16
double pyramid loading 251, 251*t*
duration (time)
   daily training sessions 121, 128, 128*t*
   interval training 289
   macrocycles 160-161
   peaking 224
   preparatory phase 166
   taper 213, 213*t*

duration (training variable)
   as component of volume 71
   energy sources and 22, 24*f*
   intensity zones 74-76, 74*t*
   in interval training 288
   in speed and agility training 315, 316
dynamic stretching 125

E
elastic bands, for strength training 239
endurance. See also aerobic endurance; anaerobic endurance
   detraining effects on 174-176
   muscle fiber type and 235
   strength and 229-230
   types of 265-267
endurance training. See also aerobic endurance training; anaerobic endurance training
   in daily training sessions 126
   intensity zones for 295-299, 295*f*
   microcycles for 138
   misconception about 53
   needs analysis of 195
   periodization of 109-110, 294-300, 296*f*
energy systems. See also specific systems
   energy provision of 19, 20*f*
   exercise duration and 22, 24*f*
   glycolytic 21-22
   in interval training 285*t*, 286*t*
   microcycle intensities and 155*f*, 156-159, 157*f*, 157*t*, 158*f*, 159*f*
   overlap of 22-25
   oxidative 22
   phosphagen (ATP-PC) 20-21
   in specific sport activities 22, 23*f*, 25, 25*t*-27*t*, 27
   in speed development 303-304
environment
   intensity and 81-82
   in tactical training 60-61
   in technical or tactical errors 67
EPOC (excess postexercise oxygen consumption) 16-17
ergogenesis 25*t*-27*t*, 158, 286*t*
evaluations
   of athletes 40-41, 118-119, 199-201, 202*t*, 254-255, 259
   of training system 7
   as transition phase purpose 177
   using technology 292-293, 293*f*, 294*f*
   Yo-Yo Intermittent Recovery Test 287, 287*t*

evident fatigue 129
evolutionary standards 201
evolution training zone 77-78
excess postexercise oxygen consumption (EPOC) 16-17
exercise economy 55-56, 273-274
exercise order
   in speed and agility training 315-316
   in strength training 249-250, 249*t*
exercises
   compensation (accessory) 194
   defined 54
   for general physical development 54
   for sport-specific training 54-55
   in strength training program 254
   variation in 39
   in warm-ups 125
exhibition competitions 170-171, 215-216
exponential tapers 214, 214*f*
external load 83

F
fartleks 281-283, 285, 286*t*
fast exponential tapers 214, 214*f*
fast-twitch muscle fibers. See muscle fiber types
fatigue
   adaptation and 8, 12, 151
   annual plan and 182
   athlete readiness and 190
   defined 128
   injury risk and 5
   model training and 134-135, 135*t*
   speed and 301-302, 309-310
   in speed and agility training 322
   in supercompensation 15-16
   tapers and 209-210, 210*f*
   in technical or tactical errors 67, 68
   in technical training 60
   training session plans and 129-130
   types and phases of 128-129
feedback, in speed and agility training 314
female athletes. See gender differences
figure skating monocycle 100*f*
fitness–fatigue relationship 209-210, 210*f*
fixed work-to-recovery ratios 84
flat loading 47, 47*f*

flat pyramid loading 250, 251*t*
flexibility training, in microcycles 138
football. *See* American football; soccer
force 231, 232
force development (RFD) 233, 266, 276
force–velocity curve
   aerobic endurance and 266, 266*f*
   muscular strength and 232-233, 232*f*, 233*f*
Fosbury flop 56-57
free sessions 121
free weights 239
frequency
   calculating 84-85
   defined 84
   in interval training 289
   in speed and agility training 315
   in strength training 250
   supercompensation and 17-18, 18*f*
   during taper 212-213
   training load increases and 79-80
   variation in 39

G

Galen 91-92
game plan 61-63
GAS (general adaptation syndrome) 12-13, 13*f*
gender differences
   individualization and 38
   in strength-training cessation 262
   $\dot{V}O_2$max 268
general adaptation syndrome (GAS) 12-13, 13*f*
general fitness. *See* multilateral physical development
general physical training (GPT) 52-53, 53*f*, 54, 166-168, 167*t*. *See also* multilateral physical development
general speed phase 107-108
general strength 237
Germany, in periodization history 92
glucose uptake 16
gluteal amnesia 125
glutei activation exercises 125
glycogen stores 21-22, 76
glycolytic system
   described 21-22
   in intensity zones 75
   in metabolic adaptation 10
microcycle intensity and 158, 158*f*
   in speed development 303
goals and objectives
   in annual plan 197-198, 198*t*
   of competitive training phase 94, 94*f*, 169, 222*t*
   in daily training sessions 126
   as paramount to training 3
   of physical training 4-5, 29, 52, 165
   of preparatory training phase 94, 94*f*, 166, 167*t*
   in strength training 254
   of tapers 209
   of training plan 115-116
Golgi tendon organ 234
GPS technology 292-293
GPT. *See* general physical training (GPT)
Greece, ancient 91, 115
grouping method of planning 217-218, 218*f*
group sessions 120
gymnastics monocycle 100*f*

H

Handbook for the Athletic Coach (Philostratus) 115
health maintenance 5
health status, and work capacity 37
heart rate-based recovery periods 85
heart rate-based training 76-78, 77*t*, 82
heavy loads 243
Henneman size principle 233
high-intensity exercise endurance (HIEE). *See* anaerobic endurance; anaerobic endurance training
high performance phase 118
hormone response, in strength training 249
hypertrophy
   in metabolic adaptation 10
   strength training and 235, 236
hypertrophy phase 260

I

IAT (individual anaerobic threshold) 76-77
immediate training effect 11
index of overall demand (IOD) 86
individual anaerobic threshold (IAT) 76-77
individualization
   of annual plan 98, 184
gender differences and 38
   versus standardization 65
   of tapers 211, 213
   of technique 57
   training capacity and 36-37
   of training load 37
   variation in 38-40
individual sessions 120
initiation phase 118
injury rehabilitation 106, 177
injury risk and prevention
   1RM testing and 255, 259
   speed training and 108
   training patterns and 218
   warm-ups and 125
   in youth 5, 36
integration
   versus differentiation 63-64
   simultaneous versus sequential 101-103, 102*f*
   of training plan 110-113, 112*f*
intensity
   alternating in microcycle 155*f*, 156-159, 157*f*, 158*f*, 159*f*
   assessment of 73-74, 74*t*
   bioenergetic-based zones 74-76, 74*t*
   in competitive phase 169, 171-173
   defined 73
   endurance training zones 295-299, 295*f*
   factors in 81-82
   heart-rate zones 76-78, 77*t*, 82
   in interval training 288
   in microcycle structure 141-142, 142*f*, 142*t*, 143*f*
   power-based zones 78, 78*t*
   quantifying in microcycle 152-155, 154*f*, 154*t*, 155*f*
   rating 82-83
   relation to volume 78-79
   in speed and agility training 316-317, 317*t*, 318
   strategies for increasing 80
   in strength training 240-243, 242*f*, 242*t*
   stress and 183
   supercompensation and 17-18, 18*f*, 19*f*
   during taper 171-173, 210-211, 222
   types of 78
   variation in 39
intermittent runs (fartleks) 281-283, 285, 286*t*
intermuscular coordination 104, 261
internal load 83

interval training
    for aerobic endurance 266-267, 278-283, 280t, 281t, 283t
    for anaerobic endurance 276, 285-292, 285t, 286t, 288t
    in competitive phase 291-292, 291t
    descending ladder model 295, 295f
    energy sources and 24, 285t, 286t
    enzymatic alterations from 303-304
    for exercise economy 274
    lactate threshold and 273
    progression of 290, 290t
    rest intervals in 286-288, 288t
    training variables in 288-289
intramuscular coordination 104, 261
introduction, in training session 122
involution 15, 17
IOD (index of overall demand) 86
isometric strength training 239
Issurin, V. 101-103

J
javelin throwers
    competition phase microcycle for 146
    retrospective analysis of 195t
junior athletes. See youth

L
lactate accumulation curve 271, 273f
lactate dehydrogenase (LDH) 303
lactate threshold (LT) 24, 271-273, 272f
lactic acid
    buffering capacity 275, 304
    glycolysis and 21
    in intensity zones 75
    role in fatigue 16, 302
lactic acid training (LAT) 297-298
latent fatigue 129
LDH (lactate dehydrogenase) 303
learning sessions 120
LIEE (low-intensity exercise endurance). See aerobic endurance; aerobic endurance training
linear loading 43, 43f, 97
linear periodization 95
linear tapers 214, 214f
load progression. See training loads
long-lasting residual effect 94
long slow distance (LSD) training 277-278, 279t

long-term plans 117-118, 117f
low-intensity exercise endurance (LIEE). See aerobic endurance; aerobic endurance training
LSD (long slow distance) training 277-278, 279t
LT (lactate threshold) 24, 271-273, 272f

M
macrocycles
    competitive phase 162-163, 162f
    defined 159-160
    duration of 160-161
    preparatory phase 161-162, 161f
    for speed and agility training 319-322
    structure of 160-161, 160t
    for tapers 163
    term usage 119
    transition phase 163, 163f
main competitive subphase 171-173
maintenance phase 105, 262
maintenance standards 201
major competitions 215
maladaptation 8, 83
martial arts tri-cycle chart 186-189, 188f
MAS (maximal aerobic speed) test 282, 282t
Matveyev, Leonid P. 92
maximal aerobic capacity. See $\dot{V}O_2$max
maximal aerobic speed (MAS) test 282, 282t
maximal heart rate 76
maximal lactate steady state 271
maximum loads 243
maximum oxygen consumption training ($\dot{V}O_2$maxT) 298
maximum speed phase 108, 301, 309, 309f
maximum strength
    defined 238
    periodization phase 104, 260-261, 261f
menstrual cycle, and performance 38
mental practice (visualization) 68, 183
metabolic adaptation 10
MHC (myosin heavy chain) content 237
microcycles
    with aerobic intervals 281t
    alternating intensity in 155f, 156-159, 157f, 158f, 159f

with anaerobic intervals 283t
competition phase 146f, 147-151, 148f
in cyclic approach 219, 220f
defined 119, 137
developmental 146, 147f
intensity variation in 141-142, 142f, 142t, 143f
with LSD emphasis 279t
peaking-unloading 147
quantifying training in 152-155, 154f, 154t, 155f
recovery-regeneration 146-147, 151, 151f, 152f, 152t
sessions per week in 140-141, 140f, 141f
for speed and agility training 322, 323f
for stress management 184, 184f
structure of 137-139
total training demand in 142f, 143-144, 143f, 144f, 145f
minimum effective volume 72, 72f
mitochondrial density, in $\dot{V}O_2$max 270-271
mixed sessions 120-121
MK (myokinase) 303
models of performance 56-57
monocycle plans
    athlete readiness and 98, 182
    for biomotor abilities by sport 100f, 101f
    chart of 184-186, 185f
    in history of periodization 92
    model plan 177-178, 177f, 178f
    stress curve for 182-183, 183f
monotonous program overtraining 38
morphological adaptations 235-237
motivation, in speed and agility training 314
motor unit activity, in strength 233-234, 236
movement economy 55-56, 273-274
movement time 106-107, 106f
multilateral physical development. See also general physical training
    defined 4
    research studies in 30-32, 33
    versus specialization 29-36, 30f
multiple daily training sessions 132-133, 141
multiple-peak plans
    athlete readiness and 98, 182
    for biomotor abilities 99-100

multiple-peak plans *(continued)*
 chart of 191-192, 191f
 model plan 181, 181f
muscle activation, in sprinting 305-306
muscle damage 16
muscle endurance 238
muscle fiber types
 endurance training and 266, 270
 in speed development 304-305, 305f
 strength, strength training and 235, 236-237, 237t
muscle hypertrophy
 in metabolic adaptation 10
 strength training and 235, 236
muscular balance 260
musculoskeletal adaptation 110
myokinase (MK) 303
myosin heavy chain (MHC) content 237, 304, 305f

N

neurological adaptation 235-236
neuromuscular adaptation 10
neuromuscular inhibition 234-235
neuromuscular system
 in anaerobic endurance 276
 in speed development 304-306
Newton's second law 231, 232
nonprogressive tapers 214
nutrition
 in integrated training plan 111-113, 112f
 recovery and 14
 for stress management 183
 for young athletes 186

O

objectives. *See* goals and objectives
OBLA (onset of blood lactate accumulation) 24, 272, 272f
off-season (term) 94-95, 174
Olympic lifts
 in strength training 255
 velocity of 247t
Olympic traditions 3, 91-92
1RM testing 255, 259
onset of blood lactate accumulation (OBLA) 24, 272, 272f
overall demand 86
overreaching
 adaptation and 8
 concentrated loading as 44-45, 45f
overtraining
 adaption and 8

 in competitive season 291-292
 linear loading and 43
 program monotony and 38
 volume and 83
oxidative system
 described 22
 intensity zones 75-76
 in metabolic adaptation 10
 microcycle intensity and 158, 159f
 in speed development 303
oxygen transport, in $\dot{V}O_2$max 270

P

pace training 279-280, 280t, 281t
partial intensity 82
passive rest 177
PCr (phosphocreatine). *See* phosphocreatine
peaking
 in competitive phase 150-151
 defined 208
 duration of 224
 factors affecting 208, 208f
 in macrocycles 162-163, 162f
 training conditions for 207-208, 207f, 208f
 zones of 223, 224t
peaking curve 189
peaking index 188f, 189-190, 190t, 191t
peaking-unloading microcycles 147
perception, in agility 311f, 312
performance model analysis 193-195, 194f
performance oxygen uptake 271
performance plateaus
 program monotony and 38
 standard loading and 8, 9f, 43
performance prediction 196-197, 197t
performance standards 199-201, 202t
periodization. *See also specific biomotor abilities, cycles, or phases*
 of annual plan 93, 93f, 98, 98t, 202
 of biomotor abilities 93, 99-101, 99f
 defined 91, 97
 history of 91-92
 integrated 110-113, 112f
 versus loading 97-98
 load undulation in 96, 96f, 97f
 phases of 94-95
 term origin 91
 terms misused 94, 95-97

peripheral fatigue 128-129
personality development training 5
phases of training. *See also specific phases*
 adaptation and 10-11
 duration by annual plan type 182, 182t
 sequence of 94-95, 94f
 for strength training 259-263, 259t
 term usage 94
Philostratus, Flavius 91, 115, 137
phosphagen (ATP-PC) system
 described 20-21
 in intensity zones 75
 microcycle intensity and 158, 158f
 in speed development 303
phosphocreatine (PCr)
 in intensity zones 75
 in metabolic adaptation 10
 in sprint training 303
phosphorylase (PHOS) 303
physical perfection 3
physical skill classification 5-6
physical training
 as cornerstone 51
 exercises for 54-55
 general 52-53, 53f
 goals of 4-5, 29, 52, 165
 sequence of 52, 52f
 sport-specific 53-54, 53f
planning. *See* training plans
Plisk, S.S. 46, 46t
plyometric training
 for change-of-direction speed 313
 for exercise economy 274
postactivation potentiation 123, 124
postactivation potentiation complex 249-250, 249t
power
 defined 106, 237-238
 gains from taper 215
 maximun versus average output 233
 muscle fiber type and 235
 strength and 233
power-based training zones 78, 78t
power training
 barbell velocity in 247-248, 247t
 in competitive phase 169, 171
 detraining 176
 in general subphase 167
 microcycles for 158, 158f

periodization of 106-107
  tapers in 172-173, 172f
preadaptation 10
precompetitive adaptation 11
precompetitive subphase 170-171
precontest arousal sessions 135, 135t
predetermined heart rate 85
preparation model 202-203, 204t, 205t
preparatory training phase
  adaptation and 10-11
  in bi-cycle plans 179
  duration of 166
  general subphase 166-168
  macrocycles for 161-162, 161f
  in monocycle plans 178
  objectives of 94, 94f, 166, 167t
  physical training in 52, 52f
  specific subphase 168-169
  stress curve in 183, 183f
  training load models in 43, 47, 47f
  in tri-cycle plans 180
preparedness
  described 207-208
  tapers and 209-210, 210f
  term usage 94
  training load and 42
progressive overloading
  adaptation and 83-84
  GAS theory and 12-13, 13f
  in strength training 238
progressive tapers 214
psychological factors
  in performance 5
  in technical or tactical errors 67
  warm-ups and 124
psychological training 111-113, 112f
pulmonary system, in $\dot{V}O_2$max 268-269
pyramid loading 250-251, 251t

Q
quickness (term) 311

R
rate coding
  in metabolic adaptation 10
  strength, strength training and 234, 236
rate of force development (RFD) 233, 266, 276
reactive agility 107, 108-109
readiness
  described 208
  tapers and 209-210, 210f
readiness curve 189

readiness index 188f, 189-190, 190t, 191t
recovery. See also active rest or recovery
  in competitive phase 149, 150
  glycogen resynthesis 21-22
  in supercompensation cycle 14
  during taper 222, 223t
  training frequency and 39
recovery-regeneration microcycles 146-147, 151, 151f, 152f, 152t
relative density 85
relative intensity 78
relative strength 238
relative volume 85
relaxation techniques 183
repetition method 281
repetitions, in strength training 243, 243t, 244f
repetition sessions 120
residual fatigue 209
resting metabolism 17
rest intervals
  anaerobic endurance training 286-288, 288t
  speed and agility training 317-318
  strength training 248-249, 294
  training frequency 84-85, 84t
retaining load 42
retrospective analysis 195-196, 195t
RFD (rate of force development) 233, 266, 276
Rome, ancient 91-92, 115
rowers
  performance prediction for 197, 197t
  quantifying training for 153, 154f, 154t
running economy 55-56, 273-274
Russia, in periodization history 92

S
scientific disciplines
  axillary 4, 4f
  sport science 6-7
Selye, Hans 12-13, 13f
sets, in strength training 248-249
size principle 233
skeletal muscle, in $\dot{V}O_2$max 270-271
skewed pyramid loading 251-252, 252t
skill acquisition. See also tactical training; technical training
  in long-term plan 118
  in training sessions 120, 134, 134t

skill perfection
  in daily training 120
  under fatigue 134-135, 135t
  technical, tactical abilities 63-67, 64f, 65f, 66f
slow exponential tapers 214, 214f
slow-twitch muscle fibers. See muscle fiber types
soccer
  annual plan model for 321f
  competition frequency in 221
  endurance training for 110, 111f
  energy sources in 27
  interval training in 291, 291t
  macrocycle for 160t
  monocycle for 100f
  rest intervals in 286-288
  speed training for 108
  Yo-Yo Intermittent Recovery Test 287t
special endurance training 110, 290, 290t
specialization. See sport-specific physical training
specific endurance 110
specific speed phase 108-109
specific strength 237
speed
  defined 301
  energy systems in 303-304
  fatigue and 309-310
  neuromuscular systems in 304-306, 305f
  phases of 301-302
  strength and 229, 231-233, 232f, 233f, 301, 308, 309
  technical skill in 306-309
speed endurance 301-302
speed training
  in competitive phase 169, 171
  in daily training sessions 126
  in general subphase 167
  methods of 310, 310t
  microcycles for 138, 158, 158f
  needs analysis of 195
  periodization of 107-109, 319-322, 320f, 321f, 323f
  principles of 313-314
  tapers in 172-173, 172f
  training variables in 315-318, 317t
sports, sporting activities
  age for specialization 34, 34t-35t
  bi-cycle model for 101f
  biomotor abilities of 230f
  energy sources for 22, 23f, 25, 25t-27t, 27
  intensity of 81

sports, sporting activities (continued)
   monocycle models for 100f, 101f
   preparatory phase objectives for 167t
   strength, strength training for 231, 241t
   tactical classification 59-60
sport science 6-7
sport-specific physical training (SSPT)
   adaptation in 33
   age for by sport 34, 34t-35t
   in competitive phase 169
   defined 4
   exercises for 54-55
   versus general physical training 29-36, 30f, 53-54, 53f
   in long-term plan 118
   as preparation subphase 168-169
   speed and agility training 313-314
   strength training 255
sprint phases 307-309, 307f, 308f, 309f. See also speed; speed training
SSC (stretch shortening cycle) 234
stability, versus variability 64-65
stable adaptation 11
standardization 65
standard loading 8, 9f, 43
standards of performance 199-201, 202t
start phase of sprint 307, 307f, 308f
static stretching 125, 127-128
step loading 44, 44f, 47, 47f, 161, 161f
step tapers 214, 214f
stimulating load 42
Stone, M.H. 46, 46t
strategies, defined 58-59
strength
   change-of-direction speed and 313
   defined 231
   factors affecting 233-235
   role in performance 229-231, 230f
   speed and 231-233, 232f, 233f, 301, 308, 309
   types of 237-238
strength training
   adaptations to 235-237, 237t
   for aerobic endurance 273, 274, 283-284, 284f
   for anaerobic endurance 293-294

   barbell velocity in 247-248, 247t
   buffer in 245, 245f, 246f
   in competitive phase 169, 171
   in daily training sessions 126
   detraining 176
   exercise order in 249-250, 249t
   frequency in 250
   gains from tapers 215
   in general subphase 167
   heavy versus explosive 232-233
   intensity in 240-243, 242f, 242t
   loading patterns in 250-253, 251t, 252t, 253t
   macrocycle model 160t
   methods of 239
   in microcycles 138
   needs analysis of 194
   periodization of 103-106, 259-263, 259t
   program implementation 253-259
   records and logs of 256, 256t, 257f, 258f
   repetitions in 243, 243t, 244f
   sets and rest intervals in 248-249
   specificity of 255
   training to failure 240
   volume in 240, 240t, 241t
stress
   periodization and 182-184, 183f, 184f
   work capacity and 37
stretching
   cool-down 127-128
   warm-up 125
stretch reflex 306
stretch shortening cycle (SSC) 234
supercompensation
   benefits of 13
   cycle and adaptation 12-14, 14f
   fatigue and 151
   intensity and frequency in 17-18, 18f, 19f
   phases of 15-18, 15f
supermaximum loads 242-243
supplementary training sessions 130, 130t
swimmers
   bi-cycle chart for 186, 187f
   bi-cycle model for 101f
   preparatory model for 202-203, 204t
synchronous motor unit firing 234, 236

T

tactical abilities
   defined 5

   perfecting 63-67, 64f, 65f, 66f
   retrospective analysis of 196
tactical errors 67-68
tactical training
   for adverse conditions 60-61
   in daily training sessions 126
   defined 59
   energy distribution in 60
   factors in 59
   game plan 61-63
   in long-term plan 118
   specificity of 59-60
   tactical thinking 61
   for team cooperation 61
tactics
   defined 58-59
   sports classified by 59-60
tapers
   defined 209
   factors affecting 210-213, 212t, 213t
   goal of 209
   individualization of 211, 213
   macrocycles for 163
   in main competitive subphase 171-173, 172f, 173f
   peaking and 208
   performance gains from 215
   premise of 209-210, 210f
   strategies and benefits 211, 222, 223t
   for stress management 183
   types of 214, 214f
T:C ratio 45, 213
team sports
   competition frequency in 221
   competitive microcycle for 147-150, 148f, 149f
   competitive phase planning in 218-219
   endurance training for 284-285, 294-295
   exhibition games 170-171, 215-216
   general subphase for 167
   interval training for 304
   macrocycle issues in 322
   microcycle intensities for 155f, 156, 157-158, 157f
   peaking index and 190
   quantifying training in 153, 155f
   stress management in 184, 184f
   tactical training for 61-63
   tapers in 173, 173f, 213
technical errors 67-68
technical skills (technique)
   defined 4-5, 55
   perfecting 63-67, 64f, 65f, 66f

retrospective analysis of 196
sprinting 306-309
in training activities 313
technical training
   in daily training sessions 126
   exercise economy and 55-56
   individualization of 57
   learning process in 58
   in long-term plan 118
   model techniques and 56-57
   technique evolution and 58
technique. See technical skills; technical training
temperature, and warm-ups 123, 124
tempo training 107-108, 279-280, 280t, 281t
tennis multiple-peak chart 191-192, 191f
testosterone
   in biological age 36
   cortisol ratio (T:C ratio) 45, 213
tests and testing. See athletic testing and monitoring
tetra system 137
theoretical knowledge 5, 68-69
Tmax 279
tonnage, defined 71
total training demand 142f, 143-144, 143f, 144f, 145f
track and field. See also javelin throwers
   competition frequency in 221t
   peaking zones for 224t
training
   versus competitions 218
   defined 4
   objectives of 4-5, 29, 52, 165
   quality of 7, 8f, 313
   scope of 3
   sequential model of 30, 30f
   supercompensation in 12-19, 14f, 15f
   system of 6-7, 7f
training age 36
training effect
   categories of 11, 12t
   term usage 94
training factors
   physical training 51-55
   pyramid 51f
   tactical training 58-68
   technical training 55-58
   theoretical training 68-69
training history, and work capacity 36-37
training impulse (TRIMP) 82
training loads
   adaptation and 8-9, 9f

classification of 42
concentrated loading 44-45, 45f
conjugated sequence loading 45-46, 46t
external versus internal 83
flat loading 47, 47f
historical increases in 42, 42t, 79
individualized 37
linear loading 43, 43f, 97
in macrocycles 161-162, 161f
in microcycles 138
versus periodization 97-98
readiness and 208, 208f
sequence of 42-43, 48-49, 48f
standard loading 8, 9f, 43
step loading 44, 44f, 47, 47f
strategies for increasing 80
in strength training 240-243, 242f, 243t, 245, 245f, 246f, 250-253, 251t, 252t, 253t
tapering 209-210
undulation of 96, 96f, 97f, 98
training logs
   in long-term plans 119
   in strength training 256, 257f, 258f
training model development 40-41, 41f
training phases. See phases of training
training plans. See also daily training sessions
   importance of 115-116
   model approach to 134-135, 134t, 135t
   multiple daily sessions 132-133
   records of 256, 256t
   required components 116-119
   sample plan 130-131, 131f
   types of 119
training principles. See individualization; multilateral physical development; training loads; training model development
training sessions. See daily training sessions
training tolerance
   individualization and 36-37
   training plans and 93-94
training variables. See complexity; frequency; intensity; volume, volume load
transition phase
   in bi-cycle plans 179
   detraining and 174-176, 175t, 263
   macrocycles for 163, 163f
   in monocycle plans 178

passive vs. active recovery in 176-177
purpose of 94-95, 105-106, 174, 177
in tri-cycle plans 180-181
tri-cycle plans
   athlete readiness and 98
   chart of 186-189, 188f
   in history of periodization 92
   model plan 179-181, 180f
TRIMP (training impulse) 82
type I and II muscle fibers. See muscle fiber types

U

undulatory loading 96, 96f, 97f, 98
undulatory periodization 95-96
unloading. See tapers
unofficial competitions 170-171, 215-216

V

variables of training. See complexity; frequency; intensity; volume, volume load
variation in training
   individualization and 38-40
   versus stability 64-65
   in training session structure 134-135
Virgil 115
visualization 68, 183
$\dot{V}O_2$max
   athlete comparisons 271, 272f, 274
   gender differences in 268
   interval training and 303-304
   lactate threshold and 24
   in metabolic adaptation 10
   physiological factors in 268-271, 268f
   training zone for 298
$\dot{V}O_2$maxT 298
volleyball
   long-term training model 117f
   sample objectives for 198t
   Yo-Yo Intermittent Recovery Test 287t
volume, volume load
   adaptation and 83-84
   assessment of 71
   in competitive phase 169, 171-173
   defined 71
   historical increases in 42, 42t, 72, 79-80
   increases in training 71-72, 72f, 73f, 80

volume, volume load *(continued)*
   in interval training 289
   quantifying in microcycle 153
   rating 82-83
   relation to intensity 78-79
   relative versus absolute 85
   in speed and agility training 317t, 318
   in strength training 240, 240t, 241t
   during taper 171-173, 211, 212t, 222

W

warm-ups 122-125, 123t
wave loading 252, 252t
weighted objects, for strength training 239
weight-training machines 239
women. See gender differences
work, defined 19
work capacity
   individualization and 36-37
   training plans and 93-94
workload. See training loads
work-to-rest intervals. See rest intervals

Y

youth
   age for specialization 34, 34t-35t
   annual plans for 98
   competition frequency for 220, 220t
   injury risk and prevention in 5, 36
   multilateral development in 29-32, 30f
   nutrition for 186
Yo-Yo Intermittent Recovery Test (YYIRT) 287, 287t

About the Authors

Tudor O. Bompa, PhD, revolutionized Western training methods when he introduced his groundbreaking theory of periodization in his native Romania in 1963. After adopting his training system, the Eastern Bloc countries dominated international sports through the 1970s and 1980s. In 1988, Bompa began applying his principles of periodization to the sport of bodybuilding. He has personally trained 11 Olympic medalists (including four gold medalists) and has served as a consultant to coaches and athletes worldwide.

Bompa's books on training methods, including *Theory and Methodology of Training: The Key to Athletic Performance* and *Periodization of Training for Sports*, have been translated into 19 languages and used in more than 180 countries for training athletes and educating and certifying coaches. Bompa has been invited to speak about training in more than 30 countries and has been awarded certificates of honor and appreciation from such prestigious organizations as the Ministry of Culture of Argentina, the Australian Sports Council, the Spanish Olympic Committee, NSCA (2014 Alvin Roy Award for Career Achievement), and the International Olympic Committee.

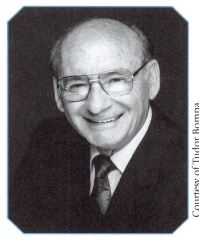
Courtesy of Tudor Bompa.

A member of the Canadian Olympic Association and the Romanian National Council of Sports, Bompa is a professor emeritus at York University, where he taught training theories since 1987. In 2017, Bompa was awarded the honorary title of *doctor honoris causa* in his home country of Romania. He and his wife, Tamara, live in Sharon, Ontario.

Carlo A. Buzzichelli is a PhD candidate at the Superior Institute of Physical Culture and Sports of Havana (Cuba), a professional strength and conditioning coach, the director of the International Strength and Conditioning Institute, a consultant for the Cuban track and field Olympic team, an adjunct professor of theory and methodology of training at the University of Milan (Italy), and a member of the President's Program Advisory Council of the International Sports Sciences Association (ISSA). Buzzichelli has held seminars and lectures at various universities and sport institutes worldwide and was an invited lecturer at the 2012 International Workshop on Strength and Conditioning of Trivandrum (India), the 2015 Performance Training Summit of Beijing (China), the 2016 International Workshop on Strength and Conditioning in Bucharest (Romania), and the 2017 Track and Field National Team Coaches Forum in Havana.

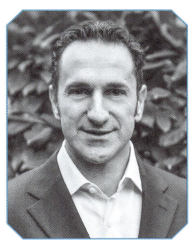

Buzzichelli's coaching experience includes the 2002 Commonwealth Games, the 2003 and 2017 World Track and Field Championships, and the 2016 Summer Olympics. As a strength and conditioning coach for team sports, his senior teams have achieved a first place and a second place in their respective league cups, and his junior teams have won two regional cups. As a coach of individual sports, Buzzichelli's athletes have won 23 medals at national championships in four different sports (track and field, swimming, Brazilian jiujitsu, and powerlifting), set nine national records in powerlifting and track and field, and won 10 medals at international competitions. In 2015, Buzzichelli coached two Italian champions in two different sports; in 2016, two of his athletes earned international titles in two different combat sports.

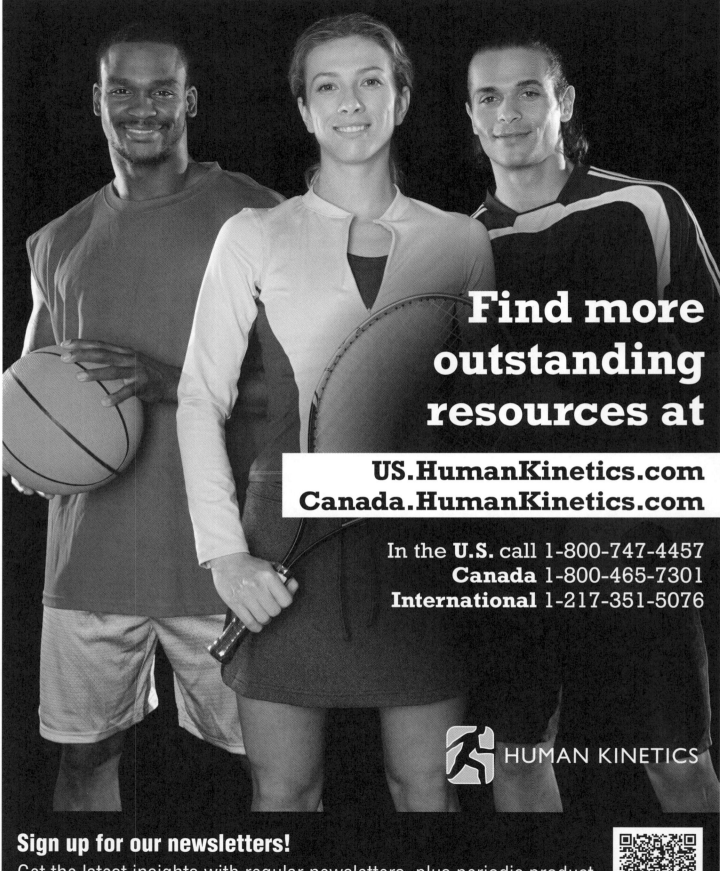